93897

Bereavement

REACTIONS, CONSEQUENCES, AND CARE

Marian Osterweis, Fredric Solomon,
and Morris Green, *Editors*

Committee for the Study of Health Consequences
of the Stress of Bereavement

Institute of Medicine

ST. PATRICK'S SEMINARY LIBRARY
MENLO PARK, CALIFORNIA
94025

NATIONAL ACADEMY PRESS
Washington, D.C.   1984

BF
575
G7
B475
1984

National Academy Press • **2101 Constitution Ave., NW** • **Washington, DC 20418**

NOTICE: The project that is the subject of this report was approved by the Governing Board of the National Research Council, whose members are drawn from the Councils of the National Academy of Sciences, the National Academy of Engineering, and the Institute of Medicine. The members of the Committee responsible for the report were chosen for their special competences and with regard for appropriate balance.

This report has been reviewed by a group other than the authors according to procedures approved by a Report Review Committee consisting of members of the National Academy of Sciences, the National Academy of Engineering, and the Institute of Medicine.

The Institute of Medicine was chartered in 1970 by the National Academy of Sciences to enlist distinguished members of appropriate professions in the examination of policy matters pertaining to the health of the public. In this, the Institute acts under both the Academy's 1863 congressional charter responsibility to be an adviser to the federal government, and its own initiative in identifying issues of medical care, research, and education.

This volume is the final report of a study conducted under Contract No. 278-82-0020 (OD) with The National Institute of Mental Health of the Alcohol, Drug Abuse, and Mental Health Administration, Department of Health and Human Services. The study also received support from the Kenworthy-Swift Foundation, New York.

Library of Congress Cataloging in Publication Data
Main entry under title:
Bereavement: reactions, consequences, and care.

   Includes bibliographies and index.
    1. Bereavement—Psychological aspects.   2. Bereavement—Psychosomatic aspects.   3. Psychotherapy.
4. Medical care.   I. Osterweis, Marian.   II. Solomon, Fredric.   III. Green, Morris.   IV. Institute of Medicine (U.S.)
BF575.G7B475 1984   155.9'37   84-14870

ISBN 0-309-03438-8

Copyright © 1984 by the National Academy of Sciences
No part of this book may be reproduced by any mechanical, photographic, or electronic process, or in the form of a phonographic recording, nor may it be stored in a retrieval system, transmitted, or otherwise copied for public or private use, without written permission from the publisher, except for the purposes of official use by the United States Government.

First Printing, September 1984
Second Printing, February 1985

Printed in the United States of America.

Cover Photograph: EDVARD MUNCH. *Evening (Melancholy: On the Beach)*, 1896. Color woodcut, 16¼ x 18". Collection, The Museum of Modern Art, New York. Abby Aldrich Rockefeller Fund. © The Museum of Modern Art, New York, 1985.

INSTITUTE OF MEDICINE

Committee on Health Consequences of the Stress of Bereavement

*MORRIS GREEN, M.D., Lesh Professor and Chairman, Department of Pediatrics, Indiana University School of Medicine, Indianapolis, Indiana (Chairman)

*ERIC CASSELL, M.D., Clinical Professor of Public Health, Cornell University Medical Center, New York, New York

PAULA CLAYTON, M.D., Chairman, Department of Psychiatry, University of Minnesota, Minneapolis, Minnesota

*DAVID S. GREER, M.D., Dean of Medicine, Professor of Community Health, Brown University, Providence, Rhode Island

JULES HIRSCH, M.D., Professor and Senior Physician, Laboratory of Human Behavior and Metabolism, The Rockefeller University, New York, New York

MYRON A. HOFER, M.D., formerly Professor of Psychiatry, Associate Professor of Neurosciences, Albert Einstein College of Medicine; currently Director, Department of Developmental Psychobiology, Columbia Presbyterian University Hospital, New York State Psychiatric Institute, New York, New York

JIMMIE HOLLAND, M.D., Chief, Psychiatry Service, Memorial Sloan-Kettering Hospital, New York, New York

MARDI HOROWITZ, M.D., Professor of Psychiatry, University of California, San Francisco, California

BERTON H. KAPLAN, PH.D., Professor, Department of Epidemiology, School of Public Health, The University of North Carolina at Chapel Hill, Chapel Hill, North Carolina

MARIE KILLILEA, Assistant Professor, Department of Mental Hygiene, Johns Hopkins School of Hygiene and Public Health, Baltimore, Maryland

*ARTHUR KLEINMAN, M.D., Professor of Medical Anthropology, Department of Social Medicine, Harvard Medical School, Boston, Massachusetts

*GERALD L. KLERMAN, M.D., Director of Psychiatric Research, Massachusetts General Hospital, Boston, Massachusetts

*Member, Institute of Medicine

iii

Members (cont'd)

GERALD KOOCHER, PH.D., Director of Training in Psychology, Children's Hospital Medical Center, Boston, Massachusetts

*IDA M. MARTINSON, R.N., PH.D., Professor, Department of Family Health Care, University of California, San Francisco, California

*JACK H. MEDALIE, M.D., M.P.H., Chairman and Dorothy Jones Weatherhead Professor of Family Medicine, Case Western Reserve University, Cleveland, Ohio

JOAN W. MULLANEY, D.S.W., Dean, National Catholic School of Social Service, Catholic University of America, Washington, D.C.

*ROBERT F. MURRAY, JR., M.D., Professor of Pediatrics, Medicine and Oncology, Howard University College of Medicine, Washington, D.C.

GEORGE H. POLLOCK, M.D., President, The Institute for Psychoanalysis, Chicago, Illinois

THEODORE SHAPIRO, M.D., Professor of Psychiatry in Pediatrics, Director of Child and Adolescent Psychiatry at Payne-Whitney Clinic, Cornell University Medical College, New York, New York

ROBERT S. WEISS, PH.D., Professor of Sociology, University of Massachusetts, and Lecturer in Sociology, Harvard Medical School, Boston, Massachusetts

WILLIAM WENDT, S.T.D., Executive Director, St. Francis Center, Washington, D.C.

Institute of Medicine

President
FREDERICK C. ROBBINS, M.D.

Study Staff, Division of Mental Health and Behavioral Medicine

MARIAN OSTERWEIS, PH.D., Study Director

VICTORIA SOLSBERRY, M.S.W., Research Associate

JANICE L. KRUPNICK, M.S.W., Staff Consultant

FREDRIC SOLOMON, M.D., Director, Division of Mental Health and Behavioral Medicine

PATRICIA A.R. WILLIAMS, Study Secretary

RACHEL HUGHES EDMUNDS, Division Secretary

*Member, Institute of Medicine

iv

Acknowledgments

This study was initially requested and funded by the Office of Prevention of the National Institute of Mental Health, with additional support from the Kenworthy-Swift Foundation, New York, for the work on children's reactions to bereavement. Stephen Goldston, Ed.D., Director of the Office of Prevention, National Institute of Mental Health, lent enthusiastic support to the project from its inception to its completion. Two other NIMH staff members were especially helpful in various phases of this study: Morton Silverman, M.D., Chief, Center for Prevention Research, and Barbara Silver, Ph.D., Special Assistant, Office of the Director.

The project was launched at the Institute of Medicine by Delores Parron, Ph.D., who served as project director from October 1982 to January 1983.

Useful background papers or critical reviews of chapters were provided by the following people: Jack Barchas, M.D., Stanford University Medical School; Maurice Eisenbruch, M.D., Harvard Medical School; Glen Elliott, Ph.D., M.D., Stanford University Medical School; Barry Garfinkel, M.D., University of Minnesota Medical School; John Mason, M.D., Veterans Administration Medical Center and Yale University; Phyllis Silverman, Ph.D., Massachusetts General Hospital, Institute for Health Professions; Albert Solnit, M.D., Yale University School of Medicine; Marvin Stein, M.D., Mount Sinai Medical Center, New York.

We especially wish to thank:

Janice L. Krupnick, M.S.W., staff consultant, who not only prepared the chapter on children's reactions to bereavement, but also assisted in the drafting and revising of the chapters on adults' reactions to bereavement and on interventions;

Leonard Rosenblum, Ph.D., Downstate Medical Center, New York, who prepared the chapter on monkeys' responses to separation and contributed to the biology chapter;

Linda Starke, who provided major editorial assistance to the staff and the committee as the report was being written; and

Pamela Steele, who designed this book and researched illustrations.

Contents

Introduction

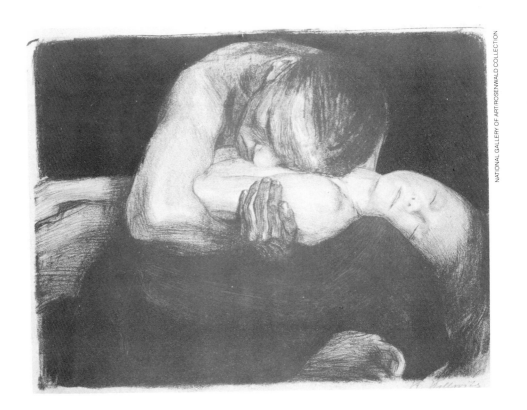

NATIONAL GALLERY OF ART/ROSENWALD COLLECTION

The influence of bereavement can be found in the works of many great artists, including painters, poets, sculptors, and musicians. Grief provides a powerful theme in Pieta *by Käthe Kollwitz, who was greatly affected by the loss of several siblings as well as her son.*

CHAPTER 1

Introduction

The father, Hermann Castorp, could not grasp his loss. He had been deeply attached to his wife, and not being of the strongest himself, never quite recovered from her death. His spirit was troubled; he shrank within himself; his benumbed brain made him blunder in his business, so that the firm of Castorp and Son suffered sensible financial losses; and the next spring, while inspecting warehouses on the windy landing-stage, he got inflammation of the lungs. The fever was too much for his shaken heart, and in five days, notwithstanding all Dr. Heidekind's care, he died.

Thomas Mann, *The Magic Mountain*[7]

Thistance passage, from the 1924 book that assured the German novelist's reputation in America, was written 30 years before health scientists began to investigate systematically what it seemed to say: That one who is bereaved can weaken and even die of his grief.

Epidemiologists were among the first to study the effects of death on survivors. They looked at rates of death and disease among bereaved persons; then they compared these rates with those for persons who had not lost a family member through death.

What they learned generally lent scientific credence to what poets, novelists, and playwrights had long suggested. Bereavement affects people in different ways, and for some, especially those whose health is already compromised, bereavement can exacerbate mental and physical health problems, or even lead to death. Hermann Castorp's troubled spirit and shaken heart did, it seems, appear in the epidemiological statistics.

For most people bereavement is a fact of life. Only those who themselves die young escape the pain of losing someone they love through death. Every year an estimated eight million Americans experience the death of an immediate family member. Every year there are 800,000 new widows and widowers. There are at least 27,000 suicides in this country annually, and probably many more, since suicide is underreported. Each year approximately 400,000 children under the age of 25 die. Just as each type of relationship has special meaning, so too does each type of death carry with it a special kind of pain for those who are left behind. As one psychiatrist said, "When your parent dies, you have lost your past. When your child dies, you have lost your future."[9]

The anguish of those left behind has always concerned society, and every culture has mourning rituals to deal with that pain. Today scientists, policymakers, educators, and the public are all concerned with the nature of bereavement and its toll on survivors. Biologists and behavioral scientists now advance theories to account for the impact of grief and propose strategies to ease both its acute pain and its longer-term effects.

The shapers of public policy and educators in the health professions also are becoming more concerned about bereavement's toll. There is strong and growing public interest in preventing stress-related illness, including that which may be precipitated or exacerbated by grief. Health professionals, technically better equipped than ever before, often are seen as having lost the compassion that once was the foundation of the healing arts. If compassion and understanding can be imparted through training, future clinicians could better deal with the realities of death, the fears of patients, and the grief of bereaved families.

This widening interest in bereavement is at least partly an outgrowth of recent social developments. First, achievements in medical science have shifted the customary causes and locations of death. Most people now die of chronic diseases in institutions rather than from acute infections at home. New technology also maintains the uncertainty of death for longer periods. If someone whose life is prolonged is comfortable and in reasonably good spirits, the effect can be regarded as positive. But if life is prolonged for someone who is unconscious or in pain, or whose personality and mental function have been dramatically altered by the illness or treatment, then such extensions of life may make the anticipation of death and the subsequent bereavement more difficult for survivors.

The second development, due primarily to geographic mobility, is a diminished access of the bereaved to traditional social supports. Contrary to popular stereotypes, extended family contact is frequent.[10] However, over a five-year period, one-fourth of the population moves to a different location,[1] making face-to-face contact limited. This places great demands on the nuclear family for ongoing emotional and social support when a member of such a family dies, both because other family members may live far away and because bereaved persons who are new to a community lack strong links to other people or institutions that could assist them.

MANDATE AND PROCESS OF THE STUDY

At the request of the Office of Prevention of the National Institute of Mental Health, the Institute of Medicine (IOM) appointed a committee to study the factors that affect the bereavement process and its impact on general and mental health. This study is related to a series of recent activities in the Division of Mental Health and Behavioral Medicine of the IOM dealing with the relationship between psychosocial stress and physical disease and the place of behavioral interventions within general health care.[2,3,5,6] The particular framework of the bereavement study grew out of the Institute's report on stress and human health.[2]

Almost uniformly researchers and the public identify death of a close family member as the most potent stressor in ordinary life. However, few earlier studies focused specifically on bereavement and none have provided a comprehensive synthesis of the evidence that attempts to assess and explain bereavement's impact. Thus the current study was mandated to address the following questions:

- What can be concluded from available research evidence about the health consequences of bereavement?
- What further research would be especially important and promising to pursue?
- Based on both research evidence and informed judgment, are there preventive interventions that should be recommended for more widespread adoption in the health care system? Which ones are not yet ready for such adoption but should be tested promptly for their value?

Committee members included clinicians and researchers from many disciplines, including psychiatry, psychology, social work, nursing, medicine (internal medicine, family practice, and pediatrics), the neurosciences, epidemiology, sociology, anthropology, and the ministry.

To supplement an analysis of the literature on bereavement, committee members and staff visited eight intervention programs around the country. Particular programs were chosen because of their extensive experience or innovative approaches to intervention with the bereaved or because of their research on the topic. The sites were not selected as models to emulate, nor were they in any sense representative of the universe of programs, although an attempt was made to visit programs with various distinguishing characteristics.*

REPORT OVERVIEW

While recognizing the similarities between bereavement and other stressful events and acknowledging that many different kinds of losses occasion grief, this report focuses principally on reactions to the death of a closely related family member.

One objective is to synthesize the evidence from many disciplines and thereby better describe the nature and consequences of bereavement, examine its underlying biologic and psychologic mechanisms, and study the factors that may protect some individuals but leave others at risk for poor outcomes.

Another objective, however, is simply to provide practical help whenever possible. Thus, the report discusses when and how to help the bereaved, and how effective the various interventions are. Recommendations for clinical practice and for promising research appear throughout.

Part I of the report focuses on bereavement reactions and consequences. In Chapter 2, the epidemiologic studies of the health consequences of bereavement are reviewed. The somewhat conflicting evidence linking bereavement with increased rates of mortality, morbidity, symptom development, and the use of health services is discussed. The epidemiological evidence for increased mortality and morbidity is not as clearcut as once thought. As is true of most potentially stressful events, the association between bereavement and enduring negative consequences is not randomly distributed in the population. Instead, there are factors that predispose some people to increased risk of mortality (premature death), some types of morbidity (illness, either physical or psychiatric), and behavior that may ultimately damage their health. Some of these factors can be identified before or very soon after bereavement, thereby raising the possibility of early preventive intervention with those at high risk.

*See Footnote on page 11.

Chapters 3 through 5 deal with psychosocial reactions of adults and children to bereavement. Unlike Chapter 2, which focuses on easily measured and quantifiable outcomes, these chapters draw primarily on clinical observations and theoretical constructs from the psychiatric literature. Chapter 3 describes the grieving process in adults and the several conceptual frameworks that have been used to try to account for the basic process and outcomes (both normal and abnormal). Chapter 4 focuses on reactions to particular types of losses—of a spouse, a child, a parent, a sibling, and death by suicide. The nature, meaning, and functions of each type of relationship are discussed in an effort to explain particular psychosocial reactions to loss. This chapter includes suicide as an example of a particularly stressful type of death that is believed to complicate the bereavement process.

Bereavement in childhood is considered especially hazardous in both the short and long term. Chapter 5 examines the large body of literature on the nature of grieving in children and discusses the implications for subsequent development. Here, the report tries to offer guidance about how to talk to children about death and how to recognize when children may need professional help with their grief.

Part II of the report examines bereavement from the perspectives of the biologic and social sciences in an effort to further understand the emotional reactions and health consequences that may ensue. Biological and behavioral scientists have studied the effects of various naturally occurring and laboratory-induced stressors on animals and humans. Bereavement has been simulated by separating infant animals from their mothers. Human bereavement has been studied in parents anticipating the death of a child, in recently bereft parents and spouses, and in subjects who have acute grieving responses revived in laboratory settings. In all these situations, alterations in cardiovascular, endocrine, and immune system functioning have been recorded. The medical importance of such changes is not known, however; some of these changes might be adaptive and some could be precursors of actual disease. Nor has it been determined to what extent the physiologic reactions to bereavement are special compared to other stressors, or whether they are unique. These and other issues are discussed in Chapter 6.

Chapter 7 reviews the research on the emotional and behavioral responses of monkeys to separation. Laboratory studies such as these permit the controlled manipulation of environmental factors in order to examine the effects of various antecedent and post-separation conditions on responses and outcomes. These animal studies provide partial models for human behaviors and may even provide clues for developing effective preventive intervention strategies with the bereaved.

Chapter 8 discusses the sociocultural context of and influences on grief and mourning. Sociologists and anthropologists have long been interested in the effects of bereavement on social group functioning and in the possible protective role played by sociocultural factors. Clearly there is a wide variation in cultural norms for outward expressions of mourning. The extent to which internal grieving processes also vary in different cultural groups is a controversial question still to be resolved.

Various approaches to assisting the bereaved are discussed in Part III of the report. Because health professionals and institutions are frequently involved with families prior to death, the committee holds that they also have some obligations to families after death. The nature of these roles and responsibilities are discussed in Chapter 9, and suggestions are presented for improving follow-up activities with bereaved individuals.

Chapter 10 examines several of the more formal approaches to bereavement interventions. The goals and methods of four major types of interventions are described—mutual support groups, hospices, various professional psychotherapeutic approaches, and drug therapies. The scant research on the efficacy of each is presented.

Although most chapters contain their own conclusions and recommendations, Chapter 11 integrates these and returns to the three questions the committee was asked to consider.

Because of its broad scope, this report should appeal to many audiences. The synthesis of findings from the many disciplines that study bereavement and the recommendations for future research should provide useful information to investigators as well as to government agencies and private foundations wishing to fund promising research in this area. The committee has added its own collective thinking to the research evidence in an effort to provide useful advice to clinicians as well as to the general public. This volume should also be valuable to students of the major health professions who wish to learn more about bereavement. Finally, it should be of interest to policymakers and lay and professional people interested in designing preventive intervention programs to assist the bereaved.

BEREAVEMENT AND STRESS THEORY

This report examines bereavement from a number of disciplinary perspectives and conceptual frameworks. The broadest of these is "stress theory," which seeks to explain the relationships between a stressor, the physiologic and emotional reactions to it, and the resulting health consequences, if any.

Since World War II, scientists from many disciplines have conducted numerous studies of the effects of stressful life events on health and well-being.[2] Significant research advances in this field have followed from the work of Holmes and Rahe,[4] who developed a quantitative technique for assessing the relative stress imposed by various types of life events, including loss and bereavement. They considered loss of a spouse the most severe change in adult life; other life events (both positive and negative), such as sickness of relatives, marrying, moving, or loss of a job, were also considered stressful but were weighted less heavily. Although both the reliability and validity of the original scale (and numerous other life-events scales modeled after it) have been challenged,[8] the findings from hundreds of studies have generally supported the proposition that life stressors of all types place individuals at greater risk for a variety of physical illnesses and mental disorders.[2]

Viewed in this context, bereavement represents one specific type of a life-event stressor. Though usually considered to have the most powerful impact of all stressful life events, in many respects bereavement is not unique. Loss through death, like loss through divorce or loss of a job, results in perturbations in physiologic functioning, emotional distress, and social disorganization, including the need to redefine one's place in society. As with other stressors, the consequences of bereavement are not uniform. The sudden and unexpected suicide of a young husband and father, for example, is likely to have much more profound effects on surviving family members than the long anticipated death of a beloved grandparent after a protracted illness. Furthermore, although the death of someone close is stressful by definition, many factors can modify that stress and affect long-term outcomes.

Although clearly not unique in all respects, some aspects of loss through death are distinctive. Even superb coping abilities cannot alter the finality of death. This helplessness and total inability to control the event of death may make bereavement a particularly stressful life event.

DEFINITIONS

With so many different disciplines studying a subject, it is not surprising that the same terms are variously employed to describe the process and its consequences. In this volume the following definitions are used:

- *bereavement*: the fact of loss through death.
- *bereavement reactions*: any psychologic, physiologic, or behavioral response to bereavement. The term ''reaction'' is not meant to suggest

automatic, reflex responses nor to imply that any particular reaction is universal.

- *bereavement process*: an umbrella term that refers to the emergence of bereavement reactions over time.
- *grief*: the feeling (affect) and certain associated behaviors, such as crying.
- *grieving process*: the changing affective state over time.
- *mourning*: in the social science sense, the social expressions of grief, including mourning rituals and associated behaviors. This definition of mourning is a departure from Freud's usage, where the term refers to an internal psychologic state and process.

Although these definitions are used consistently in this volume, the committee recognizes that they differ from the usage of some disciplines, especially some of the mental health professions. Wherever possible, the text specifies particular affects in order to avoid confusion between grief and mourning and also couples these basic terms with adjective modifiers to make their meaning clearer in the context of particular discussions.

REFERENCES

1. Bureau of the Census. *Statistical Abstract of the United States: 1982–83*. Washington, D.C.: U.S. Department of Commerce, 1982.
2. Elliott, G.R., and Eisdorfer, C. (Eds.) *Stress and Human Health: A Study by the Institute of Medicine, National Academy of Sciences*. New York: Springer, 1982.
3. Hamburg, D., Elliott, G., and Parron, D. *Health and Behavior: Frontiers of Research in the Biobehavioral Sciences. A Report of the Institute of Medicine*. Washington, D.C.: National Academy Press, 1982.
4. Holmes, R.H., and Rahe, R.H. The social readjustment rating scale. *Journal of Psychosomatic Research* 11:213–218, 1967.
5. Houpt, J., Orleans, C., George, L., and Brodie, H.K. *The Importance of Mental Health Services to General Health Care*. Cambridge, Mass.: Ballinger Publishing, 1979.
6. Institute of Medicine. *Sleeping Pills, Insomnia, and Medical Practice*. Washington, D.C.: National Academy of Sciences, 1979.
7. Mann, T. *The Magic Mountain* (1924) (H.T. Lowe-Parker, translator). New York: Alfred A. Knopf, 1963.
8. Rabkin, J.G., and Streuning, E.L. Life events, stress and illness. *Science* 194:1013–1020, 1976.
9. Schiff, H.S., quoting Eliot Luby. *The Bereaved Parent*. New York: Penguin Books, 1977.
10. Shanas, E., Townsend, P., Wedderburn, D., Friis, H., Milhaj, P., and Stehouwer, J. *Old People in Three Industrial Societies*. London: Routledge and Kegan Paul, 1968.

FOOTNOTE

The eight sites visited and the rationales for selecting them were:

- *The Children's Hospital National Medical Center, Emergency Room* (Washington, D.C.). This setting was chosen because of its written protocol for dealing with dead-on-arrival cases (DOAs), which specifies how parents of children should be assisted in the immediate period of crisis and seeks to alleviate staff stress as well. The potential for more widespread use of such protocols was of particular interest to the Committee.
- *The Children's Hospital National Medical Center, Neonatal ICU* (Washington, D.C.). As regional referral center for seriously ill newborns, Children's Hospital is experienced in assisting parents who are anticipating the death of their infants. The nature of anticipatory bereavement reactions, the use of multi-disciplinary teams, and attempts to follow up with parents subsequent to bereavement were of particular interest.
- *The St. Francis Center* (Washington, D.C.). This center includes professional counseling and lay assistance programs for people prior to or following bereavement, as well as educational programs for professionals and lay people. Of special interest were the Center's extensive links to the Washington community and its nationwide leadership role in death education.
- *The Hospital for Sick Children* (Washington, D.C.). As a chronic care facility for very sick and handicapped children, this site provided an opportunity to learn about the effects of lengthy anticipatory bereavement reactions on parents and siblings, the effects of bereavement on staff who typically have cared for children for years prior to their deaths, and approaches to assisting both parents and staff.
- *The Center for Preventive Psychiatry* (White Plains, N.Y.). This center is one of very few in the country devoted specifically to the care of children who have experienced major life crises, including bereavement. It was chosen for a site visit in order to gain a better understanding of children's reactions to bereavement including the effects of situational factors and preventive intervention strategies on long-term outcomes.
- *The Center for the Study of Neuroses, Langley-Porter Institute* (San Francisco, Cal.). This center, which is part of the University of California Medical Center, is one of very few places in the country that is conducting systematic research on the efficacy of particular psychotherapeutic interventions on the course and outcomes of adult bereavement. When the IOM study began, very little of this research had been published.
- *Boulder County Hospice* (Boulder, Col.). This particular hospice was chosen for a site visit because of its extensive attention to the care of bereaved relatives, and its leadership role in developing educational materials and in training professionals and lay hospice volunteers around the country.
- *Palliative Care Service, Royal Victoria Hospital* (Montreal, Canada). In addition to its bereavement service component, the Palliative Care Service is one of very few hospices worldwide that has engaged in research on bereavement. It is currently in the final stages of a very large study of the impact of hospice versus traditional care on bereaved families, and of the relative efficacy of trained volunteers versus trained nurses on the course of bereavement.

A detailed summary of the site visits ("Site Visit Case Studies") is available from the National Academy Press, 2101 Constitution Ave., NW, Washington, DC 20418.

Epidemiologic Perspectives on the Health Consequences of Bereavement

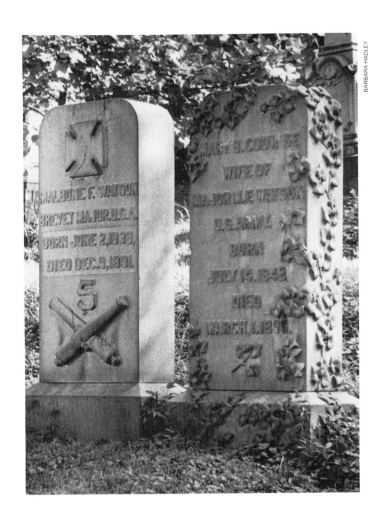

BARBARA HADLEY

Epidemiologic studies now confirm what has long been suspected and can be observed in any cemetery: the death of a close family member may result in premature death for some survivors. Following the death of a spouse, young and middle-aged widowers are particularly vulnerable and remain at risk for a number of years.

CHAPTER 2

Epidemiologic Perspectives on the Health Consequences of Bereavement

This chapter reviews and evaluates the epidemiologic evidence that adults are at greater risk for a variety of adverse health consequences following bereavement. The health consequences of bereavement during childhood are discussed in Chapter 5.

Epidemiology is the medical science that studies the distribution of disease in populations. Epidemiologic research attempts to determine the incidence, prevalence, and timing of health-related phenomena, and to identify risk factors that alter the probability of such occurrences. The identification of risk factors, even in the absence of full understanding of the etiology of disease, has in the past contributed to the development of public health measures for control and prevention. The application of such methods to bereavement phenomena will, it is hoped, also lead to intervention strategies that can reduce long-term negative outcomes, as well as to research that increases understanding of the bereavement process.

It has been hypothesized that bereavement:

- predisposes people to physical and mental illness;
- precipitates illness and death;
- aggravates existing illness;

This chapter is based on material prepared by committee members Gerald L. Klerman, M.D., and Paula Clayton, M.D.

- brings on a host of bodily complaints and physical symptoms;
- leads to or exacerbates health-threatening behaviors such as smoking, drinking, and drug use;
- causes increased use of health services.

To test these hypotheses, observations of bereaved individuals must be compared with those of nonbereaved individuals matched for such relevant characteristics as age, sex, social class, and race. However, the collection of reliable information about bereavement is not easy. There is difficulty even in establishing baseline rates of bereavement for any given population in any given time period. Although mortality rates are readily available for the general population and for specific subgroups, rates of bereavement cannot be readily extrapolated from death rates because the number of surviving family members will vary depending on many different factors.

Estimates of one-year incidence rates of bereavement in the general population range from 5 to 9 percent. For example, Imboden et al.[35] found in a population of 455 healthy men (employees at an Army base, average age 35) that 8.9 percent had lost a family member to death within one year. Frost and Clayton[23] reported a 6 percent one-year incidence of bereavement of first-degree relatives among 109 people with an average age of 61. Pearlin and Lieberman[59] report that death of a parent occurs in 5 percent of the population annually.

These estimates of bereavement rates in the general population provide some basis for determining whether there is a relationship between bereavement and ill health. If it is found that sick populations have higher rates of bereavement in the year preceding their illness, that would suggest a possible relationship between bereavement and the subsequent development of illness. Paykel et al.,[58] for example, found a one-year incidence rate of 5 percent in a healthy population, compared with 18 percent in a population of clinically depressed people whose bereavement occurred in the year preceding their diagnosis.

Retrospective studies, which rely on extrapolations of base rates calculated from previous reports, are generally less accurate than prospective studies which match a population at risk with a concurrent control group. For this reason, greater weight is given in this chapter to prospective studies. Among such studies, three designs have been used: (1) studies of whole population groups, (2) studies of bereaved samples compared with control groups, and (3) case control studies.

Prospective studies of whole populations, such as the one by Helsing and Szklo,[31] are the most powerful designs, because they enable assessment of individuals before they are bereaved and therefore the observations made are not influenced by the state of bereavement. Very large samples are required for such studies because the rate of bereavement for an immediate family member in a general adult population is only about 5 percent per year.

Because of the complexity and logistical difficulties of doing prospective studies of whole populations, the more commonly used approach is to study samples of recently bereaved people, and to compare them to a control group matched for relevant characteristics. Such groups are followed in order to observe the subsequent occurrence of symptoms, particular behaviors, and health changes. This design has been used most powerfully by Clayton in a series of studies on the bereavement experience of widows.[9,10,12]

In the third type of design—case control—individuals with a particular condition (e.g., depression, ulcerative colitis) that is believed to be associated with bereavement are compared with an appropriate control group. This approach is used because of the low frequency of both bereavement and the conditions that may be precipitated by it. Assuming that approximately 5 percent of the population is bereaved in a given year and that only a small portion of the bereaved develop a depression or other specific disorder, it would be necessary to follow an extremely large sample prospectively to determine whether bereavement is associated with a greater risk of that illness. Thus several researchers have worked backwards from a disorder to ask how many people with the disorder were recently bereaved. If the proportion is higher than the rate for the same age and sex group in the general population, it suggests that the bereaved are at risk for that condition.

The somewhat conflicting results found in epidemiologic studies are accounted for in large part by differences in the study designs just discussed, in sample sizes and characteristics (including, for example, controlling for length of widowhood and remarriage), and in changes in populations over time. These differences make it hard to compare studies and to establish precise rates of bereavement or its health consequences. In addition, as is true of all research on humans, perfect experimental controls are never possible; there will always be some uncontrolled variables.

THE QUESTION OF OUTCOMES

Another major problem in bereavement research is the lack of agreement about what constitutes normal or abnormal outcomes and the absence of reliable criteria for assessing them. Among the normal outcomes that have been proposed are reduction of depression-like symptoms, return to usual level of social functioning, remarriage (in the case of spouses), reduction in frequency of distressing memories, the capacity to form new relationships and to undertake new social roles, and other functional outcomes such as return to work. Numerous scales and indices have been used to measure reduction of symptoms and various aspects of social and emotional recovery and adjustment, but their reliability and validity often have not been ascertained. Some other outcomes, although easy to measure, are conceptually faulty, especially if they are the only measure used. Kinship patterns and related social roles, for example, can never be fully reestablished because of the irreversibility of the death. Remarriage may sometimes be a useful outcome measure of conjugal bereavement; for elderly women, however, it is unrealistic to expect high rates of remarriage because there are not enough elderly men available in the population.

Clinicians have described a number of processes associated with poor outcomes, including absent, delayed, prolonged, or chronic grief. The nature of these reactions is covered in detail in Chapter 3, and the therapeutic implications are discussed in Chapter 10. It is commonly assumed, particularly by clinicians, that the absence of grieving phenomena following bereavement represents some form of personality pathology and will have later adverse consequences. But the empirical research in support of this assumption has not been undertaken. Individual variation in response to bereavement is expected, but the amount of grief that is too much or too little in terms of psychologic well-being has not been definitively determined. Until the criteria for distinguishing normal from abnormal and too much grief from too little have been agreed on, definitive epidemologic research on the frequency of these outcomes cannot be conducted.

THE CONSTELLATION OF DISTRESS AND GRIEF

Human experience through the centuries has recorded the near-universal occurrence of intense emotional distress following bereavement, with features similar in nature and intensity to those of clinical depression. These features include crying and sorrow, anxiety and agitation, sleeplessness, lack of interest in things, and frequent gastrointestinal complaints, such as loss of appetite. Grieving individuals are also often seriously impaired in their social functioning.

There is considerable controversy about whether it is appropriate to consider this constellation of depression-like symptoms to be an illness. This issue was raised most pointedly by Engel in "Is Grief a Disease?"[20] The current consensus is that although individuals experiencing grief are distressed, they are not ill or diseased. A number of considerations lead to this conclusion. For one thing, society does not consider them to be sick, nor do bereaved individuals consider themselves ill; they believe they are undergoing a "normal" period of distress. In this sense bereavement may be compared to pregnancy. Both are naturally occurring conditions for which many individuals seek medical attention. Grieving individuals may seek medical attention and may be prescribed tranquilizers, sleeping pills, and sedatives, but they seldom seek psychiatric care.

Second, although there are similarities between the behavior and distress of grieving individuals and those who are clinically depressed, there are also some important differences. Most grieving people do not report gross motor retardation or suicidal thoughts. A persuasive distinction between grief and depression was made by Freud in his classic paper on *Mourning and Melancholia*.[22] He contended that most people in the grieving state feel there has been a loss or emptiness in the world around them, while depressed patients feel empty within. A pervasive loss of self-regard and self-esteem is common in depressed patients but not in most grieving individuals. Therefore the almost universal conclusion among clinicians and theorists is that grief and clinical depression, although they share some subjective and objective features, represent different conditions.

That grief is not generally considered an illness is also reflected in the American Psychiatric Association's Diagnostic and Statistical Manual[1] (DSM-III) by the category "uncomplicated bereavement." The description of this "diagnosis" acknowledges a depression-like syndrome as normal for three months following bereavement. As discussed later in this chapter and elsewhere in this report, however, three months seems substantially shorter than the time needed by most people to begin to regain their psychologic equilibrium.

Despite the general agreement that grief is not an illness, many theorists, particularly those of psychoanalytic background, regard the grief situation as the prototype for understanding the dynamics of clinical depression, particularly depression precipitated by loss—either through bereavement or through separation, disappointments, or "symbolic" losses. Moreover, in animal research, particularly in the primate studies described in Chapter 7, experimentally induced separation has been found to produce a characteristic syndrome of behaviors. Whether this represents a true animal model of clinical depression remains unresolved.

Until the patterns of normal bereavement reactions are understood, it is not possible to develop sound criteria for abnormal reactions. For example, since the bereaved suffer from and report significant depressive symptoms, how many of them have enough symptoms to be diagnosed as "depressed"? In prospective studies of older widows and widowers,[3,13,14] Clayton and her colleagues found that 35 percent at one month, 25 percent at four months, and 17 percent at one year could be classified as depressed based on a constellation of symptoms. Forty-five percent were depressed at some point during the year and 13 percent were depressed for the entire year. When a consecutive series of younger widowed people was added to the sample, 42 percent at one month and 16 percent at one year met the criteria; 47 percent of the sample were depressed at one of the two points and 11 percent were depressed for the entire year. Among a control group who had not lost a first-degree relative in the preceding year, 8 percent reported a depressive syndrome at some time during the year, a one-year incidence figure that can be compared with 47 percent in the widowed population. It should also be noted that, of the many widowed who did not meet the criteria for the syndrome of depression, many did have individual symptoms in varying combinations, durations, and sequences.

ADVERSE HEALTH CONSEQUENCES OF BEREAVEMENT

Mortality

Notwithstanding methodological shortcomings in both retrospective and prospective controlled studies, it is clear from the epidemiologic evidence that some people are at increased risk for mortality following bereavement. The most important evidence is from studies that demonstrate an increase in overall mortality among the recently bereaved (see Table 1 for a summary of the studies discussed in this section).

Kraus and Lilienfeld[39] reported one of the earliest systematic studies on mortality in the bereaved. They retrospectively calculated mortality rates for widows and widowers, matching data from the National Office of Vital Statistics for 1956 with data from the 1950 census. Death rates of widowed subjects were compared to the rates for married men and women matched for age, sex, and race. The mortality ratios of widowed to married were strikingly higher at younger ages; as age increased the differences in mortality between the widowed and married decreased for men and women and for all races. Mortality rates for males who were widowed were consistently higher than those of female widowed.

Specifically, younger widows and widowers (ages 20–24) had the highest ratio of mortality for eight causes of death: vascular lesions of the central nervous system, arteriosclerotic heart disease, non-

TABLE 1 Summary of Epidemiologic Evidence for Mortality Following Bereavement

Author(s) and Date	Country	Research Design	Number and Type of Subjects	Mortality Risk
Kraus and Lilienfeld, 1959[39]	USA	Retrospective from vital statistics	Bereaved spouses from all deaths in US in 1949–1951 vs. matched married controls	Elevated for widows and widowers. Risk of mortality 7× greater for widowed under age 45 than for controls. Risk for men greater than for women.
Young, Benjamin, and Wallis, 1963[77]	UK	Cohort of widowers	4,486 recent widowers over age 55 compared with death rates for married men of same age. Followed for 5 years.	Significantly higher death rates for widowers in 1st 6 months following bereavement than for married. No differences after 6 months.
Cox and Ford, 1964[17]	UK	Retrospective from vital statistics	60,000 widows followed for 5 years after application for widow's pension.	Some elevation of mortality rate in 2nd year following bereavement; none in 1st, 3rd, 4th, or 5th year.
Rees and Lutkins, 1967[63]	UK	Cohort of bereaved relatives	903 bereaved relatives vs. 878 nonbereaved matched controls followed for 6 years.	Significantly higher mortality for bereaved spouses in 1st year. Insignificant differences in 2nd and 3rd years. In general, mortality rate for men higher than for women; rates for bereaved relatives higher than nonbereaved for all types.
Clayton, 1974[9]	USA	Cohort of widows and widowers	109 widows and widowers and matched controls followed for 4 years.	No increased risk of mortality.
Shepherd and Barraclough, 1974[66]	UK	Cohort of bereaved spouses	44 spouses of suicides vs. nonspecified, nonsuicide widow group. Age unspecified.	No difference in mortality and remarriage rates between suicide widows and nonsuicide widows in 1st year. 23% mortality over 58-month period.

TABLE 1 Summary of Epidemiologic Evidence for Mortality
Following Bereavement—(*Continued*)

Author(s) and Date	Coun-try	Research Design	Number and Type of Subjects	Mortality Risk
Gerber et al., 1975[25]	USA	Cohort of bereaved spouses	169 bereaved spouses and matched married controls followed for 4 years.	No deaths in either group during 1st year. Slightly higher percentage of deaths among bereaved in 2nd and 3rd years.
Ward, 1976[75]	UK	Cohort of bereaved spouses	87 widowers and 279 widows compared with known age- and sex-specific rates.	No increased risk of mortality
Helsing and Szklo, 1981[31]	USA	Prospective population study	12-year prospective study of 92,000 people. Matched pair analysis of bereaved and married spouses.	No increased mortality in 1st 6 months. Highly significant increase thereafter for widowers, especially those who did not remarry. No excess mortality for widows.
Levav, 1982[41]	UK	Reanalysis of Rees and Lutkins[63] cohort focusing on parents	35 bereaved parents vs. 29 controls followed for 5 years.	Highly significant difference between bereaved and nonbereaved cumulative death rate over 5 years (34.3% vs. 6.9%).

rheumatic chronic endocarditis and other myocardial degeneration, hypertension with heart disease, general arteriosclerosis, tuberculosis, and influenza and pneumonia. When all these disease groups were combined, the mortality rate was at least seven times greater among the young widowed group (under age 45) than for the matched young married control group. The mortality rate for death from cardiovascular disease was 10 times higher for young widowers than for married men of the same age. Kraus and Lilienfeld concluded that as a group, the recently bereaved were at greater risk for mortality. Although provocative, these data did not take into account either the duration of widowhood or the fact that widows and widowers who do not remarry may have been in poorer health.

Cox and Ford[17] reanalyzed government records of 60,000 widows receiving pensions for the first time in 1927, and then identified from vital statistics those who died over the next five years. They compared the actual and expected numbers of deaths for the first five years of widowhood. Only during the second year following bereavement was there some excess in mortality, and it appeared most pronounced in women between the ages of 60 and 68.

Several studies of relatively small cohorts of widows and widowers[9,10,25,75] found no significant increase in mortality in the first or subsequent years following bereavement. However, Young et al.[77] found that among recent widowers over the age of 55, mortality rates were significantly higher for the first six months of bereavement than in married controls of the same age. No differences were found after six months.

Rees and Lutkins,[63] in a prospective study, followed a cohort of 903 relatives of 371 residents of a village in Wales who had died during the previous year. These 903 persons were compared with a cohort of 878 nonbereaved individuals matched for age, sex, and marital status. These cohorts were followed for six years. Mortality rates were slightly higher for all types of bereaved relatives, but significant differences were only found among spouses during the first year. The mortality rate for the bereaved spouses was significantly greater than for the control spouses—12 percent of bereaved spouses died compared with 1 percent of nonbereaved spouses.

The most definitive study on mortality after bereavement was conducted by Helsing and his colleagues.[30-32] In a 1963 health census conducted in Washington County, Maryland, data were obtained on 91,909 persons—98 percent of the noninstitutionalized population. The population was followed prospectively to 1975. The widowed population in 1963 was matched to a married population of the same race, sex, year of birth, and geographic category of residence. Any member of the married population who became widowed after entry into the study was withdrawn from that category and enrolled in the widowed population as of the date of death of the spouse.

Widowed men aged 55–74 exhibited a highly significant increase in mortality. Those younger, 19–54, also showed a difference in the relative risk of death, but because there were so few deaths in this group the differences did not achieve statistical significance. Interestingly, widowers over 75 did not have a significantly increased mortality. This finding is consistent with Clayton's[11] observation that older widowed men who survive their spouses may be in better health than married men of the same age. There was no evidence that men's mortality was higher in the first year than in subsequent years of the study; for women, however, the data suggest that the risk of mortality is greatest in the second year following bereavement.

Although there were some differences in the mortality rates by age among females, and for widows as compared with married women, when education, social class, cigarette smoking, and other potential risk factors were controlled the differences disappeared. Control of these factors did not affect the significance of the mortality rates in men.[32]

At least half the men who were widowed before the age of 55 remarried during the course of the study. As would be expected, given the demographic composition of the population,[16] remarriage among women was far less common, with the remarriage rate in any age group being similar to that among males 20 years older. The differences in mortality rates between the widowed males who remarried and those who did not remarry were substantial. In fact, age-specific mortality rates among widowed males who remarried were lower than the rates among married males. The ratio of remarried/not remarried mortality rates for males ranged from about 1:8 to 1:2; the small numbers of widowed females who remarried plus the already low mortality rate among the widowed females made their remarried/not remarried ratios meaningless. Clearly, remarriage must be taken into account in any mortality study of bereavement. It should be noted, however, that it is not known whether marriage itself protects against ill health or whether good health is what permits remarriage.

Helsing and his colleagues[32] also found that there was a significant mortality difference for both sexes by change of address after widowhood. This high mortality rate among subjects who moved was due largely to those who moved into nursing homes, retirement homes, and chronic care facilities (presumably indicators of poor health). Finally, living alone was also associated with a higher mortality than living with others.

It has often been suggested that vulnerability to illness and death is increased following the suicide of someone close. Shepherd and Barraclough[66] reported that spouses of suicides have no increased mortality in the first year of bereavement. Over a longer period, 58 months, there were 10 deaths in 44 spouses (23 percent), a trend that indicates survivors of suicidal deaths are at greater risk of mortality than survivors of other deaths. Compared with mortality rates of the married rather than widowed, this excess mortality is even more significant. Half the spouses who subsequently died were seriously ill at the time of the suicide. The authors felt that in addition to contributing to their own deaths the consequences of these illnesses might have precipitated the suicide. This is an example of the complicated interactions that arise in studying mortality following bereavement, and is consistent with similar findings about poor health and mortality in the Ward[74,75] data.

The mortality studies reviewed in this section provide examples of somewhat different results due to the methodological and population variations mentioned earlier. Unless differences are very great they will not reach statistical significance in small samples. Comparisons of the retrospective study from vital statistics by Kraus and Lilienfeld[39] and the prospective study by Helsing and Szklo[31] reveal somewhat different findings with regard to mortality rates and specific causes of death. These may be attributable to differences in sample characteristics— Kraus and Lilienfeld studied only widowers who had not remarried, whereas Helsing and Szklo included widowers who had remarried and examined the interaction between remarriage and mortality. The different findings may also be traced to changes in general mortality characteristics (such as reduction in cardiovascular death rates) during the 20 years between these two studies, or to differences stemming from retrospective and prospective study designs.

These differences notwithstanding, the weight of the evidence indicates that, up to age 75, widowed men are about one-and-one-half times more likely to die prematurely than their married counterparts. Although especially pronounced during the first year, the mortality rate for men who do not remarry continues to be elevated for many years. For widows, there is no increase in risk the first year, but several reliable studies find excess mortality in the second year.

It should be noted that there are very few studies dealing with mortality following any bereavement other than conjugal loss. The effect of the death of parents, children, or siblings has been virtually unstudied. With regard to parents, there is one highly controversial study. Levav[41] reanalyzed the data from Rees and Lutkins,[63] focusing specifically on bereaved parents in the original sample. The 35 bereaved parents were compared with 29 control parents. When the accumulated deaths were compared over the five-year study period it was found that 34.3 percent of bereaved parents had died compared with 6.9 percent of nonbereaved parents. Although loss of a child is generally considered hazardous,[11] these mortality figures seem very high, perhaps because of some unspecified characteristics of the particular population that was studied. The effects of this type of loss are discussed in detail in Chapter 4.

Death by Suicide. National statistics for the United States in the years 1949–1951 established that suicide rates were higher among the widowed than the married.[51] Since that time numerous studies from vital statistics and from survey data (e.g., Kraus and Lilienfeld,[39] Bock and Webber,[2] Stroebe et al.,[69] and Helsing et al.[30]) have confirmed this increase, especially among elderly men. Among women the suicide rate is not as high for widows as for the divorced or separated.

Several hypotheses have been tested in recent studies, including that bereavement itself and the circumstances of widowhood predispose people to suicide, that those who remain widowed (that is, do not re-marry) following the death of their spouse have preexisting characteristics (such as alcoholism and depression) that predispose them to suicide, and that the nature of the death of the spouse (especially suicide) predisposes the surviving spouse to suicide.

MacMahon and Pugh[43] found that the suicide rate among a widowed population was 2.5 times higher in the first six months after bereavement and 1.5 times higher in the first, second, and third years after bereavement than in the fourth or subsequent years, thus suggesting that bereavement itself is a powerful etiologic factor in death by suicide. These figures were based on a study of 320 widowers and widows who had committed suicide (excluding homicide-suicide combinations) in Massachusetts between 1948 and 1952. The suicide sample was compared with a control group of widows and widowers matched for age, sex, and race who died from causes other than suicide. The age-standardized suicide rate for widowed men was 3.5 times higher than among married men and for women the rate was twice as high. Generally, men were found to have a higher suicide rate than women.

In a striking study, Bunch et al.[6] reported that half of 75 people who committed suicide in West Sussex, Great Britain, had experienced maternal bereavement within the last three years. This high maternal bereavement rate in suicides was compared to a 20 percent rate among controls who were matched for age, sex, marital status, and geographical location. Moreover, 22 percent of the suicides, compared with 9 percent of the controls, had experienced loss of their fathers within the previous five years. In addition, although married suicides and controls were not significantly different with respect to loss of a mother, the single male suicides showed greater recent maternal bereavement (60 percent) than the single male controls (6 percent). The authors hypothesize that single men may be a high-risk group for suicide following their mother's death because of a higher proclivity of males to act out via self-destructive impulses, whereas women more easily seek out medical and psychiatric help.

In a small study, Murphy and Robins[49] found that among a group of alcoholics who committed suicide, 17 percent (5 out of 31) had experienced the death of someone close in the previous year. An additional 41 percent of the alcoholics who committed suicide had experienced another type of loss such as separation or divorce. Thirty-two percent of these other types of loss occurred within six weeks of the suicide. In a later study[64] it was found that in a group of people who were diagnosed after their suicides as having had an affective disorder (chiefly depression), 5 percent (3 out of 60) had experienced bereavement in the year before they killed themselves. An additional 12 percent with affective disorders had experienced other types of losses. The authors' main conclusion was that alcoholics were a high-risk group for suicide after the loss of an affectional relationship.

Morbidity and Health Care Utilization

There is considerable controversy over the nature and extent of morbidity associated with bereavement and the concomitant burdens on the health care system. General health status, specific medical and psychiatric disorders, health-related behavior, and health care utilization have all been studied in an attempt to determine the impact of bereavement on health and the use of services. The findings from these studies, however, are frequently inconsistent and inconclusive, in part because of very small sample sizes in many studies.

Psychiatric Morbidity.   An increase in psychiatric morbidity in the first year of bereavement could be signaled by higher rates of emotional and mental symptoms sufficient for diagnosable mental disorder; consumption of pills or alcohol; and use of psychiatric services, both inpatient and outpatient. As described earlier in this chapter, all studies have documented that distress and depressive symptoms dominate the emotional life of the bereaved during the first year. But how often do the bereaved meet criteria for true psychiatric illness?

Stein and Susser[68] studied widowhood and mental illness among outpatients in Salford, England. They looked at the transition into widowhood and first entry into psychiatric care and compared the widows with a general population control group. Significantly more widows entered psychiatric care in the first year after the death of a spouse than in subsequent years. Thus, widows who enter psychiatric care are more likely to do so early in widowhood than later. This is the only study with controls, though not age-matched, showing a relationship between widowhood and psychiatric care.

Parkes and Brown,[56] in a prospective study, followed for four years a group of Boston widows and widowers under the age of 45. They found higher rates of depressive symptoms among the widowed and more use of counseling by the young widowed than by controls. Other studies also mention this use of counseling,[62] but the appropriate data are sparse.

Data on psychiatric hospitalization are also very limited. Clayton's prospective studies of the widowed[9,10] found that psychiatric hospitalization occurred in three (2 percent) of the bereaved and one of the controls. Two were alcoholics and the third was previously diagnosed as depressed.

Of all the psychiatric conditions, clinical depression would appear to be the one most likely to occur with greater frequency among the bereaved. As noted earlier in this chapter, Clayton and others have found that a fairly substantial proportion of bereaved individuals—estimated at approximately 17 percent—still have a constellation of depressive symptoms such that they could be diagnosed as depressed at one year. Conceptually this makes sense. Loss through death would be expected to be an important life stressor precipitating clinical depressive disorders, particularly in those predisposed by virtue of family history, personality, or previous life experience.

In view of this, it is surprising how few studies have systematically attempted to test this commonly believed clinical hypothesis. Of the three studies reported, only Paykel et al.[58] found an increased risk of clinical depression following bereavement. The authors studied life events in 185 depressed outpatients and inpatients and a group of matched community controls. Sixteen of the depressives and four of the control group reported the death of an immediate family member in the six months prior to the onset of the illness or the interview. There were five patients who had experienced the death of a child, which is surprisingly high but is consistent with other research indicating that this type of bereavement is extremely traumatic.

Hudgens et al.[34] studied 40 hospitalized patients with affective disorders and 40 matched nonpsychiatric hospital controls for precipitating events and found no deaths of spouses in either group. In the year preceding, 13 percent of the psychiatric patients and 3 percent of the controls had lost a first-degree relative, a difference that was not significant. When the sample was expanded to 100 psychiatric patients and 100 controls, 7 percent of the former and 3 percent of the latter experienced the death of first-degree relatives, though none was a spouse.[48]

Frost and Clayton[23] evaluated 344 psychiatric inpatients for bereavement in the six months preceding admission. These patients were matched with nonpsychiatric hospitalized patients. In each group, 2 percent reported the death of a first-degree relative. Three psychiatric patients (less than 1 percent) had experienced the death of a spouse within six months of the current admission to the hospital; there were no deaths of spouses in the control group.

Many of the bereaved subjects in all these studies reported marked increases in their consumption of pills, alcohol, and tobacco, which could indicate psychiatric morbidity, and some reported initial use of these substances following bereavement.

Parkes[53] observed that sedative drugs were prescribed seven times more frequently for widows under the age of 65 during the first six months of bereavement than in the period preceding the death. For widows aged 65 and older, there was no significant increase in the prescription of sedatives.

In their later study, Parkes and Brown[56] observed that 25 percent (17) of the 68 widows in Boston under the age of 45 years reported an increase in the consumption of tranquilizers, alcohol, and tobacco during the 13-month period after bereavement. Twenty-eight percent of bereaved subjects reported an increase in smoking, compared with 9 percent of controls. Increased consumption of alcohol was reported by 28 percent of the bereaved women versus 3 percent of the controls. A first use of tranquilizers was reported by 26 percent of the widows and 4 percent of the controls. There was no statistically significant difference between bereaved subjects and controls in the use of sleeping pills.

Maddison and Viola[44] reported a marked increase in both sedative (tranquilizers) and hypnotic (sleeping pills) drug intake in their sample of 374 widows aged 45–60 years old, compared with controls, during the 13 months after bereavement. They also noted increased alcohol consumption and tobacco use among the widows versus the controls.

There was a small but significant difference in the consumption of sleeping pills between the 90 widows and widowers (average age 61 years) and the matched controls in Clayton's[9] study. There were no differences between the two groups, however, in consumption of tranquilizers or other medicine taken for general health.

In a study of recently widowed persons over the age of 55 and a control group of married individuals, Thompson et al.[70] report both increased and new medicine use among the widowed. Fifty-four percent of the medicines used by the widowed were analgesics, sedatives, sleep medication, or antidepressants.

Self-Reported Symptoms and Health Status. Many investigators have asked the bereaved about physical and other symptoms following bereavement. These include crying, changes in sleep patterns or appetite, difficulty in breathing, sighing, palpitations, inability to concentrate, and a host of other signs of distress. Unfortunately there are only a few studies that assessed self-reported symptoms before and after bereavement. Self-reports of symptoms and of perceived changes in health status are likely to be exaggerated by the general distress of bereavement such that these reports are not ideal measures of actual health status. They may be better indicators of general distress, especially if repeated measures are done over time.

Crisp and Priest[18,61] administered a brief self-rating inventory intended to cover a full range of neurotic symptoms to samples of bereaved and controls between the ages of 40 and 65 who were registered with a group practice in southwest London. Although their numbers were small, they found minimal differences between the bereaved widows and the controls. They commented that the bereaved subjects on the whole withstood the stress in a "robust way."

Heyman and Gianturco,[33] as part of a continuing Duke Center Longitudinal Study for Aging, reported on the reactions to widowhood in the elderly. They found little difference in before-and-after scores of either sex on health, leisure activity, financial security, or ratings for anxiety or hypochondriasis. There was a small increase in depression in the women after bereavement, but it was felt that this depression was mild and that all the widows kept active contact with their friends despite depression.

Parkes[54] studied a group of London widows, average age 49 years, who had visited their doctors during the first month of bereavement. At 13 months, six widows (27 percent) reported that their health was definitely worse. In the later study, in Boston, Parkes and Brown[56] found that in terms of self-reported physical symptoms, widows and their controls were not significantly different, but widowers reported more severe symptoms and more anxiety than controls. No excess of psychosomatic illness was found. There were no differences in general health or in "health worries."

In a retrospective mail survey of 375 widows aged 40–60 (132 in Boston, Massachusetts, and 243 in Sydney, Australia), Maddison and Viola[44] found significant differences between widows and matched controls in reports of several symptoms and complaints. Among widows considered to be at high risk, Raphael[62] found marked deterioration in health in the first year following bereavement as evidenced by numerous physical symptoms, diminution of work capacity, weight loss, and health-damaging behaviors.

Parkes and Weiss[57] report marked differences between well-matched young widowed spouses and married controls in self-reported symptoms, reflecting the somatic effects of anxiety. There were no significant differences in the worsening of chronic symptoms, perceived general health, or health worries between the groups. However, Thompson et al.[70] found that recently widowed elderly individuals reported worsening of existing illness as well as new illnesses more frequently than controls.

These prospective studies document less physical distress than had been expected. The literature suggests that the young widowed have more anxiety symptoms than their married counterparts. Except for those already ill, older men and women reported little change in their general health status following bereavement.

Specific Medical Disorders. The hypothesis that bereavement predisposes to, precipitates, or exacerbates medical illness and thus increases morbidity has been proposed for several disorders, including acute closed-angle glaucoma, cancer, cardiovascular disorders, Cushing's disease, disseminated lupus erythematosus, idiopathic glossodynia, pernicious anemia, pneumonia, rheumatoid arthritis, thyrotoxicosis, tuberculosis, and ulcerative colitis (see Klerman and Izen[38] for a detailed review of this literature).

The evidence linking each of these diseases to bereavement and grief is meager. Not only is much of the evidence based on clinical case reports of small numbers of patients, but many studies use "loss," "stress," or "depression" broadly defined as the condition preceding the disorder. Bereavement as a specific stressor and the "depression of grief" as distinct from other types of depression are often not distinguished, thus rendering it difficult to draw definitive conclusions about the association between bereavement and specific diseases. Adequate testing of the hypothesized associations requires prospective studies with large samples.

Nonetheless, an extensive literature in the psychosomatic tradition suggests that bereavement is a contributing factor to somatic disease in individuals who are already predisposed to that disease because of genetic susceptibility, physiologic responsiveness, or preexisting psychologic susceptibility.

For example, studies of hyperthyroidism (thyrotoxicosis or Graves' disease) in children[45,46] and in adults[37] suggest that traumatic events, especially loss, may activate the disease in susceptible individuals. In the case study reports of children with hyperthyroidism, loss of a parent by divorce, separation, or death was found to be a common antecedent to depression, which in turn may activate the disease in those children who are genetically predisposed or physiologically vulnerable. In adults who are already excessively anxious or depressed, a "normal life stress," such as bereavement, can contribute to the development of hyperthyroidism. However, as Kleinschmidt et al.[37] caution, affective states and disorders are unlikely to cause the disease without some genetic or physiologic vulnerability as well.

Parental loss has also been proposed as a precipitator of diabetes in children[40] but probably only in genetically or physiologically predisposed individuals. There is also some evidence of an association between psychologic trauma and exacerbation of diabetes in some adult patients (see, for example, Grant et al.[26] and Treuting[71]). In many discussions of this issue, however, bereavement as a specific stressor is not separated out from other stressors, nor is it clear what makes some individuals vulnerable to an altered course of their disease when they are under stress.

Bereavement has been implicated as a contributor to many different kinds of cancer. As with studies of other diseases, most of the cancer studies are retrospective and often do not distinguish among various losses that precede the disease. Schmale and Iker[65] reported an association between loss and several cancers, especially cancer of the cervix. Several studies by Greene[27-29] suggest a high incidence of leukemia and lymphoma among individuals with a recent loss (actual or psychic). Men who are separated from their mothers or mother figures appear to be particularly vulnerable. Once again, however, these findings remain inconclusive because of lack of control groups, small sample sizes, and a failure to distinguish actual bereavement from other losses.[47] Although the link between bereavement and the development of various types of cancer has not been confirmed by rigorous epidemiologic studies, there is currently great interest among researchers in exploring the immunologic mechanisms that could contribute to the development of cancer. These are discussed in Chapter 6.

The most extensive evidence of a link between disease in a specific organ system and bereavement exists for the cardiovascular system. Sudden cardiac arrhythmias, myocardial infarction, and congestive heart failure are the most frequently mentioned conditions in that system. Studies have shown that patients with congestive heart failure[8] and with essential hypertension[76] are particularly prone to exacerbation of their condition in response to threatened or actual loss of human relationships.

In a study of 170 sudden and rapid deaths during psychologic stress, Engel[21] found that 39 percent of the women and 11 percent of the men died immediately following the death of someone close and another 23 percent of women and 20 percent of men died within 16 days of such a death. Although Engel did not have access to clinical data for all the people in his sample, he suggests (based on what he did have and on the literature) that most of these sudden deaths were due to cardiac arrest in individuals with preexisting cardiovascular disease. As Parkes and Weiss[57] conclude:

> It certainly seems unlikely that bereavement causes arteriosclerosis since that condition takes many years to develop, but it seems very likely that a person who already has arteriosclerosis affecting his or her heart is at special risk after bereavement. The added burden of bereavement on that heart may be sufficient to produce a myocardial infarction and to reduce the person's chances of surviving an infarction should one occur.

Beyond case reports there are two additional sources of data regarding specific morbidity following bereavement that lend credence to the hypothesized association. Several of the studies discussed in the section on mortality examined specific causes of death. For example, Helsing et al.[30] found that widowed women who died had a higher percentage of deaths from cirrhosis of the liver than would have been expected. In men there were increased death rates from infectious diseases, accidents, and suicides, but no increase from cardiovascular disease. Kraus and Lilienfeld[39] found for the young widowed who had not remarried greatly increased mortality rates for several kinds of cardiovascular and infectious diseases. And in diagnosis-specific health care use studies, Parkes[52] found that increased rates of physician visits in the first six months following bereavement were due largely to increased consultations for vascular and articular conditions, especially osteoarthritis in a widowed population under 65 years of age.

Aside from psychosomatic mechanisms involving physiologic changes, Jacobs and Ostfeld[36] suggest that excess mortality, and presumably morbidity, in the recently bereaved may be mediated by behavioral changes that compromise health maintenance or chronic disease management. Increased alcohol consumption and cigarette smoking, common behavioral changes in the bereaved, may exacerbate or precipitate illness. Excess mortality, especially among bereaved men, is explained in large part by deaths from suicide, cirrhosis, and cardiac arrest. All three conditions have clinical antecedents (depression, alcoholism, and cardiovascular disease) that could be detected before or very shortly after bereavement, thus identifying three high-risk groups for whom early intervention might be useful.

Health Care Utilization. Use of health services can be an indicator of medical morbidity or a measure of the burden, including costs, of bereavement on the health care delivery system. The second is straightforward. As a proxy for actual medical disease, however, the use of health services, especially physician visits, is imperfect; it is well established in the health services research literature that a substantial proportion of visits are precipitated by psychosocial concerns and nonorganic symptoms rather than by diagnosable illness.

Given that bereavement often results in significant distress, depression-like symptoms, and increased use of drugs, and is sometimes associated with increased morbidity and mortality, significant increases in the use of health services would be expected. Yet most studies conducted in the United States show no increase in physician visits or hospitalization following bereavement.[14,56] On the average, Americans make almost five physician visits each year.[50] Among the bereaved it appears that although some visits are related to their reactions to loss, the actual number of visits does not increase. Most of the evidence from England,[52,54] however, and one U.S. study of elderly widows in a prepaid health plan[76] do show an increase in physician visits for some people following bereavement. This discrepancy suggests that payment method may have a powerful effect on people's decisions to visit a physician, with fee-for-service systems inhibiting health care utilization.

Possible Consequences Beyond the First Year

The form that grief takes, its outward expressions, and the length of the recovery process all are influenced by the social and cultural context within which bereavement occurs (see Chapter 8). Although most studies report a decrease in the reported distress and other manifestations of grieving by the end of the first year, persistent experiences of distress are frequently observed. Many people who are grieving report "it is always with you." The significance of these reactions is not clear. True delayed grief—in the sense of physiologic disruptions, social withdrawal, and persistent sadness and yearning that emerge only after a period of absent grief—is so rare that little research has been conducted on it. Yet, distortions of personality and alterations in the quality of social functioning that are related to the distress associated with memories of the dead person have been observed by many clinicians, particularly for patients in psychotherapy.

A number of observers have proposed that failure to cope adequately during the usual bereavement period predisposes a person to later psychiatric and medical problems. Although there are no systematic data available to support or refute this hypothesis, its proponents put forth two alternative explanations of the process. The first predicts that later health problems are a consequence of the duration and intensity of distress—the more prolonged and intense the distress, the greater the burden on an individual's adaptive capacity.

In contrast, many psychiatric and mental health professionals believe that the grieving process is adaptive and that "failure to grieve" or an interruption of the grieving process leaves an individual vulnerable to later illness. This hypothesis is usually attributed to Erich Lindemann in his writings on the survivors of the Coconut Grove Disaster[42] and is a view held widely in mental health circles. Mental health professionals generally encourage emotional expression during the bereavement process. Although some believe in prescribing medications to facilitate grieving, others are hesitant to recommend the use of drugs, including tranquilizers and antidepressants, lest the adaptive function of grieving be suppressed.[19] These issues are discussed further in Chapters 3, 5, and 10.

As discussed earlier in this chapter there is some evidence suggesting that mortality rates remain high for certain categories of bereft individuals beyond the first year—perhaps into the sixth year after their loss. There is also some indication of an increase in medical illnesses in the second and third years following bereavement, but adequate studies have not been performed to verify this hypothesis.

RISK FACTORS

Many factors relating to characteristics of the bereaved individual, the nature of the relationship to the deceased, the nature of the death, and the early reactions to bereavement have been hypothesized as placing individuals at risk for one or more adverse outcomes or as protecting individuals from them. These variables are listed in Table 2, with an indication of the chapters in which they are discussed in detail. Because research in this area has not been systematic, few definitive conclusions can be offered.

Characteristics of Bereaved Individuals

Some studies have reported that men do more poorly than women following conjugal bereavement.[25,56,60,72] Other studies[4,12,67] have not. If premature death is the outcome studied, certainly men do worse; if remarriage is the outcome, men do better. The physical and psychologic outcomes are unclear because most prospective studies have not had large enough samples of men to draw any conclusions about their relative risk of illness.

It is generally held that bereavement reactions are more intense and have more enduring consequences for younger people, particularly for children but also for adolescents and young adults. Older individuals

TABLE 2   Report's Discussion of Variables Associated With Health Outcomes of Bereavement

Variables Associated With Health Outcomes	Chapter[a]				
	3. Adults' Reactions	4. Specific Losses	5. Particular Types	8. Socio-cultural	10. Inter-ventions
Characteristics of bereaved individuals					
Sex	x	x	x		x
Age			x		
Prior physical health	x		x		x
Prior mental health	x		x		x
Personality factors	x				x
Alcohol abuse	x				x
Socioeconomic status			x	x	
Sociocultural factors				x	
Relationship to the deceased					
Kinship		x	x		
Ambivalence, dependence	x		x		x
Nature of the death					
Suddenness	x	x	x		
Suicide		x	x		
Behaviors and attitudes appearing early in the grieving process					
Consumption of alcohol, drugs	x	x			x
Smoking	x	x			x
Perceived social support	x	x	x	x	x
Suicidal thoughts	x				
Morbid guilt	x	x	x		

[a]Chapters 6, 7, and 9 do not discuss these variables in any detail.

appear to experience fewer, less intense consequences, perhaps because experiencing the death of someone close, family, or friends is common over the age of 60. Another possibility is that older individuals already have passed through the period of highest risk for psychiatric problems, such as alcoholism, depression, and anxiety disorders.

It seems clear that poor prior physical or mental health is a risk factor. Those who are physically ill before a bereavement are more likely to be ill after it too, with more physician visits and perhaps even with greater risk of death in the first year.[76] Those with a previous psychiatric disorder or with a history of misuse of drugs will be at risk psychiatrically.

Most researchers and clinicians in this field would hypothesize that personality variables probably affect outcome; unfortunately only one study has examined this systematically. Vachon and her colleagues[73] used Cattel's 16 Personality Factor Questionnaire[7] to test whether specific aspects of personality were related to level of distress and adjustment to bereavement. They found that widows with enduring high distress scores were characterized as emotionally less stable, more apprehensive and worrying, and highly anxious. Widows with low distress scores were more likely to be emotionally stable, mature, conscientious, moralistic, conservative, controlled, and socially precise. These and other assessments were done both six months and two years after the bereavement. Ideally, these personality variables should be tested before the terminal illness or when a spouse first becomes ill, as distress itself could confound the personality inventories.

In addition to the previously mentioned high suicide rate among alcoholics shortly after bereavement, alcoholics are more likely than nonalcoholics to be doing poorly one year following bereavement. When psychiatric hospitalization occurs, the diagnosis is likely to be alcoholism.[49,64]

The association between socioeconomic status and bereavement outcomes has not been adequately studied. Whether individuals with low incomes do any worse following bereavement than the more well-to-do is not known. A frequent concomitant of bereavement, however, especially for widows, is financial difficulty brought on by the loss of the major wage earner and perhaps by large medical bills as well. Recent work by Vachon et al.[73] has shown that poor outcome in middle-aged widows was associated with financial problems.

Relationship to the Deceased

Each kinship relationship has particular difficulties associated with it following bereavement (see Chapter 4). In addition to kinship, the nature of the relationship with the deceased has been hypothesized to influence outcomes. The literature on conjugal bereavement is replete with data indicating that individuals who had highly ambivalent relationships with their spouses do worse following bereavement than people whose relationships did not have these characteristics (see Chapters 3 and 4). There also is evidence to suggest that spouses who are unable to function independently do poorly following bereavement,[57] although there is some controversy about the meaning and predictive value of this variable.

Nature of the Death

Sudden death is frequently hypothesized to be more traumatic for the survivors and to lead to poorer outcomes than deaths that have been anticipated. There are marked variations in the criteria used to assess suddenness of death. Clayton et al.[15] defined it as an illness of five days or shorter duration. Parkes[55] classified survivors as having "short" preparation if they had less than two weeks' warning that a spouse's condition was likely to prove fatal, or less than three days' warning that death was imminent. Gerber et al.[25] defined "acute illness death" as one occurring without warning and prior knowledge of the condition, or a death after a medical condition of less than two months' duration with the absence of multiple attacks and hospitalization.

Contrary to commonly held views, most of the research literature indicates that sudden death, however defined, does not produce more disturbed survivors. In Parkes' data[55] the young widowed who experienced a sudden death had a poorer outcome, as did widows in the study by Vachon et al.[73] However, studies by Clayton et al.[15] and by Fulton and Gottesman[24] did not find this to be true. In a study by Gerber et al.[25] of older men and women, there was a negative correlation between length of illness and outcome; that is, the longer the terminal illness, the more likely there was to be a poor outcome for the surviving spouse.

The time course of the loss is a risk factor that deserves further attention. Common wisdom holds that time to say goodbye and to express love will facilitate grieving by lessening later feelings of anger and guilt. However, it may be that the moment of death is always a surprise no matter how much warning there has been. Perhaps a very lengthy terminal illness produces its own stresses and strains that complicate bereavement. Perhaps suddenness of death interacts with age of the deceased or age of the survivors in ways that have not yet been uncovered. As discussed in Chapter 10, suddenness of death may have important implications for the design of strategies to assist the bereaved.

A number of studies have been undertaken of suicide's impact on family members and other survivors. Given the high rate of assortative mating (i.e., people with similar characteristics tending to marry each other; depressed people are particularly likely to marry other depressed people), the impact of death by suicide is likely to be associated with a propensity for psychiatric illness in the spouse, particularly for alcoholism and depression. In general, as discussed in Chapters 4 and 5, death by suicide renders survivors vulnerable to increased psychologic distress and, especially in the case of children, may leave them vulnerable to suicide as well.

Risk Factors Appearing After the Death

All bereavement studies report that among people already using alcohol, drugs, or cigarettes, consumption of these substances increased after a death. Some people, however, begin using these substances following bereavement. Even without a chronic dependency developing, increased use of these substances might lead to deterioration in health and well-being. Certain individual symptoms during the early bereavement period may also predict poor outcome. These include suicidal thoughts (particularly after the first month), psychomotor retardation, and morbid guilt.

As discussed in several later chapters, there is mounting evidence to suggest that social support has a positive effect on general health status and may serve as a protective factor to buffer or modify the impact of adversity and stressors, not only on the mental health of an individual, but also upon his or her physical health.[5] Perceived lack of social support is one of the most common risk factors cited in the bereavement literature. The perception by the recently bereaved that there is no one to talk to or lean on appears to be a reliable predictor of poor outcome.[73]

Research testing the magnitude of these hypothesized risk factors is difficult because of lack of agreement on relevant outcome measures. Different risk factors are likely to be involved in different outcomes; until these conceptual and methodological problems are resolved, risk factor studies and predictive studies will be seriously handicapped.

CONCLUSIONS AND RECOMMENDATIONS

Research to date has demonstrated some important effects of bereavement on health and has generated a number of intriguing findings that deserve further study.

• Following bereavement there is a statistically significant increase in mortality for men under the age of 75. Although especially pronounced in the first year, the mortality rate continues to be elevated for perhaps as long as six years for men who do not remarry. There is no higher mortality in women in the first year; whether there is an increase in the second year is unclear.

• There is an increase in suicide in the first year of bereavement, particularly by older widowers and by single men who lose their mothers. There may be a slight increase in suicide by widows.

• Among widowers, there is an increase in the relative risk of death from accidents, cardiovascular disease, and some infectious diseases. In widows, the relative risk of death from cirrhosis rises.

- All studies document increases in alcohol consumption and smoking and greater use of tranquilizers or hypnotic medication (or both) among the bereaved. For the most part, these increases occur in people who already are using these substances; however, some of the increase is attributable to new users.
- Depressive symptoms are very common in the first months of bereavement. Between 10 and 20 percent of men and women who lose a spouse are still depressed a year later.
- Although these observations suggest several types of associations between bereavement and specific diseases—including exacerbation of existing cardiovascular disease, vulnerability to certain infectious diseases, precipitation of depression leading to suicide, and health-damaging behavioral changes—the epidemiologic evidence linking bereavement to specific diseases is sparse. Few well-controlled studies have been conducted.
- Although some studies have shown an increase in self-reported physical symptoms and perceived deterioration in health status, other studies have not. It appears that it is only in prepaid health care delivery systems that utilization of services increases in the year following bereavement.
- Risk factors for poor outcome include poor previous physical and mental health, alcoholism and substance abuse, and the perceived lack of social supports. It is unclear whether sudden death or lingering illness produces more disturbing outcomes.
- Perceived adequacy of social support and remarriage protect the bereaved from adverse outcomes.

Some promising areas require further investigation. Systematic research is needed on the consequences of bereavement following loss of parents, children, and siblings for people of all ages. To date, most epidemiologic research has focused on conjugal bereavement.

As part of a comprehensive program of bereavement research, systematic epidemiologic studies should be conducted of the period of anticipation prior to the death of someone close. Advances of medical science lead increasing numbers of individuals with chronic illnesses, particularly cardiovascular disease, cancer, Alzheimer's disease, and other central nervous system diseases, to experience long periods of illness and disability prior to their death. The epidemiologic hypothesis would be that anticipation of disruption of the attachment bond is a source of intense emotional distress that places family members and others at risk for adverse health consequences during this period. Clinicians, clergy, and others are familiar with the emotional distress and strain that chronic illness places on family members, but the committee could find no systematic epidemiologic study that attempted to document the frequency of this or the increased risk for some adverse consequences.

During the intense distress following a death, further phenomenologic studies are indicated to identify people who do not manifest emotional symptoms. Health care professionals, and increasingly the educated public, commonly believe that the failure to manifest distress is "abnormal" and will have adverse consequences. The available research evidence does not allow support or refutation of this hypothesis, which needs to be tested before intervention strategies can be recommended for such individuals.

More research is needed on the relationship between bereavement and disease in order to understand the extent to which bereavement is a specific or nonspecific stressor and to understand its role in precipitating, predisposing to, or exacerbating disease. A fundamental research problem has to do with the definition of outcomes. There is no agreement on the criteria for adequate recovery. Pending development of such criteria from empirical studies, it is difficult to identify and measure risk factors that should be paid attention to in preventive interventions.

REFERENCES

1. American Psychiatric Association. *Diagnostic and Statistical Manual* (Third Edition). Washington, D.C.: APA, 1980.
2. Bock, E.W., and Webber, J.L. Suicide among the elderly: isolating widowhood and mitigating alternatives. *Journal of Marriage and the Family* 34:24–31, 1972.
3. Bornstein, P.E., Clayton, P.J., Halikas, J.A., Maurice, W.L., and Robins, E. The depression of widowhood after thirteen months. *British Journal of Psychiatry* 122:561–566, 1973.
4. Bowling, A., and Cartright, A. *Life After Death: A Study of the Elderly Widowed.* London: Tavistock, 1982.
5. Broadhead, W.E., Kaplan, B.H., James, S.A., Wagner, E.H., Schoenback, V.J., Grimson, R., Heyden, S., Tibblin, G., and Gehlback, S.H. The epidemiologic evidence for a relationship between social support and health. *American Journal of Epidemiology* 117:521–537, 1983.
6. Bunch, J., Barraclough, B., Nelson, B., and Sainsbury, P. Suicide following death of parents. *Social Psychiatry* 6:193–199, 1971.
7. Cattell, R.B., Eber, H.W., and Tasuoka, M.M. *Handbook for the 16 Personality Factor Questionnaire.* Champaign, Ill: Institute for Personality and Ability Testing, 1970.
8. Chambers, W.N., and Reiser, M.F. Emotional stress in the precipitation of congestive heart failure. *Psychosomatic Medicine* 15:38–60, 1953.
9. Clayton, P.J. Mortality and morbidity in the first year of widowhood. *Archives of General Psychiatry* 125:747–750, 1974.
10. Clayton, P.J. The sequelae and nonsequelae of conjugal bereavement. *American Journal of Psychiatry* 136:1530–1543, 1979.

11. Clayton, P.J. Bereavement. In: *Handbook of Affective Disorders* (Paykel, E.S., ed.). London: Churchill Livingstone, 1982.
12. Clayton, P.J., and Darvish, J.S. Course of depressive symptoms following the stress of bereavement. In: *Stress and Mental Disorder* (Barrett, J.E., ed.). New York: Raven Press, 1979.
13. Clayton, P.J., Halikas, J.A., and Maurice, W.L. The depression of widowhood. *British Journal of Psychiatry* 120:71–78, 1972.
14. Clayton, P.J., Herjanic, M., Murphy, G.E., and Woodruff, R.A. Mourning and depression: their similarities and differences. *Canadian Psychiatric Association Journal* 19:309–312, 1974.
15. Clayton, P.J., Parilla, R.H., Jr., and Bieri, M.D. Methodological problems in assessing the relationship between acuteness of death and the bereavement outcome. In: *Psychosocial Aspects of Cardiovascular Disease: The Life-Threatened Patient, The Family, and The Staff* (Reiffel, J., DeBellis, R., Mark, L., Kutscher, A., Patterson, P., and Schoenberg, B., eds.). New York: Columbia University Press, 1980.
16. Cleveland, W.P., and Gianturco, D.T. Remarriage probability after widowhood: a retrospective method. *Journal of Gerontology* 31:99–102, 1976.
17. Cox, P.R., and Ford, J.R. The mortality of widows shortly after widowhood. *Lancet* 1:163–164, 1964.
18. Crisp, A.H., and Priest, R.G. Psychoneurotic status during the year following bereavement. *Journal of Psychosomatic Research* 16:351–355, 1972.
19. Editorial. Is Grief an Illness? *Lancet* 2:134, 1976.
20. Engel, G. Is grief a disease? *Psychosomatic Medicine* 23:18–23, 1961.
21. Engel, G. Sudden and rapid death during psychological stress. *Annals of Internal Medicine* 74:771–782, 1971.
22. Freud, S. *Mourning and Melancholia* (1917). *The Standard Edition of the Complete Psychological Works of Sigmund Freud*, Vol. 14 (Strachey, J., ed.). London: Hogarth Press and Institute for Psychoanalysis, 1957.
23. Frost, N.R., and Clayton, P.J. Bereavement and psychiatric hospitalization. *Archives of General Psychiatry* 34:1172–1175, 1977.
24. Fulton, R., and Gottesman, D.J. Anticipatory grief: a psychosocial concept reconsidered. *British Journal of Psychiatry* 137:45–54, 1980.
25. Gerber, I., Rusalem, R., Hannon, N., Battin, D., and Arkin, A. Anticipatory grief and aged widows and widowers. *Journal of Gerontology* 30:225–229, 1975.
26. Grant, I., Kyle, G.C., Teichman, A., and Mendels, J. Recent life events and diabetes in adults. *Psychosomatic Medicine* 37:121–128, 1974.
27. Greene, W.A. Psychological factors and reticuloendothelial disease. *Psychosomatic Medicine* 16:220–230, 1954.
28. Greene, W.A. Disease response to life stress. *Journal of the American Medical Women's Association* 20:133–140, 1965.
29. Greene, W.A., Young, L.E., and Swisher, S.N. Psychological factors and reticuloendothelial disease. *Psychosomatic Medicine* 18:284–303, 1956.
30. Helsing, K.J., Comstock, G.W., and Szklo, M. Causes of death in a widowed population. *American Journal of Epidemiology* 116:524–532, 1982.
31. Helsing, K.J., and Szklo, M. Mortality after bereavement. *American Journal of Epidemiology* 114:41–52, 1981.
32. Helsing, K.J., Szklo, M., and Comstock, G.W. Factors associated with mortality after widowhood. *American Journal of Public Health* 71:802–809, 1981.
33. Heyman, D.K., and Gianturco, D.T. Long-term adaptation by the elderly to bereavement. *Journal of Gerontology* 28:359–362, 1973.

34. Hudgens, R.W., Morrison, J.R., and Barchka, R.G. Life events and onset of primary affective disorders. *Archives of General Psychiatry* 16:134–145, 1967.

35. Imboden, J.B., Canter, A., and Cluff, L. Separation experience and health records in a group of normal adults. *Psychosomatic Medicine* 25:433, 1963.

36. Jacobs, S., and Ostfeld, A. An epidemiological review of the mortality of bereavement. *Psychosomatic Medicine* 39:344–357, 1977.

37. Kleinschmidt, H.J., Waxenberg, S.E., and Cuker, R. Psychophysiology and psychiatric management of thyrotoxicosis: a two year follow-up study. *Journal of the Mount Sinai Hospital* 23:131–153, 1965.

38. Klerman, G.L., and Izen, J. The effects of bereavement and grief on physical health and general well-being. *Advances in Psychosomatic Medicine* 9:63–104, 1977.

39. Kraus, A.S., and Lilienfeld, A.M. Some epidemiological aspects of the high mortality rate in the young widowed group. *Journal of Chronic Disease* 10:207–217, 1959.

40. Leaverton, D.R., White, C.A., McCormick, C.R., Smith, P., and Sheikholislam, B. Parental loss antecedent to childhood diabetes mellitus. *Journal of the American Academy of Child Psychiatry* 19:678–689, 1980.

41. Levav, I. Mortality and psychopathology following the death of an adult child: an epidemiological review. *Israeli Journal of Psychiatry and Related Sciences* 19:23–38, 1982.

42. Lindemann, E. Symptomatology and management of acute grief. *American Journal of Psychiatry* 101:141–148, 1944.

43. MacMahon, B., and Pugh, T.F. Suicide in the widowed. *American Journal of Epidemiology* 81:23–31, 1965.

44. Maddison, D.C., and Viola, A. The health of widows in the year following bereavement. *Journal of Psychosomatic Research* 12:297–306, 1968.

45. Morillo, E., and Gardner, L.I. Bereavement as an antecedent factor in thyrotoxicosis of childhood: four case studies with survey of possible metabolic pathways. *Psychosomatic Medicine* 41:545–555, 1979.

46. Morillo, E., and Gardner, L.I. Activation of latent Graves' Disease in children. *Clinical Pediatrics* 19:160–163, 1980.

47. Morrison, F., and Paffenbarger, R. Epidemiological aspects of biobehavior in the etiology of cancer: a critical review. In: *Perspectives in Behavioral Medicine* (Weiss, S., Herd, A., and Fox, B., eds.). New York: Academic Press, 1981.

48. Morrison, J.R., Hudgens, R.W., and Barchka, R.G. Life events and psychiatric illness. *British Journal of Psychiatry* 114:423–432, 1968.

49. Murphy, G.E., and Robins, E. Social factors in suicide. *Journal of the American Medical Association* 199:303–308, 1967.

50. National Center for Health Statistics, U.S. Department of Health and Human Services. *Health United States, 1980.* Washington, D.C.: U.S. Government Printing Office, 1980.

51. National Office of Vital Statistics. *Mortality from Selected Causes by Marital Status—United States, 1949–1951, Vital Statistics—Special Reports*, Vol. 39, No. 7. Washington, D.C.: U.S. Public Health Service, May 8, 1956.

52. Parkes, C.M. Effects of bereavement on physical and mental health: a study of the medical records of widows. *British Medical Journal* 2:274–279, 1964.

53. Parkes, C.M. Recent bereavement as a cause of mental illness. *British Journal of Psychiatry* 110:198–204, 1964.

54. Parkes, C.M. The first year of bereavement: a longitudinal study of the reaction of London widows to the death of their husbands. *Psychiatry* 33:444–467, 1970.

55. Parkes, C.M. Determinants of outcome following bereavement. *Omega* 6:303–323, 1975.
56. Parkes, C.M., and Brown, R. Health after bereavement: a controlled study of young Boston widows and widowers. *Psychosomatic Medicine* 34:449–461, 1972.
57. Parkes, C.M., and Weiss, R.S. *Recovery from Bereavement*. New York: Basic Books, 1983.
58. Paykel, E.S., Myers, J.K., Dienelt, M.N., and Klerman, G.L. Life events and depression: a controlled study. *Archives of General Psychiatry* 21:753–760, 1969.
59. Pearlin, L., and Lieberman, M. Social sources of distress. In: *Research in Community Health* (Simms, R., ed.). Greenwich, Conn.: Jai Press, 1979.
60. Pihlblad, C.T., and Adams, D.L. Widowhood, social participation and life satisfaction. *Aging and Human Development* 3:323–330, 1972.
61. Priest, R.G., and Crisp, A.H. Bereavement and psychiatric symptoms: an item analysis. *Psychotherapy and Psychosomatics* 2:166–171, 1973.
62. Raphael, B. Preventive intervention with the recently bereaved. *Archives of General Psychiatry* 34:1450–1454, 1977.
63. Rees, W., and Lutkins, S.G. Mortality and bereavement. *British Medical Journal* 4:13–16, 1967.
64. Robins, L.N., West, P.A., and Murphy, G.E. The high rate of suicide in older white men: a study testing ten hypotheses. *Social Psychiatry* 12:1–20, 1977.
65. Schmale, A., and Iker, H. The psychological setting of uterine cervical cancer. *Annals of the New York Academy of Sciences* 125:794–801, 1965.
66. Shepherd, D., and Barraclough, B.M. The aftermath of suicide. *British Medical Journal* 2:600–603, 1974.
67. Singh, B., and Raphael, B. Postdisaster morbidity of the bereaved: a possible role for preventive psychiatry? *Journal of Nervous and Mental Diseases* 169:203–212, 1981.
68. Stein, Z., and Susser, M. Widowhood and mental illness. *British Journal of Preventive and Social Medicine* 23:106–110, 1969.
69. Stroebe, M.S., Stroebe, W., Gergen, K.J., and Gergen, M. The broken heart: reality or myth? *Omega* 12:87–106, 1981–82.
70. Thompson, L., Breckenridge, J., Gallagher, D., and Peterson, J. Effects of bereavement on self-perceptions of physical health in elderly widows and widowers. *Journal of Gerontology* (in press), 1984.
71. Treuting, T.F. The role of emotional factors in the etiology and course of diabetes mellitus: a review of the recent literature. *American Journal of Medical Science* 244:93–109, 1962.
72. Vachon, M.L.S. Grief and bereavement following the death of a spouse. *Canadian Psychiatric Association Journal* 21:35–44, 1976.
73. Vachon, M.L.S., Sheldon, A.R., Lancee, W.J., Lyall, W.A.L., Rogers, J., and Freeman, S.J.J. Correlates of enduring distress patterns following bereavement: social network, life situation, and personality. *Psychological Medicine* 12:783–788, 1982.
74. Ward, A.W.M. Terminal care in malignant disease. *Social Science and Medicine* 8:413–420, 1974.
75. Ward, A.W.M. Mortality of bereavement. *British Medical Journal* 1:700–702, 1976.
76. Wiener, A., Gerber, I., Battin, D., and Arkin, A.M. The process and phenomenology of bereavement. In: *Bereavement: Its Psychosocial Aspects* (Schoenberg, B., Berger, I., Weiner, A., Kutchner, A.H., Peretz, D., and Carr, A.C., eds.). New York: Columbia University Press, 1975.
77. Young, M., Benjamin, B., and Wallis, G. The mortality of widowers. *Lancet* 2:454–456, 1963.

Adults' Reactions to Bereavement

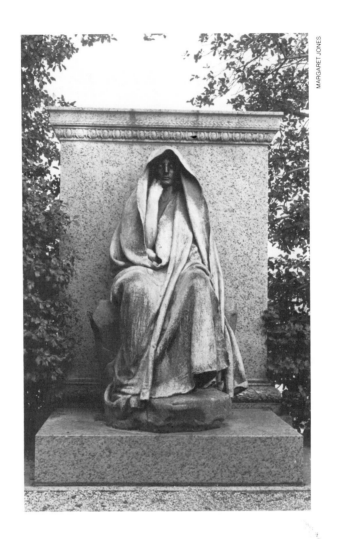

MARGARET JONES

People express grief in many different ways. Henry Adams, after his wife's suicide in 1885, commissioned the sculptor Augustus Saint-Gaudens to create the memorial pictured here. Placed in a setting designed by Stanford White, the Adams Memorial is located in Rock Creek Cemetery, Washington, D.C.

CHAPTER 3

Adults' Reactions to Bereavement

Adulthood is the most common time for bereavement, with losses occurring with ever-increasing frequency as people age. Whereas loss through death may be a relatively uncommon event for the young person, bereavement and grief are frequent companions of old age. It has been asserted that "grief as a result of loss is a predominant factor in aging."[7]

This chapter deals with the basic psychologic reactions of adults to bereavement. Unlike Chapter 2, the findings presented here are based mostly on clinical observation and inference. The focus is on the phenomenology of grief—changes in emotions, thought processes, behavior, interpersonal interactions, and physical symptoms that characteristically follow loss—and on several different theoretical models that try to account for these phenomena and for individual variations.

Reactions to bereavement cover a wide, often confusing range. The bereavement experience may include not only sadness, an expected response, but also numerous other unanticipated emotions, experiences, and behaviors that can puzzle the bereft, their friends and relatives, and the health professionals called upon to assist them. Increased knowledge about the various processes and outcomes associated with bereavement is likely to help avert some of the misunderstanding that can make the experience more difficult.

This chapter is based on material prepared by Victoria Solsberry, M.S.W., research associate, with the assistance of Janice Krupnick, M.S.W., consultant.

THE PHENOMENOLOGY OF GRIEF

Despite some earlier descriptions of bereavement reactions,[13,14] the first systematic study of bereavement was not conducted until 1944. Drawing on clinical observations of survivors of the Coconut Grove fire, Lindemann[26] detailed the symptomatology of grief. He described uncomplicated grief as a syndrome with a predictable course and distinctive symptoms, including (1) somatic distress, (2) preoccupation with the image of the deceased, (3) guilt, (4) hostility, and (5) loss of usual patterns of conduct. A sixth reaction, displayed by persons with a possibly pathologic response, was appearance of traits of the deceased (such as mannerisms or symptoms associated with a prior illness).

Since that time numerous clinicians and researchers, including Pollock,[34] Clayton et al.,[10] Glick et al.,[18] Parkes,[31,32] Parkes and Weiss,[33] and Raphael,[39,40] have sought to corroborate these earlier observations and to describe the grieving process in adults. They have systematically observed and measured changes in emotions, thought, and behaviors, and the emergence or intensification of physical complaints following bereavement.

Despite the nonlinearity of the grieving process, most observers of it speak of clusters of reactions or "phases" of bereavement that change over time. Although observers divide the process into various numbers of phases and use different terminology to label them, there is general agreement about the nature of reactions over time. Clinicians also agree that there is substantial individual variation in terms of specific manifestations of grief and in the speed with which people move through the process.

Noting recent misapplications of Kubler-Ross's[25] stages in the acceptance of one's own impending death, the committee cautions against the use of the word "stages" to describe the bereavement process, as it may connote concrete boundaries between what are actually overlapping, fluid phases. The notion of stages might lead people to expect the bereaved to proceed from one clearly identifiable reaction to another in a more orderly fashion than usually occurs. It might also result in inappropriate behavior toward the bereaved, including hasty assessments of where individuals are or ought to be in the grieving process.

Changes in Emotions and Thought Processes

There is general agreement that forewarning of death permits the soon-to-be-bereaved to structure the event cognitively and to reconcile differences with the dying person in a way that can serve to alleviate some of the feelings of anger and guilt that commonly appear after bereavement. There is disagreement, however, about whether the emotional responses to an impending death, which may resemble postdeath reactions in many ways, are comparable to grief following loss and about whether these reactions soften the blow of the actual death. Some observers of the bereaved (e.g., Bowlby,[4] Brown and Stoudemire,[5] and Bugen[6]) have found that grieving begins when a person learns of a terminal diagnosis. In their experience, anticipatory grieving allows people to begin to let go of the relationship. The clinical observations of Parkes and Weiss[33] and Vachon et al.,[44] however, have led them to conclude that persons threatened with loss typically intensify, rather than give up, attachment behaviors.

The most frequent immediate response following death, regardless of whether or not the loss was anticipated, is shock, numbness, and a sense of disbelief. Subjectively, survivors may feel like they are wrapped in a cocoon or blanket; to others, they may look as though they are holding up well. Because the reality of the death has not yet penetrated awareness, survivors can appear to be quite accepting of the loss.

Usually this numbness turns to intense feelings of separation and pain in the months after the funeral. Based on her review of the literature as well as her own years of clinical experience with the bereaved, the Australian psychiatrist, Beverly Raphael,[40] describes this phase in the following way:

> The absence of the dead person is everywhere palpable. The home and familiar environs seem full of painful reminders. Grief breaks over the bereaved in waves of distress. There is intense yearning, pining, and longing for the one who has died. The bereaved feels empty inside, as though torn apart or as if the dead person had been torn out of his body.

According to clinical researchers, "searching" behaviors—including hallucinations, dreams in which the deceased is still alive, "seeing" the deceased person in the street, and other illusions and misperceptions—are frequently reported during this phase. When the lost person fails to return, however, these behaviors decrease and despair sets in.[1] Symptoms such as depressed moods, difficulties in concentrating, anger, guilt, irritability, anxiety, restlessness, and extreme sadness then become common. Offers of comfort and support are often rejected because of the bereaved person's focus on the deceased.

The bereaved may swing dramatically and swiftly from one feeling state to another, and avoidance of reminders of the deceased may alternate with deliberate cultivation of memories for some period of time. People generally move from a state of disbelief to a gradual acceptance of the reality of the loss, although, as already noted, the progression is by no means linear. The bereaved may be intellectually aware of the finality of the loss long before their emotions let them accept the new information as true. Although no two bereaved persons are exactly alike, depression and emotional swings are characteristic of most people for at least several months, and often for more than a year following bereavement.

As old, internalized roles that included the deceased begin to be given up and as new ones are tried out, the bereaved person enters the final phase of "resolution"[5] or "reorganization."[4,23] Eventually, the survivor is able to recall memories of the deceased without being overwhelmed by sadness or other emotions and is ready to reinvest in the world.

Behavioral Changes

Feeling slowed down, with accompanying postural changes, may alternate with agitation, restlessness, and increased motor activity in the early stages of bereavement. Crying and general tearfulness also are common. During the period of despair, the bereaved may lack interest in the outside world and often give up activities they used to enjoy, such as eating, watching television, or socializing.

As noted in Chapter 2, potentially health-compromising behaviors, such as smoking and drinking, may become excessive following bereavement, especially in people who tended to use these substances before experiencing loss. Such behaviors may be considered normal in the bereaved because they occur with considerable frequency. Nevertheless, they are also psychologically and physically self-destructive, potentially leading to such illnesses as lung cancer and cirrhosis of the liver. Substance abuse and other dangerous activities, such as reckless driving, may not appear to be obviously suicidal, but they can serve the same purpose as more overt efforts. Risk-taking behavior may not appear to be directly associated with bereavement; such behavior is not readily expressive of grief but may instead be part of a defensive operation.[33] So although they are endangering their lives and, in reality, struggling with grief, survivors may appear to be coping reasonably well.

Interpersonal and Social Changes

Although bereavement precipitates changes within people, it also alters their interpersonal and social experiences. Although the bereaved person may have begun to resolve the loss emotionally, shifts in social status may lead to changes not only in self-perception but also in the ways a person is perceived by others, and the changes may continue for some time. Suddenly thinking of another as a "widow" or "bereaved person" may also instigate particular stereotypes or expectations, resulting in different qualities being ascribed to the person. The nature of these interpersonal changes is largely dependent on the relationship that was lost and sometimes on the nature of the death (see Chapter 4). These changes also are influenced by the broad sociocultural context in which the person lives (see Chapter 8) and by the bereaved person's age. For example, a middle-aged widow or widower may find social life greatly curtailed because people tend to socialize in couples. An elderly person may find that most of his or her friends and relatives have died, leaving few familiar people to be with. Making new friends may be difficult. Thus, social isolation and feelings of loneliness are common, often long after the bereavement.

Physical Complaints

Because of the defense mechanisms used by a particular person, as well as cultural norms that influence the way psychologic pain is expressed, grief may be expressed more in terms of physical symptoms than psychologic complaints.[2,29,41] As noted in Chapters 2 and 8, numerous clinical observers and social scientists have found that acute grief is associated with a variety of physical complaints, including pain, gastrointestinal disturbances, and the very "vegetative" symptoms that, at another time, might signal the presence of a depressive disorder (e.g., sleep disturbance, appetite disturbance, loss of energy). Especially in the elderly, this grief-related depression may be misdiagnosed as organic dysfunction if health professionals are not aware of the nature of bereavement reactions and the history of the particular patient.

Some bereaved persons, identifying with the deceased, may take on symptoms of the illness that killed the person for whom they are grieving. In a prospective exploration of identification phenomena in the bereaved, Zisook et al.[46] found that 14 percent of their sample admitted to feeling physically ill since their loss, 15 percent felt "just like the person who died," 8 percent had acquired habits of the deceased, 12 percent felt they had the same illness, and 9 percent had pains in the same area of their bodies as the person who died.

Physical symptoms may not necessarily disguise the personal pain associated with grief, but they may divert the attention of physicians, other health professionals, friends, family, and even the afflicted person from the psychologic aspects of loss. These symptoms normally abate as the loss is resolved.

THE END OF THE BEREAVEMENT PROCESS

The committee deliberated at length about how to label and define the end of the bereavement process, designating it variously as "recovery," "adaptation," and "completion." Each term connotes something different and none of the meanings was fully satisfactory to the entire committee.

"Recovery" is an indispensable concept in understanding outcomes; it may suggest, however, either that grief is an illness or that people who "recover" are unchanged by the loss, neither of which is correct. "Adaptation" is another essential idea, but it carries with it the negative connotation often associated with "adjustment"—making the best of an unpleasant situation—and it also seems too limited. Someone could adapt to bereavement without recovering lost functions. "Completion" is helpful in denoting relative resolution, but it suggests that there is a fixed endpoint of the bereavement process after which there is no more grieving, a notion that is inaccurate. Each expression is important and useful, but no one term alone adequately describes the end of bereavement. Thus, using varied terminology provides a better perspective on the multiple issues pertaining to outcome.

In fact, as described below, a healthy bereavement process can be expected to include recovery of lost functions (including investment in current life, hopefulness, and the capacity to experience gratification), adaptation to new roles and statuses, and completion of acute grieving. Both favorable and unfavorable outcomes along several dimensions can be identified.

One of the most important dimensions is time. Despite the popular belief that the bereavement process is normally completed in a year, data from systematic studies and from clinical reports confirm that the process may be considerably more attenuated for many people and still fall well within normal boundaries. It is not the length of time per se that distinguishes normal from abnormal grief, but the quality and quantity of reactions over time. Thus a precise endpoint in time cannot be specified.

As in other areas of mental health, there is substantially better agreement about what constitutes pathology than there is about normality or health. In the bereavement literature, this is reflected in the lack of uniformity in definitions of favorable or "normal" outcomes except in the most general terms.

Favorable Outcomes

Although the bereavement process involves the completion of certain tasks and the resumption of others, all the feelings and symptoms triggered by bereavement do not simply disappear or return to exactly the same state as before. People do adapt and stabilize, yet clinical observers of the bereaved have found that some of the pain of loss may remain for a lifetime. Reactions to the loss may recur around birthdays, holidays, or other circumstances that are particularly poignant reminders of the deceased. Clinical observations of psychiatric patients show that anniversaries can trigger serious pathology in vulnerable persons,[35] but usually such responses are transitory; recurrent waves of grief are normal and usually limited both in intensity and duration. An examination of bereavement outcomes should consider not only the presence or absence of various signs and symptoms, but also the quality and personal meaning of different behaviors.

For example, readiness to invest in new relationships does not invariably indicate completion of or recovery from grief. As with many types of behavior, a given action may mean different things to different people. A seemingly quick remarriage or a decision to have another child may reflect a sense of hope or strength in one case, whereas in another such actions may stem mainly from a wish to avoid grief. Many clinical and nonclinical observers have found wide variation in the ways people grieve and adapt. A healthy outcome for one person may be different from adequate resolution for another.

It has also been found that bereavement can have positive, growth-producing effects. Pollock,[36] having studied the lives and works of many gifted artists and scientists, concluded that the successful completion of grieving might result in increased creativity. Among the less gifted, a new relationship or new satisfactions may occur following bereavement. Creativity does not always reflect a successful working through of grief, however. It may also be an attempt to cope via restitution, reparation, or discharge.[37]

Silverman and Cooperband[43] observed dramatic personal growth in some older widows who had been in traditional marriages. For women who had relied on their husbands to assume the bulk of responsibility for the couple, a myriad of new skills may be acquired as the widow is forced to assume tasks and behaviors formerly the province of her spouse.

Pathological Outcomes

Prolonged or Chronic Grief. Parkes and Weiss,[33] in a clinical study of 68 normal widows and widowers, found that prolonged or chronic grief (defined as persistent grieving without diminution in intensity despite the passage of time) is the most common type of pathologic grief. In the research of Vachon et al.,[44] it was found that prolonged severe grief (chronic grief) accounted for the poorest outcome in almost all cases. Survivors who manifested chronic grief were described by Parkes and Weiss as having become ''stuck'' in the grieving process. A certain comfort and reassurance against anxiety was observed among those who displayed this reaction. The inability to work through grief seemed preferable to the bleak hopelessness anticipated should the bereaved truly relinquish the lost relationship.

One measure of the possible frequency of prolonged or chronic grief reactions derives from the epidemiologic findings of Clayton and Darvish[9] discussed in Chapter 2. Although the vast majority of widows and widowers no longer had symptoms one year after bereavement, approximately 12–15 percent still reported symptoms that were sufficient to meet the criteria for clinical depression.

According to Parkes and Weiss,[33] in prolonged or chronic grief the normal phases may become protracted or excessively intense, making resolution and adaptation impossible for the survivor. There may be excessive anger, guilt and self-blame, or depression that lasts longer than usual. Because these types of behavior do not differ from normal bereavement responses, it can be difficult to diagnose chronic grief. One indication would be the lack of a sense of future in a person whose loss occurred several months earlier. For example, if someone who was bereaved a year ago actively resists engagement with his or her present life—wondering, it seems, ''What is there for me now?''—chronic grief could be suspected. This assessment would stem not so much from the person's sadness as from his or her active resistance to changing that feeling. Not only is there no movement, but there also is a sense that the person will not permit any movement. It is the felt intensity of anger, self-blame, or depression that makes the reactions pathologic.

Absent Grief. Not all the bereaved report feelings of distress and other symptoms of typical grief, regardless of the apparent importance of the relationship with the deceased. Bowlby, who has devoted his career to the clinical study of response to separation and loss, describes this phenomenon as follows[4]:

> After the loss they take a pride in carrying on as though nothing happened, are busy and efficient, and may appear to be coping splendidly. But a sensitive observer notes

that they are tense and often short-tempered. No references to the loss are volunteered, reminders are avoided and well-wishers allowed neither to sympathize nor to refer to the event.

Bowlby reports that the bereaved person might appear to be coping effectively, but there are clues that all is not well. For example, the bereaved may continue to experience undue anxiety when recalling memories of the deceased or may forbid references to the death. Expressions of sympathy from others may be experienced as intolerable.

Parkes and Weiss[33] conclude that absent grief is a relatively infrequent form of pathologic grieving; nevertheless, they confirm that it does occur. They describe the process as a "fending off" of threatening emotions that are too painful to bear. Examples of such painful emotions are guilt over previous death wishes or a perceived inadequacy in loving and caring for the deceased. Over the course of many years of clinical observation of the bereaved, Horowitz[20] has found that denial is a form of coping that may be temporarily useful—if reality receives more and more attention as time passes. He has observed that it is typical for most bereaved persons to go through a period of denial; denial that continues for weeks or months, however, may be cause for concern. Horowitz has found that some denial may be adaptive in reducing fear and allowing pacing of decisions, enabling the patient to feel less troubled. But extended postponing of awareness of what must be faced may lead to hazardous choices of action.

Clinical experience with bereaved psychiatric patients has led a number of practitioners to speculate on the psychologic meaning of absent grief. Deutsch,[12] basing conclusions on a limited number of patients undergoing psychoanalytic treatment, found that grief-related affects were sometimes omitted in persons who were emotionally too weak to undertake grieving. She concluded that where the intensity of affects was too great or the coping ability too weak, defensive and rejecting mechanisms came into play. Other authors have observed that a potentially hazardous outcome of this unconscious refusal to grieve may be depression, often masked by a multitude of physical symptoms. Based on their clinical experience in a major academic health center, Brown and Stoudemire[5] advise that "patients who experience persistent symptoms of major depression, often with the development of coincidental unusual physical symptoms, should be carefully considered as having an unresolved or latent grief reaction." Volkan[45] observed that patients who do not overtly manifest grieving responses will often appear in a physician's office with physical illnesses that he termed "depressive equivalents," but that today would more likely be called "somatization." He discovered that these symptoms seldom served as "substitutes'' for depression, and advised that if the physician looks closely enough and asks the correct questions, the depressive symptoms generally will also be found.

Because of pressures to return to the prebereavement state, as well as the unpleasantness for others of experiencing the grieving of the bereaved, absent grief may not be perceived as a problem. The survivor who seems to be doing so well relieves others of the burden of support. The bereaved who goes on with his or her life in a seemingly productive way without suffering the agony of grief looks to many as someone who has finished the process. Too often, however, the process may not even have been started.

Delayed Grief.   Whether delayed grief, a concept implying a long period of absent grief (perhaps months or even years) after which grief-like symptoms emerge, even exists is controversial, as noted in Chapter 2. Some experts conceptualize this unusual reaction as a bereavement response while others view it as a new episode of affective disorder.

These different perspectives naturally carry treatment implications. Those who formulate the problem as purely psychologic would be more likely to recommend psychotherapeutic intervention, whereas those who diagnose a major depressive disorder, unrelated to bereavement, might be more inclined to treat the symptoms with antidepressant medication.

EXPLANATORY MODELS OF THE BEREAVEMENT PROCESS

A number of models—in this report divided into classical psychoanalytic, psychodynamic, interpersonal, crisis, and cognitive and behavioral—have been developed to explain the observable reactions to and reported experiences of bereavement. Each conceptual framework tries to account for the various normal and pathologic processes and outcomes related to bereavement. The hypothesized mechanisms that account for different responses also provide frameworks for various intervention approaches with the bereaved (see Chapter 10).

Rather than representing rigidly different schools of thought, the various models are overlapping. They tend to differ in the amount of emphasis placed on different aspects of response and in their therapeutic techniques, although many clinicians use an eclectic approach employing concepts from several different schools of thought. Of particular note is the growing convergence between psychodynamic, behavioral, and cognitive perspectives. Although each favors particular therapeutic techniques, observations of the bereavement process have led adherents of these perspectives to agree on the importance of certain phenomena.

For example, in both the psychodynamic perspective and in cognitive theories, importance is placed on the meanings attributed to the loss and on what happens to a person's self-concept as a result. Overlap occurs in conceptualizations regarding impulses and defenses that emerge during grieving, in ideas about belief systems, and in assessments regarding a person's perceived locus of control.

In considering the essential points of each of these models, the reader should bear in mind that theoreticians from the various perspectives may use different vocabulary to describe the same basic phenomena. What is conceptualized by behaviorists as one kind of maladaptive social reinforcement, for example, may be seen by psychoanalysts as a problem with dependency.

It should also be emphasized that the different theoretical models are based on data from clinical observation rather than from rigorous statistical tests of hypotheses. There is no empirical evidence that can be called upon to assert the validity of the approaches described. However, supporters of each school of thought report substantial clinical consensus regarding both the validity and utility of the various explanatory models.

Classical Psychoanalytic Theory

The classical psychoanalytic model of bereavement rests largely on Freudian theory.[16] According to this perspective, grieving presents a dilemma because there is a need to relinquish the tie to the cherished love object if one is to complete the grieving process, but "letting go" of the deceased involves considerable emotional pain. Initially the bereaved person is likely to deny that the loss has occurred, increase his or her investment in the lost person, become preoccupied with thoughts of the deceased, and lose interest in the outside world. Eventually, however, as memories are brought forth and reviewed, the person's ties are gradually withdrawn, grieving is completed, and the bereaved regains sufficient emotional energy to invest in new relationships.

Classical analysts, basing their formulations on experiences with patients undergoing psychoanalysis, infer that relinquishing the loved object takes place largely through identification with the deceased, and they pay considerable attention to the different outcomes of identification following loss. They have found that, in cases in which the deceased was an object of hate or of the mixed emotions of intense ambivalence, identification with the lost person may become a precursor to certain kinds of depression.

Current Psychodynamic Perspectives

A number of contemporary psychoanalytic and psychodynamically oriented practitioners who have worked clinically with the bereaved have elaborated on the premises of Freud and his followers. These observers of the grieving process continue to focus their attention on internal psychic structures, defense mechanisms, and intrapsychic processes, but they also are concerned with interpersonal dynamics and the ways in which relationship issues may affect self-concept and views of others. Based on their clinical experiences, they have described additional ways in which antecedent personality and relationship variables may have an impact on grieving.

Of course, psychologic processes do not take place in a vacuum. A variety of sociocultural factors, including cultural norms, values, belief systems, and financial status, all contribute to the way a bereaved person perceives, interprets, and understands a loss. Preexisting health, as mentioned earlier, also affects responses to and the outcome of bereavement. Thus, to understand fully the individual factors that come into play, consideration must be given to psychosocial influences as well as purely psychologic, social, or cultural issues.

The Role of the Preexisting Personality. Although there are almost no systematic studies of the role played by preexisting personality variables in affecting the process or outcome of grieving,[44] clinicians generally agree that such factors do influence every aspect of the grief experience, ranging from the way the loss is initially perceived to the way it is or is not resolved. Habitual styles of perception, thought, coping, and defense determine how a person experiences and handles all life situations, and these same modes are called upon to deal with the stress of bereavement. Clinical experience has shown that people who are characteristically more flexible and able to use more mature coping strategies will deal with bereavement more effectively than others. Those who are psychologically healthier prior to bereavement are expected to experience the pain of loss, but are viewed as unlikely to become overwhelmed or unduly frightened by their feelings.

Observers with psychological training agree that personality variables also probably relate to the quantity and quality of a bereaved person's social support network, which, in turn, has been found to influence outcome. People with well-integrated personalities are expected to be better integrated socially, because their personality traits enable them to both attract and sustain supportive relationships. Preexisting personality may also be seen as a determinant of the degree to which someone can perceive and use the community support system. It may be that social variables are even more important in predicting outcome than intrapsychic conflicts, although most researchers and clinicans believe that these variables are inextricably linked.

The Activation of Latent Negative Self-Images. Clinical experience with a number of bereaved psychotherapy patients has led Horowitz et al.[22] to infer that people who are particularly vulnerable to difficulties following bereavement have latent images of themselves as bad, incompetent, or hurtful. They speculate that loss activates these once-dormant negative images and find that distorted thoughts about the self and others intensify the grieving process, frequently resulting in pathologic responses. Self-concepts that appear to complicate grieving include feeling too weak to function without the deceased (resulting in overwhelming instead of tolerable sadness), considering oneself hostile and somehow responsible for the death (leading to intensified guilt), and feeling damaged or defective (leading to a sense of emptiness and apathy).[19,21,22]

These clinical researchers have found that most people who lose a person who supplied a significant amount of gratification revert to some self-representations of weakness and helplessness. Normally, however, "these self-images may be less desperate in quality, less discrepant with other self-images, and less compelling as organizers of information than the needy self-images of a person with conflicts or developmental defects in this area."[22]

This view of pathologic grieving is based in part on the same conceptualizations that underlie cognitive therapy. In the latter, however, the focus is on the maladaptive attitudes and thoughts themselves, whereas the conceptualizations of Horowitz and his colleagues emphasize the way people think about themselves and others within the context of their interpersonal relationships.

The Ambivalent Relationship. Many clinicians, regardless of their theoretical orientation, point to the quality of the relationship with the deceased as predictive of postbereavement response. Freud,[16] basing his formulations on a limited number of bereaved psychoanalytic patients, maintained that the most "important precondition leading to depression following bereavement was an ambivalent relationship with the deceased prior to the death."

In its most general sense, ambivalence in relationships is universal and not especially significant. Few affectionate relations are uncomplicated by some hostility, and many hostile relations are tempered by affection. "When, however, the strength of these conflicting feelings increases to the point where actions seem unavoidable yet unacceptable, some defensive maneuver is undertaken . . . [e.g.] the ambivalence is repressed . . . and only one of the two sets of feelings is permitted to become conscious. Usually it is the hostility that is repressed.''[30] Because of this hostility—whether overtly expressed, secretly experienced, or unconsciously repressed—a person might feel remorseful after the death of the other.

In their clinical investigation of 68 normal widows and widowers, Parkes and Weiss[33] found that recovery after conjugal bereavement was more likely to occur in marriages that had been "happy" than in those that had been conflict-ridden. In this study, participants were separated into two categories—those who rated their marriages as having had one or no areas of conflict versus those who had two or more problem areas. Differences between the two groups were highly significant. At 13 months after bereavement, good outcomes were more than twice as likely in the no-conflict group than in the conflict group (61 versus 29 percent). At two to four years postbereavement, the widows and widowers who reported a high level of conflict (many of whom had displayed little or no distress during the first year) were almost twice as likely as their low-conflict counterparts to be depressed, anxious, guilty, in poorer health, and yearning for the dead spouse. From these data, Parkes and Weiss[33] concluded:

> Marital conflict had produced anger, and perhaps, desire for escape, but coexisting with these feelings were continued attachment to the other and even, perhaps, affection. Anger interfered with grieving, and only with the passage of time did persisting need for the lost spouse emerge in the form of sadness, anxiety, and yearning.

The Dependent Relationship. A second type of relationship that may predispose a survivor to difficulties in grieving is one that involves excessive dependency. Parkes and Weiss[33] caution, however, that it is often difficult to define what is meant by this because

> dependency is, in many ways, an unsatisfactory and ambiguous term. It can be taken to mean any situation in which one person relies on another to perform physical functions; thus an amputee can be described as dependent on his wife for functions that formerly he would have performed for himself. Or it can be used to describe any situation in which one person seeks reassurance and comfort from another, as in the case of the frightened child who clings in a dependent way to the mother. Or, as in the case of Queen Victoria, it can be used to describe intolerance of separation from another person (this was the case even during Prince Albert's life).

Researchers who assert that excessive dependency may lead to difficulty following bereavement cite as evidence the literature on the psychologic development of the young child. This material suggests that children who successfully complete the separation-individuation process are able to achieve a secure attachment with their parents and to turn to them for protection and nurturing when they feel endangered. The child who, for whatever reason, feels that this protection is not forthcoming or is questionable is said to be more likely to experience the world as a threatening place and to experience anxiety when separated from a parent. In an effort to feel secure, such children have been observed to become clingy, a tendency that Parkes and Weiss[33] infer is carried into adult relationships. They describe such adults as typically responding to real or threatened separation with fear, distress, and intense anger, and report that this group has particular difficulty in coping with bereavement.

In studies of conjugal bereavement, Parkes and Weiss[33] and Lopata[27] found that survivors in their samples who had been overly dependent tended to do poorly. The grief responses of the widows and widowers in this previously dependent group were characterized by positions of helplessness, indecisiveness, and intense yearning.

Although excessively dependent spouses may be vulnerable if left on their own, the tendency of many families to reconstitute following bereavement may offer some protection from frightening levels of increased anxiety. After a husband's death some dependent widows move in with sisters or other family members whom they have not seen or socialized with for years, although elderly widows may no longer have surviving siblings or even children to take them in. More concrete problems, such as the inability to drive a car or lack of job skills, deficits that are likely to be especially pronounced among older women, may prove to be better predictors of poor outcome among elderly widows. Older widows also fall into a "high-risk" group in terms of financial difficulties following the death of a spouse, another situation that exacerbates feelings of anxiety, depression, and social isolation.

It should also be noted that the deceased may have been an important source of social and emotional support even when ill and dying. Thus, with the death, the survivor loses not only the person depended on for many years, but also the support that enabled him or her to cope during the illness.

Interpersonal and Attachment Theory Models

Unlike the psychoanalytic models that emphasize intrapsychic dynamics, interpersonal models focus primarily on relationships—the nature of attachment bonds and the psychosocial consequences of breaking them. As already noted, the two perspectives are not mutually exclusive. Both deal with relationships, but psychoanalysts focus more on their personal meaning, while the interpersonal theorists focus more on their social meaning, on social roles, and on role transitions.

Although attachment theory grew out of and incorporates much psychoanalytic thinking, it also incorporates a number of principles from animal ethology.[4] The biologic substrate of grief reactions and the function of grief responses—namely, to revive or ensure the survival of the interpersonal relationship or the social group—are emphasized by both Bowlby[4] and Darwin.[11]

As conceptualized by Bowlby, the propensity of human beings to make strong affectional bonds to particular others is instinctive. Within this framework, bereavement can be viewed as an unwilling separation that can give rise to many forms of emotional distress and personality disturbance. Bowlby, studying young children who were placed in institutional settings away from their parents, observed that when a bond was threatened by separation, powerful attachment behaviors—including clinging, crying, and angry protest—were instigated. When the actual loss of an important relationship occurred, Bowlby found that there was a brief period of protest followed by a longer period of searching behavior. Over time, these behaviors, aimed at reestablishing the attachment bond, usually ceased and despair set in. Eventually, new attachment bonds were formed. However, in some cases chronic stress ensued, leading to emotional or physical illness.

Interpersonal theorists have focused considerable attention on conceptualizations of the phases of grieving described earlier and have observed different interpersonal behaviors in each phase. For example, they have found that people in an early state of disbelief or shock are likely to be socially withdrawn. Preoccupied with a desire to reject the new situation, a bereaved person may even attempt to care for others who are suffering.[42] In an angry, yearning phase of grief, the bereaved may actively disrupt social relationships. In a sad phase, they may seek support and allow others to feel that they are being appropriately helpful.

According to this perspective, the bereaved feel capable of engaging in new relationships only as they begin to redefine themselves. Silverman,[42] in her extensive experience with the conjugally bereaved, has observed that the bereaved "need opportunities to practice assuming, at least in part, a new identity that can involve new behavior patterns" that are aligned with the changes that have occurred. Parkes and Weiss[33] call this identity "a theory of self" that is used in thinking about ourselves, in presenting ourselves to others, and in defining our choices in the world. They found that bereaved persons sometimes chose new satisfactions that were appropriate in light of the role loss but would not have been appropriate before. Thus, one measure of a favorable outcome in bereavement is a survivor's ability to make this transition and redefine his or her role.

Crisis Theory

According to crisis theory, the death of an important other disturbs the survivor's "homeostasis" or equilibrium.[8] The bereavement is conceptualized as a stressful life event that highlights preexisting personality problems that previously may have lain dormant or did not seriously interfere with the person's ability to function. Because the crisis creates an acute situation, the bereaved may be in danger of increased disorganization. At the same time, however, because the loss intensifies and exaggerates already existing problematic ways of coping and defending, the death may provide an opportunity to recognize and work on what may have been formerly entrenched, unconscious issues. Thus, the potentially traumatic life event is viewed as presenting potential for positive growth and change.

Cognitive and Behavioral Theories

Theory emerging from cognitive therapy provides a model for understanding a variety of depressive and anxiety disorders. Developed by Beck,[3] a psychoanalytically trained psychiatrist, this model emphasizes the link between distorted thinking and psychopathology. Its focus on the relationship between disturbed thinking and dysphoric feelings parallels the thinking of some current dynamic theorists (e.g., Horowitz et al.[22]), thus reflecting some of the convergent thinking noted earlier among theorists with different orientations.

Cognitive therapists have not explicitly delineated the psychologic processes specific to bereavement, although Beck's cognitive model of depression could be applied to pathologic grief reactions. According to this conceptualization, a person's affect and behavior are based on the way he or she structures the world. People who experience episodes of clinical depression carry negative views of themselves, their futures, and their experiences. Extrapolating from this model, it could be assumed that bereavement might instigate a chain of negative thoughts that could intensify or prolong grief in those persons who had a premorbid tendency to see themselves and the world in a negative light. In such individuals, the death of someone important might be interpreted as deliberate rejection based on their inherent defectiveness. These persons might then experience themselves as social outcasts and, because of this, feel excessively sad and lonely. Negative ideas may predate the loss, at least to some degree, but the reality of the loss tends to reinforce those ideas. Thus, pessimistic expectations of the future and negative views of the self that may have existed prior to the bereavement become intensified.

According to the cognitive theory of Gauthier and Marshall,[17] grief may become distorted if attempts are made to inhibit it. For example, if a grieving person is led to believe that it is bad to think about the deceased because the pain produced by memories will be intolerable, that person may develop secondary anxiety when intense bereavement-related experiences occur. Clinical experience has led Gauthier and Marshall to infer that when intrusive thoughts about the deceased then occur, the immediate reaction is to attempt to avoid them for fear of losing control. This is said to produce ideal conditions for suppression of grief-related ideas, possibly leading to further distress because troubling trains of thought are not resolved.

Behaviorally oriented clinicians and researchers generally are less concerned with describing internal, underlying processes and personal meanings of loss than are representatives of other schools of thought. Their emphasis is exclusively on troubling, manifest behaviors that emerge following bereavement and on any environmental factors that foster or reinforce such behaviors. They regard grief as "a particular case of the more general malady of depression"[17] and devote considerably more attention to the development of models to explain the phenomena of clinical depression. Of the few who do address the subject of bereavement, the major emphasis is on developing and assessing methods of intervention.

Behaviorists who are specifically concerned with grief reactions (e.g., Mawson et al.[28] and Ramsay[38]) focus primarily on pathologic grief. They liken persistent distress of more than one year's duration that is initiated or exacerbated by bereavement to other forms of avoidance such as phobias or obsessive-compulsive behaviors. Ramsay's[38] clinical experience has led him to conclude that persons likely to become "stuck" in pathologic grief reactions are those whose prebereavement response patterns were to avoid confrontation and to escape from difficult situations. He has found that, following the death of someone important, these people fail to enter situations that could trigger their grief. In other words, they avoid stimuli that could elicit undesired responses, such as crying. Because such stimuli are avoided, however, they find it impossible to work through their grief.

Mental health professionals with a behavioral orientation also view severe or persistent grief as a function of inadequate or misplaced social reinforcement. For example, Ramsay[38] has found that persons suffering from pathologic grief have lost a major portion of the positive reinforcers in their lives. He describes a typical case of this as the widow whose reinforcement consisted of doing everything for her husband and who finds everything meaningless when he dies. According to this theory, because people feel powerless in the face of death, they conclude that all action is futile and stop responding in ways that would eventually alleviate their stress.

Gauthier and Marshall[17] have found that grief reactions may be prolonged or exacerbated if family or friends provide excessive social reinforcement for grieving behavior. They caution that if people in the social environment fail eventually to withdraw attention for grieving or do not provide consistent encouragement for more adaptive behavior, they are in effect encouraging the continuation of manifestations of grief.

CONCLUSIONS AND RECOMMENDATIONS

There is tremendous individual variation in adults' reactions to bereavement. Such factors as ethnicity and culture, preexisting personality variables, and the nature of the bereaved person's prior relationship to the deceased are major determinants of outcome.

Most clinicians recognize phases of grieving in which clusters of reactions are more or less prominent at different points in the process. Grieving may involve alternating phases of response, including periods of both numbness and distress. A variety of clinical signs and symptoms, including changes in appearance, withdrawal from social activities, and increased physical complaints, fall within the norm following the loss of someone close. The grieving process does not, however, proceed in a linear fashion. It is important to consider each person's background when assessing the relative normality of manifestations of grief and the speed with which he or she recovers.

In most instances there is satisfactory resolution following loss, in terms of an ability to return to an earlier level of psychologic functioning. The length of time this will take varies, although it is generally agreed that progress should be evident a year after a loss. Pathologic responses to bereavement include those characterized by an absence of grief, seemingly delayed grief, or excessively prolonged or intense grief. Professional help may be warranted for persons who show no evidence of having begun grieving or who exhibit as much distress at one year postbereavement as they did the first few months after the death.

Representatives of a number of theoretical schools have provided models to explain the different responses of adults to bereavement, based on their clinical observations of people who have sustained a major loss. They place varying degrees of emphasis on the intrapsychic, interpersonal, or situational factors that facilitate or impede resolution, although their models overlap on a number of points.

More empirical data on the response to loss are needed. Theoretical formulations should be translated into operational definitions, and hypothetical constructs must be broken down into particular variables that can be systematically studied. However, detailed clinical case reports should not be discouraged. Clinical observations continue to serve as a valuable source of insights into the bereavement process and to provide ideas for systematic research.

REFERENCES

1. Averill, J.R. Grief: its nature and significance. *Psychological Bulletin* 70:721–748, 1968.
2. Barsky, A., and Klerman, G. Overview: hypochondriasis, bodily complaints and somatic styles. *American Journal of Psychiatry* 140:273–283, 1983.
3. Beck, A., Rush, J., Shaw, B., and Emergy, G. *Cognitive Therapy of Depression.* New York: Guilford Press, 1979.
4. Bowlby, J. *Loss: Sadness and Depression—Attachment and Loss*, Vol. III. New York: Basic Books, 1980.
5. Brown, J.T., and Stoudemier, G.A. Normal and pathological grief. *Journal of the American Medical Association* 250:378–382, 1983.
6. Bugen, L.A. Human grief: a model for prediction and intervention. *American Journal of Orthopsychiatry* 42:196–206, 1977.
7. Butler, R.N., and Lewis, M.I. *Aging and Mental Health* (2nd edition). St. Louis: C.V. Mosby, 1977.
8. Caplan, G. Emotional crisis. In: *Encyclopedia of Mental Health*, Vol. 2 (Deutsch, A., and Fishman, H., eds.). New York: Franklin Watts, 1963.
9. Clayton, P.J., and Darvish, H.S. Course of depressive symptoms following the stress of bereavement. In: *Stress and Mental Disorder* (Barrett, J.E., ed.). New York: Raven Press, 1979.
10. Clayton, P.J., Desmarais, L., and Winokur, G. A study of normal bereavement. *American Journal of Psychiatry* 125:168–178, 1968.
11. Darwin, C. *The Expression of Emotion in Men and Animals.* London: Murray, 1872.
12. Deutsch, H. Absence of grief. *Psychoanalytic Quarterly* 6:12–22, 1937.
13. Eliot, T.D. The adjustive behavior of bereaved families: a new field for research. *Social Forces* 8:543–549, 1930.
14. Eliot, T.D. The bereaved family. *Annals of the American Academy of Political and Social Sciences* 160:184–190, 1932.
15. Engel, G.L. Grief and grieving. *American Journal of Nursing* 64:93–98, 1964.
16. Freud, S. *Mourning and Melancholia* (1917). *The Standard Edition of the Complete Psychological Works of Sigmund Freud*, Vol. 14 (Strachey, J., ed.). London: Hogarth Press and Institute for Psychoanalysis, 1957.

17. Gauthier, Y., and Marshall, W. Grief: a cognitive behavioral analysis. *Cognitive Therapy and Research* 1:39–44, 1977.

18. Glick, I.O., Parkes, C.M., and Weiss, R. *The First Year of Bereavement*. New York: Basic Books, 1975.

19. Horowitz, M. *States of Mind*. New York: Plenum, 1979.

20. Horowitz, M. Psychological processes induced by illness, injury and loss. In: *Handbook of Clinical Health Psychology* (Millon, T., Green, C., and Meagher, R., eds.). New York: Plenum, 1982.

21. Horowitz, M., Marmar, C., Krupnick, J., Wilner, N., Kaltreider, N., and Wallerstein, R. *Personality Style and Brief Therapy*. New York: Basic Books, 1984.

22. Horowitz, M., Wilner, N., Marmar, C., and Krupnick, J. Pathological grief and the activation of latent self-images. *American Journal of Psychiatry* 137:1157–1162, 1980.

23. Jacobs, S., and Ostfeld, A. The clinical management of grief. *Journal of the American Geriatrics Society* 28:331–335, 1980.

24. Katon, W., Kleinman, A., and Rosen, G. Depression and somatization: a review. *American Journal of Medicine* 72:127–135, 241–247, 1982.

25. Kubler-Ross, E. *On Death and Dying*. New York: Macmillan, 1969.

26. Lindemann, E. Symptomatology and management of acute grief. *American Journal of Psychiatry* 101:141–149, 1944.

27. Lopata, H. Self-identity in marriage and widowhood. *The Sociological Quarterly* 14:407–418, 1973.

28. Mawson, D., Marks, I., Ramm, L., and Stern, R. Guided mourning for morbid grief: a controlled study. *British Journal of Psychiatry* 138:185–193, 1981.

29. Mechanic, D. Social psychological factors affecting the presentation of bodily complaints. *New England Journal of Medicine* 286:1132–1139, 1972.

30. Moore, B.E., and Fine, B. (Eds.) *A Glossary of Psychoanalytic Terms and Concepts* (2nd edition). New York: American Psychoanalytic Association, 1968.

31. Parkes, C.M. The first year of bereavement. *Psychiatry* 33:422–467, 1970.

32. Parkes, C.M. *Bereavement*. London: Tavistock, 1972.

33. Parkes, C.M., and Weiss, R.S. *Recovery from Bereavement*. New York: Basic Books, 1983.

34. Pollock, G.H. Mourning and adaptation. *International Journal of Psychoanalysis* 42:341–361, 1961.

35. Pollock, G.H. Anniversary reactions, trauma and mourning. *The Psychoanalytic Quarterly* 34:347–371, 1970.

36. Pollock, G.H. Process and affect: mourning and grief. *International Journal of Psychoanalysis* 59:255–276, 1978.

37. Pollock, G.H. The mourning-liberation process and creativity: the case of Kathe Kollwitz. *The Annual of Psychoanalysis* 10:333–354, 1982.

38. Ramsay, R.W. Bereavement: a behavioral treatment of pathological grief. In: *Trends in Behavior Therapy* (Sioden, P.O., Bates, S., and Dorkens, III, W.S., eds.). New York: Academic Press, 1979.

39. Raphael, B. Preventive intervention with the recently bereaved. *Archives of General Psychiatry* 34:1450–1454, 1977.

40. Raphael, B. *The Anatomy of Bereavement*. New York: Basic Books, 1983.

41. Rosen, G., Kleinman, A., and Katon, W. Somatization and family practice: a biopsychosocial approach. *The Journal of Family Practice* 14:493–502, 1982.

42. Silverman, P.R. Transitions and models of intervention. *Annals of the Academy of Political and Social Science* 464:174–187, 1982.

43. Silverman, P.R., and Cooperband, A. On widowhood: mutual help and the elderly widow. *Journal of Geriatric Psychiatry* 8:9–27, 1975.

44. Vachon, M., Sheldon, A.R., Lance, W.J., Lyall, W.A., Rogers, J., and Freeman, S. Correlates of enduring stress patterns following bereavement: social network, life situation, and personality. *Psychological Medicine* 12:783–788, 1982.

45. Volkan, V. Normal and pathological grief reactions—a guide for the family physician. *Virginia Medical Monthly* 93:651–656, 1966.

46. Zisook, S., Devand, R.A., and Click, M.A. Measuring symptoms of grief and bereavement. *American Journal of Psychiatry* 139:1590–1593, 1982.

Reactions to Particular Types of Bereavement

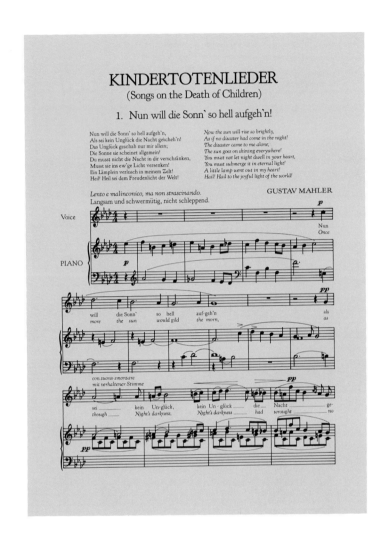

Of the many musical expressions of bereavement, Gustav Mahler's Kindertotenlieder *are among the most poignant and tender. Greatly affected by the numerous illnesses of his twelve brothers and sisters, half of whom died, Mahler chose for this song cycle the poems of Friedrich Rücket, who had lost two of his own children.*

CHAPTER 4

Reactions to Particular Types of Bereavement

$\mathbf{I}$t is generally acknowledged that the type of relationship lost influences the reactions of the survivor. Because the needs, responsibilities, hopes, and expectations associated with each type of relationship vary, the personal meanings and social implications of each type of death also differ. Thus, it is assumed that the death of a spouse, for example, is experienced differently from the death of a child.[75]

This chapter summarizes and discusses current knowledge about the various psychosocial responses to particular types of bereavement. The focus is on loss of immediate kin—spouse, child, parent, and sibling. There is also discussion of the response to suicide, often regarded as one of the most difficult types of loss to sustain. Other types of particularly difficult losses, such as multiple simultaneous deaths resulting from accidents or natural disasters and deaths caused by war and terrorism, are not discussed.

DEATH OF A SPOUSE*

The death of a husband or wife is well recognized as an emotionally devastating event, being ranked on life event scales as the most stressful of all possible losses.[29] The intensity and persistence of the pain associ-

---

*This section is based on material prepared by committee member Robert S. Weiss, Ph.D.

ated with this type of bereavement is thought to be due to the emotional valence of marital bonds linking husbands and wives to each other. Spouses are co-managers of home and family, companions, sexual partners, and fellow members of larger social units. Although the strength of particular linkages may vary from one marriage to another, all marriages seem to contain each of these linkages to some extent.

The death of a spouse ends the relationship but does not sever all relational bonds. The sense of being connected to the lost figure persists—sometimes exacerbating a sense of having been abandoned, sometimes contributing to a sense of continuing in a relationship, although with an absent partner.

There are two distinct aspects to marital partnerships. First, both husband and wife look to the other to collaborate in the setting of marital policy: How should money be used? Where should the family live? Should they have children? If so, how should they be raised? Loss of a spouse leaves the survivor to plan alone. Occasionally, when a marriage has been filled with conflict, the survivor finds rueful gratification in now being able to decide matters without argument. But most often, and especially if there are children, widows and widowers complain of having to shoulder all responsibilities alone. The burden of sole responsibility for children is especially difficult.[74]

The partnership of marriage also serves to divide familial labor. Following the death of a spouse, the survivor is left with unfamiliar tasks to be accomplished in addition to accustomed ones. The loss of the husband may mean the loss of the family's chief income producer, imposing on the widow not only sole responsibility for managing the family's finances, but also the problem of compensating for the husband's absent contribution. The sudden need to manage finances and, perhaps, enter the labor force may be particularly stressful for older widows who never received training in money matters and who frequently lack practical job skills. Early socialization for dependency on their spouses has left many elderly widows ill-prepared for earning and managing their money. Insurance and pension payments may provide a sudden augmentation of capital, but such payments constitute a one-time event that the widow may not know how to use wisely.

For most men, the loss of a wife means the loss of the partner who had taken responsibility for child care and home management. Some bereaved husbands, regarding themselves as ill-equipped to take over this role, employ housekeepers; others find some way of using the services of other women in their families; still others manage on their own, perhaps sharing responsibilities with children.

If there are children in the home, the surviving parent may feel unable to meet their children's demands for attention and understanding. The single parent can be vulnerable to overload and emotional exhaustion,[74] especially since their enormous and constant effort seems so largely unrecognized.

Companionship in many marriages consists only of sharing daily routines, outings, and bed—activities which themselves can facilitate well-being. In other marriages, however, the relationship is characterized by an intense sharing of intimate lives. In all cases, the death of a spouse necessitates finding substitute companions or tolerating a lonelier life; the loss of a spouse who had been a "best friend" represents additional impoverishment.

As already suggested, the death of one's spouse means the loss of one's sexual partner. According to the research of Glick et al.,[25] some widows totally lose interest in sex as one aspect of grief and are celibate for some time after their husbands' deaths, although with the passage of time, at least some report unsatisfied yearnings. Widowers' grieving appears less likely to involve loss of sexual yearning.

Finally, the death of a spouse is likely to alter a person's social role and standing in the community, with widows and widowers frequently excluded from the sociability of couples. Widows who had participated in leisure activities as members of a couple and widowers who had relied on their wives to arrange their social lives may find that bereavement ushers in a time of social marginality. Survivors who have trouble in establishing new friendships may be most prone to experiencing feelings of isolation; Lopata,[43] in a study of midwestern widows, found that this was especially likely among those in lower socioeconomic classes. Problems of social isolation may be particularly pronounced among elderly widows who frequently cannot afford social outings and who may live some distance from grown children. Failing health among the elderly may also make it difficult to engage in social activities following bereavement.

Redefinition of role is one of the main tasks of the bereavement process for the widowed. "Mourning . . . is not something that ends and then the widow is able to return to her life as before."[65] To the extent that a widow embraced a traditional role during marriage, she adopted an identity based on social interactions with another (her husband) and with the situation (her marriage) that were stabilized with repetition. When the "other" or the "situation" changes, the identity of the survivor must be modified. In addition, for a widow who did not work outside the home, a husband's absence leaves no object for her work, so her daily activities change. And "since marriage created a system of specialization in knowledge and skills, she [may have] definite gaps in her abilities."[43] These problems again may be particularly evident in elderly widows who are more likely to have had traditional marriages. For such women, who organized their lives around husband and family, conjugal bereavement removes the focus of their lives. With children grown and a lack of job skills or employment experience, they may feel that they have lost their purpose in life.

Bereavement may also initiate a "status passage." For example, perceived as a "sad person," the widow may remind others of the fragility of life. Or, because she is now unattached, she may be seen as a threatening sexual rival. As a single person, the newly bereaved widow may no longer have access to previously available social supports. Clarisa Start, in her first-person account, *On Becoming a Widow*,[68] recalled finding that "grief teaches you that there are two kinds of people in the world, those who are available and those who are not." In her clinical research, Golan[26] found that the new widow is sometimes forced to change roles sooner than she would like, learning to cope with the insecurity of possible incompetence, handle the anxieties involved with decision making and the stress of taking on this new role, adjust to all that the role implies in terms of status and position in the community and family, and devise new standards of well-being.

Silverman[66] has observed that conjugal loss may also initiate a process that can lead to "dramatic growth or a quiet reorientation." Golan[26] describes a process of moving from "being a wife to being a widow to being a woman." She means by this that a widow must first accept the reality of the loss, signifying that she is no longer someone's wife. In Golan's opinion, however, growth really occurs when the widow gives up her view of herself as a "partnerless half" and strives to enhance her sense of individuality.

Widowed individuals may be seen by members of the extended family as requiring concerned attention. With this increase in sympathy may come a decrease in respect; for example, the widow is now more likely to be perceived as the recipient rather than the giver of advice. Widows and widowers who once provided holiday dinners for the family may now agree to allow a sibling or grown child to assume this responsibility. Reduced standing in the family may lead to reduced confidence in the self.

There seem to be few sex differences in terms of vulnerability to distress following conjugal loss. Differences in outward expressions of grief, including more crying among widows, seem to be based primarily on the tendency for women to be more expressive than men.

There does seem to be a sex difference, however, in the recovery processes following conjugal bereavement. In their research on the first year after spousal death, Glick et al.[25] found that widows usually could not engage in new relationships soon after their husbands' deaths without feeling disloyal. In contrast, widowers did not seem to feel that a new relationship would conflict with their commitment to their deceased spouses. In fact, widowers who established a new quasi-marital relationship a few months after bereavement expected their new partners to be sympathetic to their continued grieving.

Among those past middle age, conjugal bereavement can no longer be considered untimely. Even when the death is long foreshadowed by a slow terminal illness, however, observers generally doubt the occurrence of "anticipatory grief" in the sense of an initiation of grieving and withdrawal from the dying partner. Clinical observations of grieving couples[52,71] reveal (as discussed in Chapter 3) that feelings of attachment may actually intensify (as is typically the case in response to threat) and the marital tie may be further reaffirmed by demonstrations of loyalty and commitment. Consciously admitting and planning for a husband's or wife's demise may make a spouse feel disloyal. Furthermore, following a spouse's death there are so many changes in the sense of self and situation that earlier plans may no longer seem desirable.

DEATH OF A CHILD*

Bereavement can certainly be painful whenever it occurs, but many feel that the experience of losing a child is by far the worst[27,72] because it conflicts with our life-cycle expectations. Although once common, deaths of children between the ages of 1 and 14 now account for less than 5 percent of mortality in the United States.[51] In contrast with earlier years when couples sometimes had several children die, most families today lose none. It is now expected in this country that children will live to adulthood.

Nevertheless, 400,000 children under the age of 25 die each year from accidents, diseases, suicide, or murder, leaving approximately 800,000 bereaved parents.[20] And, as life expectancy increases, the number of elderly adults who experience the deaths of their middle-aged children can also be expected to multiply.

---

*This section is based on material prepared by Victoria Solsberry, M.S.W., research associate.

In addition to being loved, children take on great symbolic importance in terms of generativity and hope for the future. Childrearing involves decisions, conscious or otherwise, about how to shape a "healthy" person who will be happy and creative as an adult. All parents have hopes and dreams about their children's futures; when a child dies, the hopes and dreams die too. Although some amount of guilt and self blame are present in most bereavement situations, they are likely to be especially pronounced following the death of a child. This guilt may itself be a psychological risk factor.[38]

Although many of the issues are the same as in other types of bereavements, the impact of a child's death may vary depending on the child's age when death occurs, with the death of a newborn feeling somewhat different from the loss of a teenager. As parents in a support group described by Macon[44] reported, "it is not necessarily 'harder' or 'easier' to lose a very young child as opposed to a teenager. It is simply a quite 'different' kind of pain."

Stillbirths

Stillbirths, like miscarriages, are regarded by some as "nonevents"[8] or "nondeaths"[54] of often unnamed "nonpersons."[40] In stillbirth, which occurs approximately once in every 80 deliveries,[41] an anticipated joyful event turns into tragedy. Stillbirth can assume two forms. The more common occurs when the baby was viable until labor, and then dies during labor or delivery. In the second type of stillbirth the fetus dies in utero and the mother is forewarned of the death, sometimes weeks before the delivery. Although this forewarning could provide parents with an opportunity for anticipatory grieving, the tendency to rely heavily on denial when told of an intrauterine death commonly precludes this. Kirkley-Best and Kellner,[35] in their clinical observations, have found that the emotional reaction to both types of stillbirth is similar—both are experienced as "the simultaneous birth and death of the child."

By the time of a stillbirth, the subtle but powerful bonding of parents, especially of mothers, to a baby has usually progressed to a stage of "primary maternal preoccupation"[77] and a narcissistic investment has been made in the child. Fletcher and Evans[22] have found that, in some cases, technology has intensified prenatal bonding. Parents who receive photographs of their infants in utero (a result of increasing use of sonograms for diagnostic purposes) may become more intensely attached to the fetuses because they have a concrete image on which to attach their dreams.

Part of what can complicate the grieving process following stillbirths is a conspiracy of silence. An assumption is often made that the mother is better off not discussing the loss, resulting in her being sedated to suppress distressing responses. When hospital personnel and friends do talk about the death, they may advise the mother that she will be able to "have another baby" or observe that "something must have been wrong with the baby, so it's better this way." Wolff et al.[78] have found from their research, however, that negative feelings may be exacerbated by such responses. Stringham et al.[70] have similarly found that the silence surrounding the bereaved mother seems to confirm feelings of guilt and underscores the "unspeakable" nature of the death.

Frequently observed responses among mothers after stillbirth include anger, loneliness, and a sudden drop in self-esteem. Gilson[24] has found that some mothers feel ashamed of their inability to do what others apparently do with ease, and their feminine identities may be threatened. Anger may be directed toward the self for failing to produce a healthy baby, toward the doctor for providing inadequate care, and toward family and friends for providing insufficient support.[70] Loneliness can emerge because the mother is "grieving the loss of someone who was unknown to one's family and friends."[70] Although the lost child had become increasingly personalized to the parents, especially the mother, throughout the pregnancy, to others the baby remained completely anonymous.

Until recent years, the intensity of the parental attachment was underestimated, resulting in stillborn babies being whisked away before being seen by the parents. Research conducted since 1970, however, indicates that visual and physical contact with the dead infant may facilitate the bereavement process.[70] An increasing number of hospitals are now encouraging parents to name and spend time with the infant, and to collect memorabilia such as pictures, locks of hair, and the nursery bracelet.

PERINATAL DEATH

Unlike stillborns, babies who live for a few days or weeks are accorded personhood. They are named, looked at, held, talked to, and talked about.

As with stillbirths, the advent of new technologies and surgical procedures can influence reactions to a child's death in the first few days or weeks of life. With the dramatic reduction in the birthweight at which babies can be saved, the death of a very tiny, sick, or deformed newborn is no longer always expected. Parents' hopes may be buoyed with the suggestion of each additional medical procedure, and the added time that the child lives increases their attachment.

This increased ability to extend life can bring additional anguish for other reasons. For example, some parents are now faced with the dilemma of whether or not to agree to surgical intervention that may extend life for only a brief period or that may result in a life of pain and disability. The decision not to intervene, assuring the child's death, has recently resulted in the highly publicized "Baby Doe" situation in which a governmental or other third party brings legal action against the parents, trying to force medical care for the infant. Being forced into an adversarial position is likely to intensify the difficulties parents have in dealing with the loss of their child. If the parents decide to intervene, the baby may die sometime later or live its life with severe handicaps; both circumstances create their own set of emotional and often financial problems for the family.

Because an infant who lives for even a short time in a hospital is known to the staff and family friends, there is usually more support available to parents in the event of death than there is for parents whose infant is stillborn. Nevertheless, many people still ignore the loss and avoid discussion of it, instigating feelings of anger in the bereaved parents.[4] Other troublesome reactions include anxiety about the ability to produce a healthy child, a sense of the unjustness of a child never having had a chance, and feelings of guilt. According to the research of Benfield et al.,[4] mothers blame themselves for such deaths far more than fathers do, assuming that they had done something during pregnancy to cause the death, such as smoking, drinking, having intercourse late in pregnancy, or not taking enough care of themselves.

According to data collected by Kennell et al.,[34] the presence of other children in a family does not diminish the mother's grief following perinatal death. Similarly, Wilson et al.[76] found that losing one of a set of twins involves as much grief as losing a single newborn. In fact, in some ways, such a loss may be even more difficult because usually less support is available. Others assume that parents are grateful that one baby survived and focus attention on the living child, although, as these researchers discovered, no matter how many children someone has, the loss of any one of them causes painful grief reactions.

Sudden Infant Death

After the neonatal period, the most common form of death in the first year of an infant's life is Sudden Infant Death Syndrome (SIDS), which claims 7,000 to 10,000 lives per year in the United States. SIDS usually occurs between the ages of one week and one year, with a peak occurring in the two- to four-month age group.

Because the cause of SIDS is largely unknown, there is no way to predict with certainty which babies are at highest risk. Although some infants experience recurrent episodes of apnea, when breathing stops for a brief period, prior to their deaths most of these infants appear healthy. The suddenness of SIDS death in seemingly healthy babies may lead to extra difficulties in the bereavement process.

Adding to parents' sorrow are misunderstandings that sometimes arise because of the absence of an immediately identifiable cause of death and the baby's appearance. The bodies of infants that are not discovered for several hours frequently appear bruised. Law enforcement officers, investigating an unexplained death, may suspect child abuse. In an attempt to help avoid upsetting encounters between police and bereaved parents, a program in Washington, D.C. (at the Children's Hospital National Medical Center in conjunction with the District of Columbia Medical Examiner's Office) has been developed to explain SIDS to homicide officers. Seminars that sensitize them to the special vulnerability of SIDS parents have changed the way couples are approached and questioned.[16]

Guilt is especially intense in SIDS cases. Based on her own clinical experience and review of the literature, Raphael[57] reports that the unexplainable nature of the death leads parents to a relentless search for a cause. They may repeatedly review their own caretaking behavior in a search for clues, or may consciously or unconsciously blame the other parent. Donnelly[20] has found that clarification of the fact that neither parent was responsible may sometimes be needed in order to preserve the marital relationship following this type of loss.

The Death of an Older Child

Deaths are less common among older children than among infants, with accidents the most frequent cause of death, especially in adolescence. In an epidemiologic study including bereaved parents, Owen et al.[51] found that the median age of the dead child was 16.6 years. Accidents accounted for 45 percent of the deaths; leukemia and other cancers accounted for another 18 percent.

Parents whose children die at an older age usually experience many of the feelings already discussed. However, older children lived long enough to develop a well-formed personality and leave their bereaved families with a larger store of memories. As with deaths of younger children, a commonly expressed emotion is anger. In a study of 14 bereaved parents, Sanders[61] found that loss of a child, compared with the loss of a parent or spouse, "revealed more intense grief reactions of somatic types, greater depression, as well as anger and guilt with accompanying feelings of despair." Parents seemed totally vulnerable, as if they had just suffered a physical blow that left them with no strength or will to fight. Describing participants in a support group for bereaved parents, Macon[44] said that "bizarre" responses, regressive behavior, and suicidal thoughts were common. In a comparison of depressed psychiatric outpatients and matched community controls, Clayton[15] discovered that the death of a child in the previous six months had occurred in a surprisingly high proportion of the depressed patients, supporting her view that the "death of a child is the most significant and traumatic death of a family member."

The course of the bereavement process for parents may be considerably longer and more complicated than was previously believed. In a study of 54 parents whose children died from cancer, Rando[56] found an intensification of grief over time, with a decrease in symptom intensity in the second year after bereavement followed by an increase in the third year. This same trend was observed by Levav[38] in his reanalysis of Rees and Lutkins'[58] data. Looking at mortality rates in bereaved parents, he found no significant increases in the first year following bereavement, but very great differences between grieving parents and controls over a five-year period.

It has been found that cause and locale of death can significantly influence the outcome of bereavement, especially in terms of the parents' need to feel a sense of control. In cases where children have long terminal illnesses, such as cancer, it may be important for parents to feel they participated in the child's care, so that after the death they can feel they did all they could. In a study of 37 families of children who had died of cancer in the previous 29 months, Mulhern and his associates[47] found significant differences in the outcomes of parents who opted for home versus hospital care for their dying child. Although preexisting personality traits may have determined which set of parents chose which locale, thus confounding the results, parents who selected hospital care emerged as significantly more anxious, depressed, defensive, socially withdrawn, and uncomfortable, and had greater tendencies toward somatic and interpersonal problems, self-doubt, and unreasonable fears. Martinson et al.[45] found no significant differences in levels of abnormal grief between "home care" and "hospital care" parents, but noted somewhat less difficulty among parents whose children had died at home. Lauer et al.[36] found that these parents were far less likely to experience marital strain than parents whose children died in hospitals.

Parents who can explain and understand why their child's death had to happen also seem to adjust better. Spinetta et al.,[67] in a study of 23 sets of parents whose children died of cancer within the previous three years, found that those who did best had a consistent philosophy of life that enabled them to accept the diagnosis and cope with its consequences. Martinson et al.[45] found that 73 percent of their sample reported deriving consolation from religious beliefs.

The death of an adult child is a topic that has been virtually neglected in bereavement research. Based on her own research and the work of others, Raphael[57] concludes that, although the child will probably have left home, "the older parent who experiences the death of an adult child is likely to be deeply disturbed by it." From his clinical observations, Gorer[27] has come to believe that "the most distressing and long-lasting of all griefs, it would seem, is that for the loss of a grown child." Gorer,[27] Raphael,[57] and Levav[38] all infer that untimeliness is what makes this form of bereavement so difficult. Older parents typically feel that it is "unnatural" for a young or middle-aged adult to die while an older parent lives on, which may be a particular form of "survivor guilt." Ambivalence may also be more of a problem, especially where it centers on a child leaving home and choosing to form a family of his or her own. Elderly parents who lose a middle-aged child may also have lost their caretaker, as a role reversal frequently occurs with the advancing age of children and parents.

Because the bulk of the information available on loss of a child of any age remains anecdotal rather than systematic, current ideas regarding this type of loss must be considered tentative rather than definitive. More empirical data are needed before any firm conclusions can be reached.

Problems in Grieving for a Child

Having a child die can have a devastating effect on a marriage. For couples with a history of good communication and for those able to develop these skills, a child's terminal illness or sudden death may strengthen the relationship. It is not uncommon, however, for marriages to break down under the strain imposed by a child's illness and death. Marital discord and divorce have been reported in 50 to 70 percent of families whose child died from cancer.[33,69] However, as noted earlier, this rate may be considerably lower for parents who cared for a child at home.

One potential factor that can exacerbate marital difficulties may be the different styles of grieving among family members. In a study of 100 parents whose children died of cancer, Martinson and her colleagues[45] found that "fathers were nearly twice as likely as mothers to reply that the most intense part of their bereavement was over within a few weeks to one month after the child's death," although their responses may have reflected the social expectation of fathers to "take it like a man." In three studies of 112 SIDS parents, DeFrain et al.[18] found no difference in the length of time it took men and women to recover from the loss. Nevertheless, DeFrain and his colleagues did note some variations in the responses of fathers and mothers, with fathers reporting more anger, fear, and loss of control than mothers, as well as a desire to keep their grieving private. The mothers responded with more sorrow and depression.

Lack of synchrony may make it difficult for couples to support or understand each other. As one grieving mother in DeFrain's study[18] reported, "I was an open, throbbing wound, and he wanted to have sex. It was very hard for me to understand that he was also in pain and that he felt our closeness would be healing." Involvement in one's own grief may diminish empathy for the other. In relationships lacking a pattern of stable communication, help from friends, relatives, or mental health professionals may be needed to facilitate mutual understanding.

Another potential complication involves the discrepancy between a parent's real feelings for his or her child and the feelings he or she believes should exist. As with any human relationship, feelings for a child are marked by ambivalence. But as Raphael[57] points out, "societal attitudes strongly suggest that all parents must be perfectly loving, and all [children] are perfectly lovable." When a child dies, guilt over negative feelings comes to the fore.

Parents who depend heavily on a child for need-fulfillment can also experience complicated responses. Some women with negative self-concepts may be able to stabilize an acceptable sense of self only by being "good mothers." The mother feels useful and competent because the child is emotionally dependent on her. A death in this type of case, especially of an only child or of a child who had been unconsciously singled out to "care for" the mother, will disturb the mother's view of herself.

For a parent whose relationship with a child had added meaning because of the parent's painful past, death brings an additional strain. In cases where the parent used the relationship with the child to rework relationship conflicts from his or her own childhood, the child's death may be experienced as the loss not only of a son or daughter, but of some other relationship from the past as well.

Parents may also feel particularly threatened by the sense of vulnerability and helplessness associated with a child's death. A feeling expressed by a significant number of parents in the study by DeFrain et al.[18] of SIDS parents was the sense of impotence. When a child dies, parents realize the limits of their protective powers and may feel haunted by this realization.

When children who have significant roles in existing parental conflict die, the bereavement process may take a pathologic course. Orbach[50] conceptualized one mother's unresolved grief as follows: "When the irrational jealousy of her husband reached a peak of accusations, she [had] prayed for her son to become ill on the premise that this would lead to increased marital unity." When the child died of leukemia, she attributed the death to the parental quarrels.

The advisability of having another child soon after a child's death is controversial. In a study of six replacement children in psychotherapy, Cain and Cain[11] found that "the parents' relationship with the new, substitute child [was] virtually smothered by the image of the lost child." Although these authors warn that attempts to replace a dead child with another are "fraught with danger," it must be remembered that these findings are based on observations of an extremely small, disturbed sample.

Lewis[40] warns that replacement pregnancies can be used to deny the fact of the first child's death and may interrupt grieving. Poznanski[55] has observed clinically that the gradual giving up of a dead child prepares parents to "reinvest their energies in other relationships." She asserts that if they are not ready to do this, they cannot raise a new child in an emotionally healthy environment.

While a number of clinicians (e.g., Cain and Cain,[11] Legg and Sherick,[37] Lewis,[40] and Poznanski[55]) recommend waiting until the bereavement process is completed before having another child, it may be that such advice is overly prescriptive. Being treated as a replacement is certainly apt to be burdensome to a child, but waiting until there is recovery may not be the solution either, especially since it is often observed that grieving for a lost child never entirely ends.

DEATH OF A PARENT DURING ADULT LIFE*

The type of bereavement most common in adulthood is the loss of a parent. In their study of life events in 2,300 persons matched for demo-

---

*This section is based on material prepared by Victoria Solsberry, M.S.W., research associate.

graphic characteristics to U.S. census data, Pearlin and Lieberman[53] found that 5 percent of the population lost a parent within one year. Despite the relative frequency and universality of the event, very little research has been done in this area. In contemporary Western society, the loss of a parent in adulthood is not expected to produce serious effects, although some studies have shown a higher tendency to thoughts of suicide, an increased rate of attempted suicide, and higher rates of clinical depression.[1,5,9,19,42] Of course, the way an adult responds to any bereavement depends on prior experiences with losses throughout life, including those during childhood. Empirical data regarding continuing effects of parental loss experienced during childhood are discussed in the next chapter.

In a study of 35 persons seeking treatment following the death of a parent, compared with 37 field subjects who had also lost a parent but who had not sought treatment, Horowitz et al.[30] found that "the death of a parent is a serious life event that can lead to a measurable degree of symptomatic distress." Furthermore, the data suggested that the death of a mother was harder to sustain than the death of a father, possibly because of her earlier status as the nurturing caretaker.[31] Another theory suggests that because in three out of four marriages the husband dies first,[39] most adults lose their fathers by death before their mothers. When the second parent dies, some adults may mourn the loss of having "parents." The death of the second parent may "leave the child bereaved for the loss of the specific relationship, stripped of all living parents, and also with a reactivated mourning process for the earlier parental death."[31]

In contrast to these findings, several studies reported that the loss of a parent in adulthood was the least disruptive and caused the least intense grief reactions.[51,61] In a sample of 39 adult sons and daughters with a median age of 48.3, Owen et al.[51] found a "striking characteristic of their response to be the absence of grief . . . adult sons and daughters reported the fewest adjustment problems . . . the smallest increase in the consumption of tranquilizers or barbiturates as well as the smallest increase in the consumption of alcohol . . . the least preoccupation with the memory of the deceased . . . and the lowest levels of physical complaints." Concurring with these findings, Sanders[61] speculated, "for the most part, these 'adult children' were caught up in their own busy world which soon engulfed them. They had families, jobs, and daily responsibilities which allowed little time to dwell upon the deceased parent." Rather than the passage of time, however, it may be other factors that account for the relatively low level of grieving in adults who lose parents. In most cases, attachment feelings have for some time been directed toward other figures, such as mates and children. Such feelings, although briefly redirected toward parents following their deaths, usually turn back toward current figures after a relatively short time.

The death of a parent may have many meanings for an adult child. For some, who perceived their mothers and fathers as caretakers, providers of praise, and permission-givers even after the parents had to be physically cared for themselves, the death may mean the loss of security.[30] For others, it is the loss of that perfect, unconditional love experienced only as a child.

A subtle role change often occurs when an adult child's parent dies. The death is often experienced as a "developmental push," propelling the adult into the next stage of life. It is well known anecdotally that many adults, upon the loss of their parents, suddenly feel the weight of responsibility as the oldest generation in the family. This, coupled with the awareness that there are no longer parents to fall back on, may effect a more mature stance in parentally bereaved adults who no longer think of themselves as children.

DEATH OF A SIBLING DURING ADULT LIFE*

A review of the literature reveals a rather striking absence of data about adults' responses to the death of a sibling. Presumably, this type of loss has been ignored because it is viewed as having less impact than the death of a spouse, child, or parent. In most cases, adult siblings no longer live together and they may not even have much social contact. Nevertheless, it is rare to find adult siblings who have completely severed ties with one another.[60] Observation suggests that many sisters and brothers continue to visit each other, share memories, reunions, and responsibility for aging parents, and psychologically influence each other explicitly and implicitly, such as in the selection of marital partners.[49] Despite an earlier view that sibling relationships were simply a function of and subordinate to a child's relationship to parents, researchers are now commenting on the special characteristics unique to the sibling bond.[49] The empathy siblings form for one another when they are young may continue into adult life, making this tie a potentially profound one.

---

*This section is based on material prepared by Janice L. Krupnick, M.S.W., consultant.

As in other types of bereavement, the quality of the preexisting relationship with the deceased is likely to color an individual's perception and experience of the loss. The seeds of the sibling relationship are planted in childhood, but the same characteristics that were salient then continue to affect the nature of the adult tie. In an exploratory study of adult sibling relationships, Ross and Milgram[60] found that shared childhood experiences and critical life events (including parental deaths) influence the level of sibling closeness in adult life. Geographical proximity can increase either closeness or distance, depending on other factors, but complete lack of closeness is unusual. Sibling rivalry, a variable that may contribute to postdeath feelings of guilt, was found to continue throughout life in varying degrees of intensity, with rivalrous feelings peaking during early adult years. In addition, sibling relationships assume great importance among the elderly, probably making sibling loss in old age a particularly significant event.

Some of Bank and Kahn's[3] observations regarding childhood bereavement could also apply to adult sibling ties. For example, they noted that sibling death may be difficult to resolve if previous identification with the deceased sibling was too close or fused, or if it was too polarized and rejecting. Although the intensity of such closeness or hostility would probably be attenuated by the time siblings reach adulthood, such feelings could complicate grief reactions.

Another factor that may influence the response to sibling loss is the cause of death. A surviving sibling may find it more difficult to accept a loss if the sister or brother died of an illness to which the survivor may also be genetically predisposed or be a carrier, which would place the bereaved's children at risk. Anxiety following a sibling's death may be particularly acute among the elderly if it exacerbates an already present fear of one's own impending death.

Bank and Kahn[3] assert that, regardless of age, death of a sibling forces brothers and sisters to reorganize their roles and relationships to one another and to their parents. Under certain circumstances, a death can jolt surviving siblings into becoming more alert, sensitive, and concerned—particularly if they conclude that they could have prevented the death had they been more caring. Death of "the most responsible" sibling can force survivors to face their need to contribute to their parents' well-being now that the deceased sibling no longer assumes this role. As with formerly traditional wives who can mature through the bereavement experience, siblings who had previously considered themselves less capable can grow through this imposed need to become a caretaker.

BEREAVEMENT FOLLOWING SUICIDE*

Bereavement is painful no matter what the cause, but bereavement following the suicide of a close friend or family member has been called a "personal and interpersonal disaster."[64] Other kinds of death that complicate bereavement include homicide, suicide, multiple simultaneous losses, and accidents in which the survivor was complicit, such as an automobile accident in which the survivor was driving. All these types of bereavement are important and merit comparative study. In this report, however, only suicide will be discussed as an example of an especially difficult loss.

It is estimated that more than 27,000 people commit suicide in the United States each year. Men are three times more likely than women to commit suicide, and whites are almost twice as likely as blacks.[48] Elderly white men have the highest suicide rate of all.[10] Many observers have commented that reported figures are extremely conservative due to the ambiguous circumstances of some deaths and to society's need to deny suicide. Even given this conservative figure, however, suicide leaves in its wake a sizable number of survivors who must deal with a complex set of feelings and social problems.

Survivors of suicide have long been thought to be at greater risk for physical and mental health problems than individuals who are bereaved from other causes of death. Indeed, as discussed in Chapter 2, there is some evidence to suggest increased mortality among the widowed whose spouses committed suicide. There also is good evidence that children whose parent committed suicide are at risk for enduring adverse consequences and for suicide itself (Chapter 5).[63]

Clinical observations of suicide survivors[12,65] reveal that they experience some reactions that are unique to this type of bereavement, as well as displaying typical bereavement reactions in exaggerated form.

While the death of a close relative by any cause may leave the survivor with feelings of abandonment and rejection that may be irrational, the feeling of rejection following suicide is almost universal. As one survivor put it: "He could not have loved me; he did not think I was worth living for."[73]

In their study of suicide survivors, Lindemann and Greer[42] found "there is a tendency . . . to look for a scapegoat. And, as is the fate of

---

*This section is based on material prepared by Victoria Solsberry, M.S.W., research associate, drawing on a paper by Barry D. Garfinkel, M.D., Director, Division of Child and Adolescent Psychiatry, University of Minnesota Medical School, Minneapolis.

most scapegoats, the victim is usually one of their own members and frequently the one least able to bear the added burden.'' This tendency to search for blame, though common following other types of deaths, is greatly increased following a suicide. The surviving spouse, parents, or even child may be blamed for not seeing the signs of the impending suicide or for not meeting the needs of the deceased.

Bereaved individuals also often blame themselves for the death, resulting in what is often called ''survivor guilt.'' In fact, blaming others may be one way of avoiding self-blame. Survivors may question what they did to add to the deceased's stress or may wonder whether they could have foreseen and stopped the act. As suicide researcher Henslin[28] points out, ''When one can exercise control over events and in so doing prevent harm to others, our culture demands that it is one's responsibility to do so. Therefore, if one could have acted to have prevented the suicide, one feels that he or she should have done so.''

People who have made repeated threats of suicide or actual attempts may leave friends and relatives in conflict when they finally succeed. Menninger[46] has clinically observed that a typical response is ''overwhelming bitterness'' at having failed in the task of keeping the vulnerable one alive coupled with a sense of relief that the ordeal is finally over. Children, especially, who have been warned that they are ''upsetting Mommy'' or accused by the parent of ''driving me crazy'' are especially vulnerable to feelings of guilt following a suicide.

In Bowlby's[7] clinical experience, repeated threats often leave the survivor frightened and frustrated, finally wishing that the other person would just ''go ahead and do it.'' Suicide also may leave survivors with feelings of rage over being abandoned, which in tandem with the sense of relief that the person's problems will no longer demand attention, can intensify survivor guilt. Feelings of anger and relief are generally unanticipated and misunderstood under the circumstances and so may lead to a sense of shame and a denial of their existence. Finally, survivors may feel anxious after the death—worried that they may mimic the deceased's self-destructive act.

The nature and intensity of the survivor's reactions will depend largely on cultural factors, the prior relationship with the deceased, the age and physical condition of the deceased, the survivor's individual personality characteristics, and the nature of the death. Henslin[28] has found that, in some ways, suicide shares with accidental death the qualities of ''suddenness, unexpectedness, and violence.'' It should be noted, however, that there are many different types of suicides and that they may involve different types of responses. For example, in the case of a terminal illness, especially among cancer patients, the sick person may have made a clear decision to abbreviate a life of pain.[17] The impact of this kind of suicide is not known; families in this situation may need information and assistance in anticipating and responding to this type of death.

Communications before the death or suicide notes that blame the survivors directly may place those left behind at even higher risk for problems with guilt and shame. Some clinical observers infer that many suicides are motivated largely by the hostile intent of producing problems, especially guilt, for the family. In a study of suicide notes, Jacobs[32] described two types that clearly made the suicide a hostile act. In one, there is an attempt to hide the intent by claiming that the suicide is aimed at "relieving" or "freeing" the survivor, whereas the other is overtly hostile.

Following suicide, denial is frequently used to mask feelings of guilt, rage, relief, and shame. Resnik,[59] in a study of nine families in which an adolescent child committed suicide, found that this denial may take the form of hostility towards the medical examiner, police, or anyone who calls the death a "suicide." Denial and anger may also contribute to a tendency to idealize the deceased.

In his research, Warren[73] found that some survivors created a "family myth," a rationalization of the true nature of the death, that is used not only for the outside world, but also for the family itself. These forms of denial serve a definite purpose for the bereaved. As Augenbraun and Neuringer[2] have observed, "if the survivor does not accept the possibility that the deceased took his own life, he can avoid facing the notion that the suicidal person willfully abandoned him," allowing him to avoid the pain associated with the deliberateness of the death. A decision to call suicide an "accident" or to attribute it to an illness is often quite conscious, however, and is sometimes told to "protect" children from the truth. Complicity by health care personnel aids this denial, although, as discussed in Chapter 5, fabrications can frighten and confuse children who may already know the real cause of death or sense that what they have been told is untrue. This undermines confidence in adults and reinforces the idea that suicide is a valid source of shame.

A common fear among survivors concerns the "heritage of insanity," leading people to wonder whether others in the family are now "doomed" to kill themselves someday. Indeed, there are data that show a far higher than chance incidence of prior suicide in families of individuals who commit suicide.[6,21] This may be due, in part, to a shared vulnerability to mental illness, specifically depression, or to specific feelings of inevitability and guilt.[73] Warren[73] has observed that a "survivor may feel or fear the inevitability of his own death by suicide at a time coinciding with the parental age at the time of suicide. This feeling of inevitability is usually unconscious, becoming more manifest as the [survivor's] age approximates that of the parent at the time of the suicide.''

Lindemann and Greer[42] have found that identification with a person who has committed suicide may lead a person to perceive this behavior as a viable solution to life's problems. The very fact that the taboo was broken by someone close may serve to legitimize the act, perhaps suggesting to the survivor that he or she will be vulnerable when overwhelmed later in life.

In summary, there are many interacting factors that influence the response to suicide. Feelings of being rejected, guilty, responsible, and socially stigmatized appear to hamper the resolution of bereavement.

The Social Stigma of Suicide

In many cultures, the social stigma of suicide has historical roots. The early Greeks, believing that those who committed suicide must have been greatly wronged to have wanted to die, considered their ghosts to be extremely revengeful, dangerous, and frightening.[14] In other cultures, the bodies of suicide victims had to be buried outside the city walls or were pulled through the streets and stoned. Suicide has also been illegal in many places, including the United States. Most modern Western civilizations no longer adhere to such beliefs and practices, but suicide is still regarded by many to be a moral rather than a mental health issue. Roman Catholics, regarding suicide as a mortal sin, used to forbid memorial mass and last sacraments for a Catholic who died in this way and insurance companies continue to deny benefits to families of people who commit suicide within two years of buying life insurance.

These social stigmata compound the problems of suicide survivors. Whether from shame or anticipation of blame from others, people are often sensitive about and reluctant to discuss the event. Those who would usually be available for support following the death of someone close may find they are unable to comfort the survivor of a suicide. Possibly threatened by the idea of being powerless to prevent a suicide, they may join in the search for a cause and may even blame the survivor for the death. This failure of the informal support system leaves many survivors socially isolated and dealing with their complex feelings and problems alone. Some find that they can escape feeling ostracized and condemned only by moving,[12] but they are then faced with the isolation and insecurity of a new home and neighborhood that can make the bereavement process more difficult. Given these circumstances, the decision of some families to deny the fact of a suicide seems understandable.

Assisting Survivors of Suicide

Survivors of suicide, more than any other bereaved group, may require some form of professional help. Based on his observations of families of adolescent suicides, Resnik[59] has found that "an early interview after the death is a therapeutic and cathartic experience" that allows the interviewer to establish rapport before defenses have been established. This allows him to provide appropriate subsequent help as the grief work progresses. In her clinical experience, Silverman[65] has found that suicide survivors are often initially wary of those who offer help. They are generally so isolated by the experience, however, that they may need more formal opportunities to ventilate their feelings and more reassurance than other bereaved persons. In recent years, mutual support groups, such as "Survivors of Suicide" and "Seasons," have been developed to bring together survivors of suicides to clarify their understandings of the loss and to find ways of dealing with the often confusing and traumatic aftermath.

Freedman et al.[23] advocate professional psychotherapeutic intervention to alleviate the effects of stress on the "survivor-victims" of suicide, to provide "an arena for the expression of hidden emotions," and to put a "measure of stability into the grieving person's life." In their clinical work with survivors they have found that "most are willing—some are passively eager—to talk," adding that therapists often serve as reality testers, "not so much the echo of conscience as the quiet voice of reason."

As is true following all types of bereavement, the degree and type of reassurance needed by a survivor depends on his individual circumstances. Augenbraun and Neuringer[2] have found that "there is little need for therapy [when] the previous relationship between suicide and survivor was positive, minimally ambivalent, and where the fact of the suicide can be ascribed to circumstances outside the control of the survivor." They add, however, that "more often, the survivor has been involved in a conflict relationship with the suicide and the act of suicide itself is in part an outcome of this conflict." More clinical research needs to be done to determine the circumstances that make survivors vulnerable to pathologic outcomes, and to determine which particular interventions are most effective under these circumstances.

Research Issues

As with so much of bereavement research, what is known about suicide survivors comes primarily from clinical case reports of small numbers of patients in treatment. The reports have not systematically examined and controlled for demographic heterogeneity of the sample, time course following suicide, possible psychiatric disorders in family members, or differences in the intensity, duration, and symptomatology of the bereavement. Yet these clinical accounts can provide the basis for further systematic investigation. Both clinical cases and systematic investigations are needed.

Unusual methodological problems create particular difficulties in designing systematic studies of bereavement associated with suicide. Ideally, suicide bereavement should be compared with bereavement following deaths that share some of the same characteristics in order to know of any unique contributions of suicide as distinct from some of its attributes. For example, suicide is a sudden death that should be compared with bereavement following other sudden deaths such as motor vehicle fatalities. As a "volitional" death, suicide is more similar to drinking oneself to death (cirrhosis) or smoking oneself to death after heart disease has been discovered than it is to deaths caused by conditions over which individuals have no control. And comparisons of survivors of other "socially unacceptable" deaths, such as Acquired Immune Deficiency Syndrome (AIDS), might permit the effects of social stigma and suicide to be separated.

In addition, the effects of suicide in different types of relationships—such as parents-to-child, sibling, conjugal, and child-to-parent—should be studied. Further research is also needed on the meanings and responses to different types of suicides, for example drug overdoses in adolescents or suicide among the terminally ill and elderly. More information on the coping styles of suicide survivors could help others deal with the loss through suicide of someone close.

Comparative studies of all these variations and characteristics of suicide are difficult, however, because of the relative infrequency of the event. As pointed out in Chapter 2, studies of relatively rare events require very large samples.

CONCLUSIONS

Although only a small number of different types of losses have been discussed in this chapter, they indicate that different kinds of relationships and different sets of circumstances influence the personal meanings and feelings associated with bereavement. More data are needed on the response to loss of various types of relationships, and under various conditions of death. Much attention has been paid to responses to conjugal bereavement in adults, but there is relatively little information on other types of losses, such as the death of siblings and parents. As the average age at death continues to rise and as medical technology allows the prolongation of lives that previously would have ended naturally, an increasing number of people will have to deal with issues raised by elderly and ailing parents, including the thorny issues surrounding assisted suicide. Responses to loss under all these circumstances deserve exploration in order to provide appropriate assistance to the bereaved.

REFERENCES

1. Anderson, C. Aspects of pathological grief and mourning. *International Journal of Psychoanalysis* 30:48–55, 1949.
2. Augenbraun, B., and Neuringer, C. Helping survivors with the impact of suicide. In: *Survivors of Suicide* (Cain, A., ed.). Springfield, Ill.: Charles C Thomas, 1972.
3. Bank, S., and Kahn, M. *The Sibling Bond.* New York: Basic Books, 1982.
4. Benfield, G., Leib, S., and Volman, J. Grief response of parents to neonatal death and parent participation in deciding care. *Pediatrics* 62:171–177, 1978.
5. Birtchnell, J. Psychiatric breakdown following recent parent death. *British Journal of Medical Psychology* 48:379–390, 1975.
6. Blachly, P., Disher, B., and Roduner, G. Suicide by physicians. *Bulletin of Suicidology* 4:1–18, 1968.
7. Bourne, S. The psychological effects of stillbirth on women and their doctors. *Journal of the Royal College of General Practitioners* 16:103–112, 1968.
8. Bowlby, J. *Attachment and Loss. Vol. III: Loss.* New York: Basic Books, 1980.
9. Bunch, J. The influence of parental death anniversaries upon suicide dates. *British Journal of Psychiatry* 118:621–625, 1971.
10. Butler, R., and Lewis M. *Aging and Mental Health* (2nd edition). St. Louis: C.V. Mosby, 1977.
11. Cain, A., and Cain, B. On replacing a child. *Journal of the American Academy of Child Psychiatry* 3:443–456, 1964.
12. Cain, A., and Fast, I. The legacy of suicide: observations on the pathogenic impact of suicide upon marital partners. *Psychiatry* 29:406–411, 1966.
13. Cain, A., and Fast, I. The legacy of suicide: observations on the pathogenic impact of suicide upon marital partners. In: *Survivors of Suicide* (Cain, A., ed.). Springfield, Ill.: Charles C Thomas, 1972.
14. Choron, J. *Suicide.* New York: Charles Scribner's Sons, 1972.
15. Clayton, P.J. Bereavement and its management. In: *Handbook of Affective Disorders* (Paykel, E.S., ed.). Edinburgh: Churchill Livingstone, 1980.
16. Cohen, G. DOA: Preliminary report on an emergency room protocol. *Clinical Proceedings of the Children's Hospital National Medical Center* 35:159–165, 1979.
17. Danto, B.L. Suicide among cancer patients. In: *Suicide and Euthanasia: The Rights of Personhood* (Wallace, S., and Eser, A., eds.). Knoxville: University of Tennessee Press, 1981.

18. DeFrain, J., Taylor, J., and Ernst, L. *Coping With Sudden Infant Death*. Lexington, Mass.: Lexington Books, D.C. Heath, 1982.
19. Deutsch, H. Absence of grief. *Psychoanalytic Quarterly* 6:12–22, 1937.
20. Donnelly, K. *Recovering From the Loss of a Child*. New York: Macmillan, 1982.
21. Farberow, N., and Simon, M. Suicide in Los Angeles and Vienna: an intellectual report. *U.S. Public Health Reports* 84:389–403, 1969.
22. Fletcher, J.C., and Evans, M.I. Maternal bonding in early fetal ultrasound examinations. *New England Journal of Medicine* 308:392–393, 1983.
23. Freedman, A., Kaplan, H., and Sadock, B. Psychiatric emergencies. Chapter 28 in: *Modern Synopsis of Comprehensive Textbook of Psychiatry, II* (2nd edition). Baltimore: Williams & Wilkins, 1976.
24. Gilson, G. Care of the family who has lost a newborn. *Postgraduate Medicine* 60:67–70, 1976.
25. Glick, I.O., Parkes, C.M., and Weiss, R. *The First Year of Bereavement*. New York: Basic Books, 1975.
26. Golan, N. Wife to widow to woman. *Social Work* 20: 369–374, 1975.
27. Gorer, G. *Death, Grief and Mourning*. New York: Doubleday, 1965.
28. Henslin, J.H. Strategies of adjustment: an ethno-methodological approach to the study of guilt and suicide. In: *Survivors of Suicide* (Cain, A., ed.). Springfield, Ill.: Charles C Thomas, 1972.
29. Holmes, T.H., and Rahe, R.H. The social readjustment rating scale. *Journal of Psychosomatic Research* 11:213–218, 1967.
30. Horowitz, M.J., Krupnick, J., Kaltreider, N., Wilner, N., Leong, A., and Marmar, C. Initial psychological response to parental death. *Archives of General Psychiatry* 38:316–323, 1981.
31. Horowitz, M.J., Weiss, D., Kaltreider, N., Krupnick, J., Wilner, N., Marmar, C., and DeWitt, K. Response to death of a parent: a follow-up study. *Journal of Nervous and Mental Diseases* (in press), 1984.
32. Jacobs, J. A phenomenological study of suicide notes. *Social Problems* 15:60–72, 1967.
33. Kaplan, D., Grobstein, R., and Smith, A. Predicting the impact of severe illness in families. *Health and Social Work* 1:71–82, 1976.
34. Kennell, J., Slyter, H., and Klaus, M. The mourning response of parents to the death of a newborn infant. *New England Journal of Medicine* 283:344–349, 1970.
35. Kirkley-Best, E., and Kellner, K. The forgotten grief: a review of the psychology of stillbirth. *American Journal of Orthopsychiatry* 52:420–429, 1982.
36. Lauer, M., Mulhern, R., Wallskog, J., and Camitta, B. A comparison study of parental adaptation following a child's death at home or in the hospital. *Pediatrics* 71:101–111, 1983
37. Legg, C., and Sherick, I. The replacement child—a developmental tragedy: some preliminary comments. *Child Psychiatry and Human Development* 7:113–126, 1976.
38. Levav, I. Mortality and psychopathology following the death of an adult child: an epidemiological review. *Israeli Journal of Psychiatry and Related Sciences* 19:23–38, 1982.
39. Lewis, A. *Three Out of Four Wives*. New York: Macmillan, 1975.
40. Lewis, E. The management of stillbirth—coping with an unreality. *Lancet* 2:619–620, 1976.

41. Lewis E., and Page, A. Failure to mourn a stillbirth: an overlooked catastrophe. *British Journal of Medical Psychology* 51:237–241, 1978.
42. Lindemann, E., and Greer, I.M. A study of grief: emotional response to suicide. *Pastoral Psychology* 4:9–13, 1953.
43. Lopata, H. Self-identity in marriage and widowhood. *The Sociological Quarterly* 14:407–418, 1973.
44. Macon, L. Help for bereaved parents. *Social Casework: The Journal of Contemporary Social Work* November: 558–565, 1979.
45. Martinson, I., Moldow, D., and Henry, W. *Home Care for the Child with Cancer*, Final Report (Grant No. CA19490), U.S. Department of Health and Human Services. Washington, D.C.: National Cancer Institute, 1980.
46. Menninger, K.A. *Man Against Himself*. New York: Harcourt, Brace, 1938.
47. Mulhern, R., Laurer, M., and Hoffmann, R. Death of a child at home or in the hospital: subsequent psychological adjustment of the family. *Pediatrics* 71:743–747, 1983.
48. National Center for Health Statistics. *Monthly Vital Statistics Report*, 31(6) Supplement. Washington, D.C.: U.S. Department of Health and Human Services (Public Health Service), September 30, 1982.
49. Neubauer, P. The importance of the sibling experience. In: *The Psychoanalytic Study of the Child*. New Haven, Conn.: Yale University Press, 1983.
50. Orbach, C. The multiple meanings of the loss of a child. *American Journal of Psychotherapy* 13:906–915, 1959.
51. Owen, G., Fulton, R., and Markusen, E. Death at a distance: a study of family survivors. *Omega* 13:191–225, 1982–1983.
52. Parkes, C.M., and Weiss, R.S. *Recovery from Bereavement*. New York: Basic Books, 1983.
53. Pearlin, L., and Lieberman, M. Social sources of distress. In: *Research in Community Health* (Simons, R., ed.). Greenwich, Conn.: Jai Press, 1979.
54. Phipps, S. Mourning response and intervention in stillbirth: an alternative genetic counseling approach. *Social Biology* 28:1–13, 1981.
55. Poznanski, E. The "replacement child": a saga of unresolved parental grief. *Journal of Pediatrics* 81:1190–1193, 1972.
56. Rando, T. An investigation of grief and adaptation in parents whose children have died from cancer. *Journal of Pediatric Psychology* 8:3–20, 1983.
57. Raphael, B. *The Anatomy of Bereavement*. New York: Basic Books, 1983.
58. Rees, W.D., and Lutkins, S.G. Mortality of bereavement. *British Medical Journal* 1:13–16, 1967.
59. Resnik, H.L.P. Psychological resynthesis: clinical approach to the survivors of a death by suicide. In: *Aspects of Depression* (Shneidman, E.S., and Ortega, M., eds.). Boston: Little, Brown, 1969.
60. Ross, H., and Milgram, G. Important variables in adult sibling relationships: a qualitative study. In: *Sibling Relationships: Their Nature and Significance Across the Lifespan*. Hillsdale, N.J.: Lawrence Erlbaum Associates, 1982.
61. Sanders, C. A comparison of adult bereavement in the death of a spouse, child and parent. *Omega* 10:303–322, 1979–1980.
62. Schiff, H.S. *The Bereaved Parent*. New York: Penguin Books, 1977.
63. Shepherd, D.M., and Barraclough, B.M. The aftermath of parental suicide for children. *British Journal of Psychiatry* 129:267–276, 1976.

64. Shneidman, E.S. Foreword. In: *Survivors of Suicide* (Cain, A., ed.). Springfield, Ill.: Charles C Thomas, 1972.
65. Silverman, P.R. Intervention with the widow of a suicide. In: *Survivors of Suicide* (Cain, A., ed.). Springfield, Ill.: Charles C Thomas, 1972.
66. Silverman, P.R. Transitions and models of intervention. *Annals of the Academy of Political and Social Science* 464:174–187, 1982.
67. Spinetta, J., Swarner, J., and Sheposh, J. Effective parental coping following the death of a child from cancer. *Journal of Pediatric Psychology* 6:251–263, 1981.
68. Start, C. *On Becoming a Widow.* New York: Family Library, 1973.
69. Strauss, A. *Chronic Illness and the Quality of Life.* St. Louis: C.V. Mosby, 1975.
70. Stringham, J., Riley, J.H., and Ross, A. Silent birth: mourning a stillborn baby. *Social Work* 27:322–327, 1982.
71. Vachon, M., Sheldon, A., Lancee, W., Lyall, W., Rogers, J., and Freeman, S. Correlates of enduring stress patterns following bereavement: social network, life situation, and personality. *Psychological Medicine* 12:783–788, 1982.
72. Videka-Sherman, L. Coping with the death of a child: a study over time. *American Journal of Orthopsychiatry* 52:688–698, 1982.
73. Warren, M. Some psychological sequelae of parental suicide in surviving children. In: *Survivors of Suicide* (Cain, A., ed.). Springfield, Ill.: Charles C Thomas, 1972.
74. Weiss, R. *Going it Alone: The Family Life and Social Situation of Single Parents.* New York: Basic Books, 1979.
75. Weiss, R. Attachment in adult life. In: *Attachment in Human Behavior* (Parkes, C.M., and Stevenson-Hinde, J., eds.). New York: Basic Books, 1983.
76. Wilson, A., Lawrence, J., Stevens, D., and Soule, D. The death of a newborn twin: an analysis of parental bereavement. *Pediatrics* 70:587–591, 1982.
77. Winnicott, D.W. Transitional objects and transitional phenomena. *International Journal of Psychoanalysis* 34:89–97, 1953.
78. Wolff, J.R., Nielson, P.E., and Schiller, P. The emotional reaction to a stillbirth. *American Journal of Obstetrics and Gynecology* 108:73–77, 1970.

Bereavement During Childhood and Adolescence

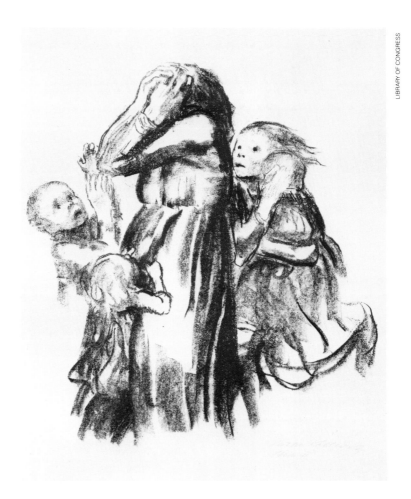

LIBRARY OF CONGRESS

As vividly depicted in the Käthe Kollwitz print entitled Killed in Action, *children are especially vulnerable to psychological problems after the death of a parent or sibling. Their vulnerability may be exacerbated by survivors who, because of their own bereavement, may not be able to provide sufficient comfort and support.*

CHAPTER 5

Bereavement During Childhood and Adolescence

It is not clear exactly how many young people are affected by the death of an immediate family member. Kliman[82] estimates that 5 percent of children in the United States—1.5 million—lose one or both parents by age 15; others suggest that the proportion is substantially higher in lower socioeconomic groups. This chapter discusses the types of bereavements considered to have the most serious implications for medical, psychiatric, and behavioral sequelae in children—namely, death of a parent or sibling. Because more of the literature in this field deals with parental than with sibling loss and because many of the reactions to both types of bereavement overlap, most of the discussion is based on studies of response to the death of a parent.

DEVELOPMENTAL CONSIDERATIONS

Individuals continue to grow and develop throughout life, but during no other period beyond childhood and adolescence are specific reactions as likely to be influenced by the level of development. Because the impact of trauma in children depends so heavily on the life stage during

This chapter was prepared by Janice L. Krupnick, M.S.W., consultant, supported in part by the Kenworthy-Swift Foundation, New York. Background materials and assistance were provided by committee members Gerald Koocher, Ph.D., and Theodore Shapiro, M.D., and by Fredric Solomon, M.D.

which the event occurs, this chapter is informed by a particular emphasis on developmental analysis. This perspective assumes that the repercussions and meanings of major object loss will be colored by the individual child's level of development. Psychiatrists and others have generally been struck by how often major childhood loss seems to result in psychopathology. Studies of adults with various mental disorders, especially depression, frequently reveal childhood bereavement, suggesting that such loss may precipitate or contribute to the development of a variety of psychiatric disorders and that this experience can render a person emotionally vulnerable for life. This special vulnerability of children is attributed to developmental immaturity and insufficiently developed coping capacities.

The tendency to impose adult models on children has generally led to a great deal of confusion and misunderstanding about children's grieving. Although sharing some similarities with adults and even with monkeys (see Chapter 7), children's reactions to loss do not look exactly like adults' reactions, either in their specific manifestations or in their duration.

For example, often what seems glib and unemotional in the small child—such as telling every visitor or stranger on the street, "my sister died"—is the child's way of seeking support and observing others to gauge how he or she should feel. Children may be observed playing games in which the death or funeral activities are reenacted in an effort to master the loss. A child may ask the same questions about the death over and over again, not so much for the factual value of the information as for reassurance that the story has not changed. A four- or five-year-old might resume playing following a death as if nothing distressing had happened. Such behavior reflects the cognitive and emotional capacity of the child and does not mean that the death had no impact.

Losses are so painful and frightening that many young children—able to endure strong emotions for only brief periods—alternately approach and avoid their feelings so as not to be overwhelmed. Because these emotions may be expressed as angry outbursts or misbehavior, rather than as sadness, they may not be recognized as grief-related. Furthermore, because their needs to be cared for and related to are intense and immediate, young children typically move from grief reactions to a prompt search for and acceptance of replacement persons. Unlike adults who can sustain a year or more of intense grieving, children are likely to manifest grief-related affects and behavior, on an intermittent basis, for many years after loss occurs; various powerful reactions to the loss normally will be revived, reviewed and worked through repeatedly at successive levels of subsequent development. Thus, in dealing with children who have sustained a loss it is important to be aware of the special nature of grieving in children and not to expect that they will express their emotions like adults or that their overt behaviors will necessarily reveal their internal distress. As noted later in this chapter, the delayed working through of bereavement may require specialized assistance if development seems blocked or psychopathologic symptoms appear.[83]

In order for complete "mourning" to occur in the true psychoanalytic sense of detaching memories and hopes from the dead person,[51,52] the child must have some understanding of the concept of death, be capable of forming a real attachment bond, and have a mental representation of the attachment figure. Although there is no doubt that even very young children react to loss, there is considerable controversy about when children have the developmental prerequisites for complete "mourning" and about the likelihood of achieving a healthy outcome if bereavement occurs prior to this time. Generally it is agreed that prior to age 3 or 4 children are not able to achieve complete mourning and it is agreed that by adolescence youngsters can mourn (but are still more vulnerable than adults because they are experiencing so many other losses and changes). The controversy centers on the years in between: can a healthy resolution be achieved and how similar are children's and adults' bereavement reactions?

A number of studies have been conducted in recent years (e.g., Anthony,[5] Bluebond-Langer,[23] Gibney,[58] Kane,[79] Koocher,[84] Menig-Peterson and McCabe,[99] Piaget,[107] Pitcher and Prelinger,[108] Spinetta,[132] Tallmer et al.[135]) to determine how children at various ages comprehend death.

A fairly standard view was put forth by Nagy[104] in 1948. Analyzing the words and drawings of a relatively large sample (378) of Hungarian children who had been exposed to considerable trauma and death in the preceding few years, she conceptualized a three-stage model of awareness and linked the stages to approximate chronological ages.

Prior to about three years of age, children's cognitive and language development is too immature for them to have any concept of death. According to Nagy's stage 1 (roughly ages 3–5), death is seen as reversible; the dead are simply considered "less alive," in a state analogous to sleep. Young children functioning at what Piaget[107] termed the "preoperational" level of development will not generally recognize the irreversibility of death.[84,86,95] In stage 2 (ages 5–9), children begin to comprehend the finality of death, but believe that it happens only to other people. In the third stage (after age 10), the causes of death can be understood, and death is perceived as final, inevitable, and associated with the cessation of bodily activities. As is true in all child development, there is considerable age variation in attainment of the different stages and children may regress when emotionally threatened.

Prior to about six months of age, infants fail to respond to separation from their mothers because they have not yet developed the capacity for memory of a specific personal relationship.[33] The development of stranger anxiety, occurring at about six to eight months, signifies that an infant has established a true object relationship with its mother or primary caretaking figure. This reaction suggests that an infant is developmentally capable of retaining memory traces of his mother and is capable of responding to her absence with displeasure[133] and depression.[40] However, it is not until three or four years of age that a child has a coherent mental representation of important attachment figures and has achieved object constancy.

Observational studies of children between about four years of age and adolescence have led psychiatrists to conflicting conclusions about the nature of children's grieving and about their ability to achieve a healthy outcome. Some psychoanalysts[3,42,75,142,143] maintain that it is not until adolescence that children have the capacity to tolerate the strong painful affects necessary for completing the separation process and that children are more likely to use immature defense mechanisms, such as denial, that interfere with adequate resolution of loss. Thus these observers view children's reactions to loss as qualitatively different from adult reactions.

Others believe that after object constancy has been achieved (at three to four years of age), bereavement need not necessarily lead to enduring psychopathology. Increasingly, it is being recognized[27,55,81] that if the child has a consistent adult who reliably satisfies reality needs and encourages the expression of feelings about the loss, healthy adjustment can occur. Furthermore, the biologic unfolding inherent in development naturally pushes children toward increasing cognitive and emotional maturity. This "developmental push" is seen as an asset that contributes to children's potential resiliency under favorable circumstances.

Some psychiatrists, most notably Bowlby,[24] emphasize the similarities between adults' and children's responses to loss and see an evolutionary basis for them. In Bowlby's view, the argument about children's capacity for "mourning" is in large part terminological, with many psychoanalysts restricting the use of "mourning" to psychological processes with a single outcome—detachment—and others using it more broadly "to denote a fairly wide array of psychological processes set in train by the loss of a loved person irrespective of outcome."[27]

Kliman suggested at one of the committee's site visits that perhaps too much concern has focused on this debate. In his opinion it would be more fruitful to have a detailed understanding of the bereavement process in children so that those who interact with children can be most responsive and helpful.

METHODOLOGICAL ISSUES

Most of the literature on bereavement in childhood is based on observations of disturbed children who are in psychotherapeutic or psychoanalytic treatment.[100] These case reports offer valuable clinical information regarding psychological symptoms and processes, but it is difficult to know the degree to which these children in treatment are representative of all bereaved children and the extent to which individual reactions may be idiosyncratic.

On the other hand, random samples of bereaved children that provide more methodologically reliable data do not offer the same depth of information. In addition, relatively few use control groups, making it impossible to know what the base rates of particular behaviors or symptoms might be in the general population. Where controls are used, it is often unclear whether they are matched for age and sex.

Most of the data on very early (below the age of five) childhood loss are not specific to bereavement but are based on observations of institutionalized children (e.g., Bowlby[24-26]) who were temporarily separated from parents. It is not clear if the children's responses in these studies were based on parental loss itself, on the multiple other losses associated with removal from the home environment, or the unfamiliar and sometimes chaotic circumstances associated with institutional placement. Because these children were not followed over a very long period of time, neither is it known whether pathologic or disturbing reactions endured.

Studies of the long-term effects of bereavement during childhood are abundant, but they are highly controversial because they almost always rely on retrospective data (see Gregory[63] for a discussion). In addition these studies often fail to consider the impact of intervening life events, rely too heavily on data based on patients' memories, and use inappropriate control groups.

A handful of prospective studies describe intermediate effects, but many of these have methodologic flaws, such as a failure to use non-bereaved control groups,[78,114] a lack of direct assessment of bereaved children,[137] and a failure to follow children over a sufficiently long period of time.[114,137] Furthermore, it is not clear that findings from studies conducted in other countries, possibly during wartime, can be generalized to American children living under less socially disruptive conditions. Different methods have been used to study outcomes of childhood bereavement and, partly because of the variation in approach, studies have yielded different results.

Few studies provide precise definitions of key terms, such as "depression," "exaggerated responses," "pathologic grief," "anger," and "sadness," so it is difficult to know whether all authors are referring to the same specific reactions. Studies on childhood loss tend to rely exclusively on interview data or material in case files; standardized instruments that permit greater generalization across studies have rarely been used in the assessment of children. In fact, such instruments have only begun to be developed in the past few years. It should be noted that, because of the way this chapter is organized, a number of studies are cited several times, perhaps giving the impression that there are more empirical data than is really the case.

OUTCOMES OF CHILDHOOD BEREAVEMENT

The death of a parent during childhood has been linked with a wide range of serious and enduring health consequences ranging from schizophrenia to major depression and suicide (see Table 1 for a summary of key findings from each of the major studies). The particular symptoms and syndromes associated with childhood bereavement are generally considered in terms of the *immediate reactions* that occur in the weeks and months following the death, the *intermediate reactions* that can appear later in childhood or adolescence, and the *long-range* or "sleeper" effects that may appear in adulthood either as enduring consequences or delayed reactions to the loss. Although these long-range effects are of most concern, the research evidence in this area is probably the weakest.

Immediate Reactions

Children, like adults, experience a range of emotional and behavioral reactions immediately following parental or sibling death. Studies of both patient and nonpatient samples report that children respond to loss with similar symptoms.

People who interact with recently bereaved children find them sad, angry, and fearful; their behavior includes appetite and sleep disturbances, withdrawal, concentration difficulties, dependency, regression, restlessness, and learning difficulties. They also note that initial symp-

TABLE 1 Major Studies of Childhood or Adolescent Bereavement

Study Author And Year of Publication	Type of Study	Methods	Description of Sample	Time of Assessment	Key Findings
Group I: Studies Using Nonpatient Samples					
Kliman, 1968[80]	Explored link between bereavement in childhood and subsequent emotional illness; clinical approach; prospective.	Interviewed 7 surviving parents about their children.	18 children (ages 1–14) from 7 families.	Interval between bereavement and first contact with the surviving parent ranged from 24 hours to 15 months. Mean interval was 8 months.	Little or no immediate tearfulness in response to the death. Neuroses frequently arose or were exacerbated following parental death. Seven of the 18 children began an unprecedented custom of frequently sharing a bed with the surviving parent. Disciplinary problems arose rapidly with 4 children who had lost a father. Identification of the child with the dead parent occurred in 7 cases.
Raphael et al., 1980[116]	Investigation of acute bereavement responses in children and their families during the crisis of parental bereavement; clinical approach; prospective.	Interviewed the surviving parent; assessed children through interview, painting, doll play, and story card sessions; systematically observed interaction between the surviving parent and the child regarding the bereavement.	Subjects included 23 children from 10 Australian families, ages 2–8. Located via funeral directors, clergy, death notices. 16 children experienced the death of a father; 7 children experienced the death of a mother.	Interviews took place 6 weeks to 3 months after bereavement.	Children displayed a preoccupation with oral-level concerns, e.g., who would feed them after death of a mother and who would pay for the food after death of a father. Even young children (age 3 years) were concerned that something could happen to the surviving parent and perceived their own vulnerability because of this. Children showed directly or indirectly some of their sad affects about the death and loss. Most children could voice a wish for the parent's return. Frequent fantasies about the death and its causes and meaning.

105

TABLE 1 Major Studies of Childhood or Adolescent Bereavement—(*Continued*)

Study Author And Year of Publication	Type of Study	Methods	Description of Sample	Time of Assessment	Key Findings
Elizur and Kaffman, 1982[45]; Elizur and Kaffman, 1983[46]	Study of social and emotional consequences of paternal death; epidemiologic approach; prospective.	Interviewed child's widowed mother and teacher, using a semistructured interview.	25 Israeli kibbutz children, ages 1–10, who lost a father in the 1973 Yom Kippur War. Sample of community children with no history of psychiatric treatment before the war.	Interviews took place $\frac{1}{2}$, $1\frac{1}{2}$, and $3\frac{1}{2}$ years after the father's death.	Over 40% of the children showed clinical evidence of "pathological bereavement" characterized by severe behavior problems and marked impairment in social functions. Only a minority did not show overt signs of emotional disturbance throughout the follow-up period. Subsequent follow-up (1983) suggested that family pretraumatic and environmental factors (e.g., marital discord in parents' prebereavement relationship) significantly determined the duration and severity of response.
Van Eerdewegh et al., 1982[137]	Studied responses of children of a consecutive sample of young widows and widowers in the community; epidemiologic approach; prospective.	Bereaved parents and controls were interviewed, using a structured interview about their children's reactions to death of the other parent.	A maximum of 3 randomly selected children per family, ages 2–17, were inquired about. All children had recently experienced parental death.	Parents and controls were interviewed at 1 month and 13 months postbereavement.	Significant increase of dysphoria (which disappeared over time), persistence of a minor form of depression, increase in bedwetting, and a significant degree of impairment in school performance. No significant increases in behavior problems and severe forms of depression. Children's general health was not affected.

106

Study	Description	Sample/Methods	Sample	Timing	Findings
Balk, 1983[8]	Investigated the perceptions of teenagers who lost a sibling during adolescence, focusing on bereavement reactions and self-concepts; epidemiologic approach; retrospective.	Subjects contacted by two organizations that support bereaved parents. Data come from a single focused interview and administration of the Offer Self-Image Questionnaire for Adolescents (a standardized instrument designed specifically for research with normal adolescents).	33 adolescents, ages 14–19, from white, middle to upper income families, who had lost a sibling. Twenty subjects were female; 24 had been younger than the sibling who died, and 20 had been of the opposite sex as the dead sibling. Most of the deaths had been unanticipated.	The death occurred on average of two years prior to the interview, with a range of 4 to 84.	One-third to one-half of the subjects reported enduring grief reactions such as confusion, depression, guilt, shock, or anger. However, moments of acute grief seemed to be transitory, and apparently became less acute as the bereaved teenager gained experience in dealing with emotional responses to the death.
Kaffman and Elizur, 1983[78]	Compared kibbutz children whose fathers died with city children raised in a regular family framework who had experienced the same event; prospective.	Interviewed mother and teacher for kibbutz sample. Interviewed only mothers for city sample.	Kibbutz sample included 8 girls and 17 boys, ages 2–10, who lost a father in the 1973 Yom Kippur War. City sample included 8 boys and 13 girls ages 2–10, who lost a father in the same war. Children in both samples were considered psychologically "normal" prior to their fathers' deaths.	Interviews conducted 18 months after notification of father's death.	In both kibbutz and urban settings the loss of a father became a serious traumatic situation for a large proportion of the children. Kibbutz society failed to provide a "protective barrier" in the case of paternal death.

TABLE 1 Major Studies of Childhood or Adolescent Bereavement—(*Continued*)

Study Author And Year of Publication	Type of Study	Methods	Description of Sample	Time of Assessment	Key Findings
		Group II:	**Studies Using Patient Samples**		
Arthur and Kemme, 1964[7]	Intensive case studies; clinical approach; retrospective.	Not clear; appears to have used interview data and review of case records.	83 emotionally disturbed children, ages $4\frac{1}{2}$–17, and their families who were in psychiatric treatment at a university-based clinic. All children had experienced the death of a parent.	Not clear.	High incidence of intellectual and emotional problems either directly or indirectly related to parental death. Children frequently manifested difficulties in abstract thinking relative to the concepts of finality and causality. Symptoms were variable. Persistence of disturbance was related to severity of preexisting pathology.
Rutter, 1966[126]	Statistical analysis of the backgrounds of parentally bereaved children; epidemiologic approach, retrospective.	Reviewed case records.	86 English children, ages 2–17, attending a psychiatric clinic in London.	Variable; 36 of the children lost one or both parents prior to age $4\frac{1}{2}$, and 50 lost one or both parents after age $4\frac{1}{2}$.	Excess of neurotic illness and delinquency among the bereaved, although disorders associated with parental loss were heterogeneous. Association between parental death and subsequent disorder was most marked in children aged 2–5. Psychiatric disturbance following parental death was usually delayed 5 or more years. Subjects who developed symptoms soon after parental death were mainly adolescents with either depressive or antisocial disorders.

Study	Approach	Method	Sample	Timing/Age	Findings
Wolfenstein, 1966[142]	Intensive case study; clinical approach; retrospective.	Observations of patients in psychoanalytic treatment.	42 parentally bereaved children and adolescents in a child guidance clinic (and some cases from private practice), supplemented by observations of nonpatient subjects (number unstated).	16 patients came under observation within 1 year of the parent's death; 8 within 3 years; and 18 from 4 to 14 years later. The age at which the children were bereaved varied from early childhood to late adolescence.	Found that adolescence constituted the necessary developmental condition for grieving (in the classical Freudian sense). In many instances, there was denial of the irrevocability of the loss due to the developmental unreadiness of children and young adolescents to grieve. Adaptive reactions to loss differed from adult grieving.
Birtchnell, 1970[14,15]	Explored possible link between early parental death and mental illness in adulthood; epidemiologic approach; retrospective.	Used case records and questionnaires.	500 Scottish psychiatric patients who were consecutive admissions to a psychiatric hospital. A control group from a local general practice matched for age and sex with the patient group.	Not clear, although the bereavements appear to have occurred several years earlier.	Death of a parent prior to age 10 appeared to be an etiologic factor in the subsequent development of mental illness. Differences between patients and controls especially striking when loss occurred prior to age 5.
Furman, E., 1974[53]	Intensive case studies; clinical approach; retrospective.	Review of case material from several therapists.	23 emotionally disturbed children who had experienced the death of a parent. Of these, 14 were in the 5×/week psychoanalytic treatment and 9 were in treatment via the parent.	Not clear; age at bereavement ranged from 10 weeks to 13 years.	Parental death can be mastered even by young children if circumstances are favorable.
Call and Wolfenstein, 1976[37]	Intensive case studies; clinical approach; retrospective.	Focused on intensive analysis of single case studies.	Total is not clear; a few psychoanalysts described experiences with analytic patients or experiences at hospitals at which they consulted.	Not clear; apparently several years had passed since the parent's death.	Below age 12 children tended to react to loss with aggression. Over age 12, they reacted with sadness, weeping, depression, psychomotor retardation, sometimes suicidal tendencies, occasional hyperactivity, or alternating manic and depressive states.

TABLE 1 Major Studies of Childhood or Adolescent Bereavement—(*Continued*)

Study Author And Year of Publication	Type of Study	Methods	Description of Sample	Time of Assessment	Key Findings
Brown et al., 1977[31]	Explored possible link between loss experience in childhood and subsequent depression in adulthood; epidemiologic approach; retrospective.	Compared three groups of women—psychiatric inpatients, psychiatric outpatients, and nonpatients. All subjects had lost a spouse, child, sibling, or parent through death.	114 English women, ages 18–65, undergoing inpatient or outpatient psychiatric treatment at time of interview, with a diagnosis of primary depression, and a random sample of 458 nonpatient women, ages 18–65.	Not clear. However, authors distinguish between those who had a recent loss (defined as occurring in the 2 years before onset of depression) and a past loss (defined as occurring any time before this).	Of past losses, only loss of mother before age 11 was associated with greater risk of depression—among both psychiatric patients and women in a random sample. Past loss of a father or sibling before age 17 (or a mother between 11 and 17, or a child or husband) was not associated with greater risk of depression. Among patients, all types of past loss by death were associated with psychotic-like depressive symptoms; other types of past loss were associated with neurotic-type depressive symptoms.
Birtchnell, 1980[18]	Drew a sample from 6,795 referrals over a 5-year period from the Scotland Psychiatric Case Register; epidemiologic approach; retrospective.	Reviewed case records.	Compared 160 Scottish female psychiatric patients whose mothers died before age 11 with 80 female controls.	Not clear, but seems to have been many years since the bereavement.	No evidence that the early death of a mother had any direct influence on development of mental illness in adult life. Within the bereaved group, the women who reported bad relationships with replacement mothers emerged as having certain clinical characteristics.

tom patterns depend largely on the age at which the child is bereaved. For example, children under age five are likely to respond with eating, sleeping, and bowel and bladder disturbances; those under age two may show loss of speech or diffuse distress. School-age children may become phobic or hypochondriacal, withdrawn, or excessively care-giving. Displays of aggression may be observed in place of sadness, especially in boys who have difficulty in expressing longing. Adolescents may respond more like adults, but they may also be reluctant about expressing their emotions because of fear that they will appear different or abnormal.[89]

Intermediate Effects

A limited number of investigators[45,46,81,116,126,137] followed cohorts of parentally bereaved children for one to six years after death. Others (e.g., Lifshitz[93]) made single assessments some years after the loss.

Medical Consequences. A few investigators have suggested a link between loss experiences and subsequent precipitation or "activation" of specific diseases, such as thyrotoxicosis, rheumatoid arthritis, and diabetes.[68,90,101] The literature on the medical consequences of bereavement in children is extremely limited, however.

Some studies found increased physical symptoms, especially abdominal pain. In a community sample of Israeli children who had lost their fathers, no objective findings about these physical symptoms were established and the investigators concluded that the responses were largely attention-seeking.[78] Van Eerdewegh et al.[137] found no increase in physician visits despite the reported increase in symptoms, possibly suggesting that grieving parents were too preoccupied with their own distress to seek help for their children.

Psychiatric Consequences. A number of psychological symptoms, most prominently neurosis and depression, appear to correlate with parental or sibling death. Signs of continuing emotional distress have been noted in both community and patient samples of children who lost a parent or sibling.

Kaffman and Elizur[45,77] found that about 40% of normal preadolescent Israeli kibbutz children who lost a father during the Yom Kippur War of 1973 continued to show severe maladaptive behavior more than three years following the death. Behavioral problems, amounting to an average of nine handicapping problems per child (e.g., soiling, social isolation, learning problems), peaked in the second year after the father's death; these represented a significant increase over prebereavement behavior. Three and a half years after the loss, 65 percent of the total clinical symptoms persisted at a medium to severe level. Assessing the children at 6, 18, and 42 months postbereavement, the authors found that nearly 70 percent of the children showed signs of severe emotional disturbance in at least one follow-up period. Fewer than one-third had achieved satisfactory family, school, and social adjustment throughout the entire three and a half years of the study. A subsequent study of this sample[46] suggested that children with preexisting emotional difficulties and those who came from families marked by marital discord were at greater risk for more severe pathologic developments than were children from stable families with no prior emotional problems.

An unevenness in the development of bereavement reactions among these Israeli children was noted. Although those with symptoms of marked emotional impairment during the early months of bereavement appeared to develop the most severe and prolonged type of pathologic grieving, others revealed no special pathology during the early months but deteriorated emotionally during the second to fourth years. Thus, the timing of severe and persistent clinical symptoms that significantly impaired the child's psychosocial functioning varied in onset and duration.

In a study comparing bereaved kibbutz and urban children, Kaffman and Elizur[78] found that 48 percent of the kibbutz children and 52 percent of those in cities showed persistent symptoms of "pathological grief" (which the authors define as "the presence of multiple and persistent clinical symptomatology of sufficient severity to handicap the child in his everyday life within the family, school, and children's group, persisting for a minimum of two months") and displayed signs of marked distress, emotional insecurity, and psychological imbalance 18 months after notification of their fathers' deaths.

That normal kibbutz children did not fare a great deal better than city children suggests that the social supports available in the kibbutz setting and the perceived less central role of the parents did not protect the youngsters from stress. Thus, while the father within a kibbutz is neither the family provider nor principal supplier of material needs, he is still a central attachment figure in his child's emotional life. These findings highlight the importance of the psychological meaning of parental loss and its impact on a child.

Such findings in general community samples are echoed in studies of psychiatric patients. Studies by both Rutter[126] and Arthur and Kemme[7] found neurotic illness was excessive in disturbed children who had lost a parent. The latter found that 52 percent of their sample were experiencing autonomy conflicts, 27 percent felt panicky over relationships and dependent on others, and 39 percent had problems in defining their relationship with the opposite-sex parent four months to two years after parental loss.

In a sample of disturbed 2½- to 14-year-olds who had lost a sibling,[36] guilt reactions, accompanied by trembling, crying, or sadness, were present in half the subjects and evident for five or more years after the death. Forty percent had prolonged or anniversary hysterical identification with the dead sibling's prominent symptoms.

A striking finding of both Van Eerdewegh et al.[137] and Rutter[126] in English psychiatric clinic samples is the high frequency of depression in adolescent boys who lost a father through death. Severe depressions were most likely in subjects whose mothers were already depressed prior to their husbands' deaths, suggesting children's emotional states may be linked to identification with the surviving parent rather than a pure response to loss. Stone[134] suggests that parental death may precipitate a depressive disorder in adolescents already at risk for manic–depressive disorder of the depressive type.

Behavioral Consequences. There is general agreement among clinicians that parental bereavement has an adverse impact on school functioning, both in academic performance and social behavior. Several studies of Australian, Israeli, and American children 13 months to 6 years postbereavement showed evidence of examination failure, school refusal, a decreased interest in school activities, and drop-out.[20,93,115,137] These findings parallel the general finding that school performance is very often a significant indicator of emotional difficulty.

Delinquency has been found to correlate with parental bereavement, particularly in adolescents.[64,115,126] In a controlled follow-up study of a sample of 264 Minnesota school children who had lost a parent, Gregory[64] found that bereaved adolescents who lived with an opposite-sex parent had higher rates of delinquency than controls.

Raphael[115] notes that loss generates longing for comforting and reassurance in girls, leading to sexualized relationships that provide a sense of ego fusion with another, whereas boys are more likely to engage in petty theft, car-stealing, fights, drug-taking, or testing of authority systems.

Long-Term (Delayed) Effects

A number of researchers have conducted retrospective studies to investigate a hypothesized link between childhood bereavement and vulnerability during adulthood to a variety of serious disorders, including neurosis, psychosis, physical illness, depression, schizophrenia, and antisocial behavior. Specific findings from these studies are contradictory, but they generally point to an increased vulnerability to physical and mental illness later in life. Findings from the one prospective study conducted by Fulton and his colleagues[12,96] also suggest that bereaved children suffer long-term vulnerabilities.

Medical Consequences.   Raphael[115] points to a number of retrospective studies suggesting that persons who have experienced such loss are more likely to demonstrate symptomatology, increased health care utilization, and complaints of ill health in adult life. She cites Seligman et al.,[128] who link early parental death with increased use of medical service by adolescents, and Schmale and Iker,[127] who found a possible association between childhood loss and development of cancer, although (as discussed in Chapter 2) the connection has not been clearly demonstrated.

Bendikson and Fulton's prospective study[12] of a cohort of 264 parentally bereaved Minnesota ninth graders also suggests a possible predisposition to later illness. When these individuals were observed in their thirties they were significantly more susceptible to serious medical illnesses than the control subjects, and experienced significantly more emotional distress. Unfortunately, the exact nature of the illnesses and distress was not specified.

Psychiatric Consequences.   Substantially more work has been done on the possible association between early loss and mental illness, with the majority of investigators reporting a positive relationship between childhood bereavement and adult-life mental illness. Most of these researchers used psychiatric patients as subjects, although community samples have also been studied in more recent years. The emphasis has generally been on the consequences of parental death, with some attempt to further specify risk factors in terms of the sex of the deceased parent and the age and sex of the bereaved child.

The evidence is contradictory, but many investigators find a significant increase of both neurosis[119] and psychosis[9] in persons who experienced early bereavement when compared with controls. Links are suggested between early loss and adult-life impairment in sexual identity, development of autonomy, and capacity for intimacy.[6,28,119] The chief disagreement is over which combination of variables puts a subject at most risk. For example, Barry and Lindemann[10] found that girls who lose a mother between birth and age 2 are at greatest risk for neurosis whereas in Norton's[106] sample, loss of the father before age 10 was most significant.

Recent studies suggest that sample characteristics may influence apparent outcome. For example, in a 1972 study comparing 500 Scottish psychiatric hospital admissions with a control group of general practice patients matched for age and sex, Birtchnell[17] found that loss of the mother before age 10 was an etiologic factor in the subsequent development of mental illness. This finding was not replicated in his later work,[18] however, which drew upon a community sample.

Individuals who lose a parent or sibling in childhood have been considered to be most at risk for subsequent depressive disorders. Based on his clinical observations, Bowlby[27] concludes that profound early loss renders people highly vulnerable to subsequent depressive disorders, with each subsequent loss triggering an upsurge of unresolved grief initially related to the early bereavement.

Research data examining the link between early loss and adult depression are only suggestive, however. In a review of controlled studies to determine if a link existed between childhood/adolescent bereavement and adult-life depression, Lloyd[94] found that 8 out of 11 studies[29,31,38,41,49,72,103,125] reported significant increases in depressive disorders among the bereaved group; childhood loss of a parent increased the risk of depression by a factor of two or three. In addition, in seven out of eight controlled studies,[11,15,31,57,102,129,141] early loss was correlated with severity of depression. Parentally bereaved subjects were more likely to experience psychotic- rather than neurotic-level depression.[31,141]

In one well-controlled study, Brown et al.[31] found that the incidence of maternal death prior to age 11 was significantly more frequent for depressed women in a community sample than for matched, nondepressed controls. They also found that 66 percent of those diagnosed as psychotically depressed had a history of early loss compared with only 39 percent of the neurotic depressives. There is also some suggestion that depressions associated with early bereavement tend to be reactive[57] rather than endogenous; studies that have included the more biologically predisposed bipolar (manic–depressive) disorders typically have not established a connection between them and early bereavement.[1,73,109]

A number of studies show a link between childhood bereavement and suicide attempts in adult life (e.g., Birtchnell,[16] Dorpat et al.,[44] Farberow and Simon,[47] Greer,[62] Hill,[71] Levi et al.[91]). Birtchnell found that twice as many depressed suicide attempters were parentally bereaved compared with nonsuicidal depressives (66.7 percent versus 33.3 percent).

Tennant et al.,[136] in a recent review of studies regarding parental death in childhood and later risk for depression, caution that the data are not conclusive. Birtchnell[18] suggests that additional factors, such as the quality of the relationship with subsequent caretakers, may be more influential in determining risk for later depression than simply the experience of bereavement in and of itself.

Evidence regarding bereavement as an etiologic factor in the development of schizophrenia is less convincing than that on depression. Dennehy,[41] Hilgard,[69] and Rosenzweig and Bray[124] report positive findings, while Granville-Grossman[61] and Gregory[65] find no significant correlation.

Behavioral Consequences. Research findings are suggestive of a link between childhood loss and subsequent criminality. In Markesun and Fulton's prospective community study,[96] men who had been bereaved in childhood had more offenses against the law when in their twenties than did controls. In samples of both male and female prisoners[30,32] the histories revealed an excess of parental death; the "affectionless criminal" appears to be most strongly represented.

Based on clinical observations of psychotherapy patients of the Barr-Harris Center for the Study of Separation and Loss During Childhood, in Chicago, Altschul and Beiser[4] have noted difficulties in parenting when the bereaved child grows up and has children of his or her own. These difficulties seem to occur more often if the loss happened when the child was between 7 and 12, and if the deceased parent was of the same sex. They hypothesize that these problems have their roots in identifications with the dead parent and in the "lack of experience with the dead parent in developmental stages that go beyond the point of loss." Because the adults who experienced childhood bereavement at times do not expect to live longer than their parents did, some avoid emotional intimacy with their children as if to prevent too much grief and suffering if they die.

Conclusions About Outcomes

It is difficult to draw conclusions about the long-term consequences of bereavement during childhood or adolescence. The data suggest potential difficulties, but there is a lack of specificity regarding what places a bereaved youth at risk.

Concerning intermediate-term consequences, the existing literature suggests that early bereavement greatly increases a child's susceptibility to depression, school dysfunction, and delinquency. Given the immaturity of the child's personality, it seems likely that even a minor depression of 13 months' duration might inhibit or interfere with normal ego development, thereby disrupting or distorting psychological growth.[137]

THE GRIEVING PROCESS IN CHILDREN

As discussed earlier in this chapter, the nature of children's reactions to loss will depend largely on their stage of emotional and cognitive development. Although specific manifestations of distress and the duration of responses vary by age and by individual, children (like adults) have been observed to go through a relatively predictable series of phases of bereavement responses.

Based on his observations of young children in a residential nursery who were separated from maternal figures, Bowlby[24-27] identified three sequential phases in response to separation and loss. When a healthy child over the age of six months was taken from his mother, a period of "protest" ensued, characterized by loud, angry, tearful behavior suggesting an expectation of and demand for reunion. This stage might last for as long as a week or more. When attempts at reunion failed to produce the desired results, a phase of "despair" set in, marked by acute pain, misery, and a sense of diminishing hope. Following this came the final stage of "detachment," during which children behaved as if they no longer cared whether or not their mothers returned; upon actual reunion, their initial reaction might be to continue avoidance behavior and withdrawal.

Elizur and Kaffman's work[45] with kibbutz children described the course of grieving during the first four years following paternal bereavement. The immediate reaction was one of pain and grief. During the first year, the children began to examine the meanings and implications of the loss and to ask realistic questions to gain understanding of "dead" and "alive." During the second year, children were generally more understanding and accepting of the loss and defensive maneuvers decreased, but they showed a significant increase in anxiety. In order to cope, they became more dependent on their mothers and were more demanding; aggressive behavior, discipline problems, and restlessness intensified. During the third and fourth years, manifestations of overdependence still characterized two-thirds of the sample, but anxiety level and augmented aggressiveness were reduced. Despite a general trend toward greater adjustment, however, 39 percent of the previously normal sample continued to show signs of emotional distress four years after their fathers had died.

Shifts in Self-Concepts Following Bereavement

A major area of concern regarding psychological functioning following bereavement relates to negative shifts in self-concepts and self-esteem. Rochlin[120-122] and Kliman[83] have observed that children often assess themselves more negatively after a parent's death than before. Children who interpret a parent's death as desertion because the parent did not love them may believe that they are unlovable, which may result in a persistent sense of low self-esteem.[37]

Following a major relationship loss, a child may see himself as help-less and vulnerable. It is possible that this image of being frighteningly small and helpless is the most disruptive and disorganizing view of the self that can emerge subsequent to parental death. Based on their exten-sive clinical experience with bereaved children, Erna Furman[54] and Rob-ert Furman[56] have observed that while there is a fairly universal ten-dency toward self-blame following bereavement, it may be that the re-sultant sense of guilt is less threatening than is the defended-against view of the self as helpless. If someone feels responsible for a death at least that person feels some sense of control over the environment. The sense of being ineffectual in controlling life events impinging on the self may lead to a kind of passivity, apathy, and depression, similar to the mental state described by Seligman in his theory of "learned helpless-ness" as the precursor of depression.[128]

Alternatively, a bereaved child may regard himself as hostile and de-structive. The tendency of children to think in egocentric, magical ways and to equate thought with deed may lead to the belief that their destructive impulses or angry feelings destroyed the parent or sibling. This can lead to a hostile image of the self, especially if there was a great deal of competition and hostility in the prior relationship, as is likely to be true of siblings.[22] Relatively universal death wishes can return to haunt the bereaved child in the form of feelings of responsibility and guilt.[122,139] Such feelings are more likely to be a problem if the death wishes were especially intense.

The Role of Identification in Grieving

Identification with a deceased person has been described as more common and dramatic in children than in adults.[13] This process may represent both an unconscious defense mechanism and a conscious at-tempt to emulate the good qualities of the deceased.[76] If done in modera-tion, such identifications can be enriching for a child.[74,83] Taken to an extreme, however, identification with a dead parent can become very frightening, as it can imply adoption of the parent's symptoms and death. Because of this fear, Wolfenstein[143] believes that genuinely adap-tive identifications in children are rare.

Johnson and Rosenblatt[76] have noted that a socially inappropriate identification with a deceased parent may be an expression of incom-plete or pathologic grief. If a child identifies too closely with adults, peers may be rejecting or critical, with a resulting loss of social sup-ports. In addition, when such replacement roles are fostered by adults they can be felt as rather frightening pressure by the child. For example, if a new widow tells her young son that he is now "the man of the house," he may feel some literal responsibility and become anxious at the prospect of having to assume all the roles of the deceased parent (e.g., surrogate marriage partner or emotional confidant to a depressed adult). If his mother later remarries, the stress on the little "man of the house" is magnified by the fact that she has chosen to "replace" him.

Likewise, a child may attempt to replace a deceased sibling as a means to help the parent(s) cope with loss feelings, thereby compromising the youngster's own identity development. Too often the tendency to idealize the dead also makes it difficult for surviving siblings to deal with their anger at the deceased or at their parents (e.g., for not preventing the death or for seeming to care more about the deceased child). This too may form a basis for overidentification, if the child attempts to secure affection by adopting the traits of the deceased.

Common Thoughts, Concerns, and Fantasies

As with adults,[88] a number of common themes emerge in bereaved children, typically associated with or underlying feelings of sadness, rage, fear, shame, and guilt.

There are at least three questions, whether directly articulated or not, that will occur to most children following a loss: Did I cause this to happen? Will it happen to me? Who will take care of me now (or if something happens to my surviving caretaker)? It is important to provide answers to these questions and to hear how the child understands those answers, because misunderstandings may give rise to feelings of anger or fear.

Perceptions that the parent or sibling's death was a deliberate abandonment, associated with feelings of rage, tend to undermine a child's badly needed sense of being cared for. This was indeed the reaction of 20 percent of the parentally bereaved patients studied by Arthur and Kemme.[7]

Worries that a dead parent might return and seek revenge,[7] concerns that what happened to the deceased parent or sibling could also happen to them or to surviving family members or caretakers, and worries that their basic physical needs for survival may not be satisfied[53,80] have all been observed. Bowlby[27] notes that fears about whom death may claim next may underlie anxious clinging or obstinate behavior. The belief that the world is a safe, predictable place may be destroyed, resulting in disruption of a child's capacity for basic trust.[7]

Common Defensive Strategies

Many of the reactions in bereaved children that have been described—denial, idealization of the dead parent, inhibition or isolation of grief-related affects, identification with the lost parent, displacement—are common defensive strategies.

Psychoanalytic writers (e.g., Altschul,[3] Deutsch,[42] Jacobsen,[75] and Shambaugh,[130]), basing their judgments on small numbers of patients, and researchers studying a sample of normal children[45] have commented on the frequent use of denial, which they believe underlies persistent fantasies of reunion with the deceased. Elizur and Kaffman[45] found that bereaved children fantasized in an attempt to maintain the illusion that the deceased parent was still nearby. Denial may help ward off painful feelings and a conscious consideration of the loss.[130] Altschul,[3] observing that such denial may continue indefinitely, feels that it is the emotional significance of the deceased person that is denied more than the reality of the death. Wolfenstein[142] has commented on a defensive (and often maladaptive) splitting of the ego in bereaved children that allows them to acknowledge a parent's death as a reality while simultaneously denying its finality. She suggests that the good moods that may be observed in bereaved children following parental death represent an affective counterpart of denial. When depressed moods occur, particularly in adolescents, they are usually isolated from thoughts of the dead parent.

A lost parent is often idealized and preserved in fantasy as the good parent while hostility is displaced onto the surviving caretaker, who is then perceived as the bad parent.[105] Arthur and Kemme,[7] assessing disturbed children, found such idealization particularly marked in girls who resented attempts to intrude on or devalue fantasized relationships with deceased fathers. In their sample, hostility toward the dead parent was denied and projected onto the surviving parent, who was blamed for the father's death. Wolfenstein[142] believes such idealization of the deceased and vilification of the surviving parent represent an attempt to undo prior feelings of hostility toward the parent who died.

Conclusions About the Grieving Process

Although many of the reactions children display in response to a loss are similar to those observed in adults, the time frame and overt process of grieving in young people are clearly different. Because of developmental differences in their cognitive abilities and personality structures, children are likely to use more primitive defense mechanisms than adults (e.g., denial and regression) in coping with their losses. These differences put children at substantial psychological risk after the death of a family member. Denial that a death has occurred, for example, may prevent a child from confronting and working through his or her feelings of loss. Troublesome behaviors and emotions related to the bereavement may emerge months, or even years, later as a child reworks his grief.[81]

VARIABLES AFFECTING PROCESSES AND OUTCOMES

In addition to psychological defenses, a number of other variables have been identified that affect the grieving process in children. These include age and emotional stability of the child, sex of the deceased and of the bereaved, the nature of the relationship between the child and the deceased, and the nature of social supports following bereavement.

Child's Age, Developmental Stage, and Emotional Stability at the Time of Bereavement

A number of clinicians and clinical researchers (e.g., Alexander and Adlerstein,[2] Bowlby,[27] Elizur and Kaffman,[46] McConville et al.,[98] Rutter,[126] Van Eerdewegh et al.[137]) report that the impact of relationship loss will be greater when it occurs at certain ages or stages than at others. Both Rutter[126] and Bowlby[27] have found that bereaved children under the age of five are more susceptible than older children to pathologic outcomes. But whereas Bowlby found that children aged six months to four years were at particular risk, Rutter concludes that the third and fourth years of life constitute a vulnerable period because he found an excess of parental deaths among psychiatric clinic patients during those years. He speculates that children under the age of one or two are less distressed than bereaved older children because there has been less time to develop ties.

Early adolescence also appears to be a vulnerable time in terms of significant relationship loss.[21] Rutter[126], Van Eerdewegh et al.,[137] and Wolfenstein[142] found that the severely depressed children in their studies mostly seemed to be adolescent boys who had lost their fathers. In contrast, Hilgard et al.,[70] using retrospective data, noted a number of outstandingly good adjustments among adults whose parental loss came between the ages of 10 and 15, preceded by a satisfactory home life.

Elizur and Kaffman's data[45,46,78] also suggest that although normal children are at risk following bereavement, preexisting emotional difficulties, in combination with other antecedent variables, may exacerbate symptoms during the early months following loss. Clarification is needed on the kinds of emotional disturbances and troubled family relationships that place children at greater risk.

Quality of Preexisting Relationship with the Deceased

As is true of adults, children's reactions to loss are more difficult to resolve when the prior relationship with the deceased person was marked by high levels of ambivalence or dependence.[115] As noted earlier, hostility toward a deceased parent or sibling may lead to defensive maneuvers, such as idealization of the deceased, which run counter to resolution and completion of grief. In addition, unlike adults or adolescents who may have a number of close relationships outside the family, a preadolescent child invests love almost exclusively in parental figures.[53] The younger the child, the more dependent he is on parents for survival. Thus, preexisting relationship and age may be interacting variables.

Sex of Deceased Parent and Bereaved Child

Studies of the impact of and interaction between the sex of the deceased parent and that of the child have produced interesting but somewhat contradictory results. Kliman[81,82] has observed that from about age three onward, while yearning for the dead parent tends to be more overt when the opposite-sex parent dies, special anxieties may develop when the same-sex parent dies, especially if the child begins to fear that he or she must in some way become the "new daddy" or "new mommy" of the family. In clinical samples, Fast and Cain[48] found that boys who lost fathers felt threatened by and therefore tried to avoid positive feelings toward their mothers, while Arthur and Kemme[7] found that girls showed a greater tendency to idealize dead fathers.

Retrospective studies of the association between early parental loss and adult-life depression in community samples[31] and studies of women psychiatric patients[14,15,17] suggest that girls are more vulnerable than boys to parental bereavement in general and more vulnerable to loss of a father during adolescence.[17,21,71]

Contrary to the findings cited above, however, Kaffman and Elizur[78] found few differences between boys and girls who lost a father, and although Rutter[127] found significantly higher levels of depression in adolescent boys who lost fathers, he concluded that, in general, "there is nothing to suggest that psychiatric disorder was more related to the death of the mother than father or vice versa."

Quality of the Child's Support System

As discussed throughout this report, social support is a modifying variable that can soften trauma. Unfortunately, children's primary source of support is usually the surviving parent, who also has been traumatically affected by the death of a spouse or child.

Widows, usually sad and anxious following conjugal bereavement, often express impatience and irritation with children who simultaneously have special needs.[27,59] After a parent dies, modes of discipline often change, with the surviving parent either becoming excessively strict or lax or being inconsistent.[27] Rutter[126] found that bereaved children frequently experienced multiple life-style changes in the context of makeshift arrangements following the death, with a few being placed in institutions. Rather than the atmosphere of stability and consistency necessary for a better outcome,[53] the common situation following a parental death may be considerable chaos, disorganization, and a sense of insecurity.

The level of trauma associated with the loss of a parent will depend in large part on relationships within the home prior to the parental death and upon the maintenance or reestablishment of the home after the death occurs. Hilgard et al.[70] interviewed a representative community sample of 65 adults between the ages of 19 and 49 who had lost a parent through death during childhood. Comparing well-adjusted subjects in the community with selected patients in a mental hospital who had suffered childhood parental losses, they identified one protective factor in father loss as being the presence of a reality-oriented, strong mother who worked and kept the home intact, instilling strength in her children both through her example and through her expectations of their performance. Elizur and Kaffman[46] agree that in the case of paternal death, the mother's assertiveness in coping with the loss and the availability of a surrogate father figure influence the course of a child's responses in the years thereafter.

Other protective factors include the presence of a mother who can use a network of support outside the home, prebereavement years spent in a home with two compatible parents who had well-defined roles so that early identifications were good, and parental attitudes that fostered independence and a tolerance for separation.[46,70] Hilgard et al.[70] note that "appropriate" grieving by the surviving parent and avoidance of excessive dependency on the children had helped their well-adjusted sample work through the loss and achieve a satisfactory adaptation following parental death.

In addition to the role of the surviving parent following a death in the immediate family, it would seem that grandparents, aunts and uncles, and perhaps close family friends, could step in to assist the bereaved child. The impact of nonparent figures on the course of children's bereavement reactions has not been documented.

Remarriage of the Surviving Parent

In a controlled retrospective study of women in a community whose mothers died before they reached age 11, Birtchnell[18] found that only those who experienced poor relationships with mother replacements emerged with major psychological problems. These women tended to manifest neurotic depressions of moderate intensity and were more prone to severe and chronic anxiety symptoms than bereaved women not characterized by such relationships.

Fast and Cain[48] identified the reluctance of the bereaved child to accept discipline or punishment from the stepparent, competition between the same-sex parent and child for the stepparent, and unfavorable comparisons of the stepparent with the deceased parent as possible sources of difficulty. Hilgard et al.[70] found that mothers of subjects in their study who remarried while in their thirties tended to marry men who made inadequate stepfathers, increasing the risk of a poor relationship with the child. They speculate that women this age who have young children have fewer choices of marital partners and may make unsatisfactory compromises.

On the other hand, some of the same situations already described as difficult seem to be associated with a parent's failure to remarry. For example, it seems likely that postbereavement bed-sharing, reported by Kliman,[80] and the emotional dependency that Hilgard et al.[70] find hazardous would pose a greater threat to the emotional stability of children when lonely, frightened, unattached parents do not have another adult with whom to share their lives.

Cultural Background

Although it has been suggested that cultural factors, such as ethnic background, social class, and religion, play a role in determining the child's understanding of and response to loss, this is an area in which very little research has been done. Based on child interview data, Tallmer et al.[135] have concluded that children from lower socioeconomic class families are more aware of at least the concept of death, due to the increased amount of violence and death in their social environments. In their studies comparing bereaved kibbutz and urban children in Israel, Kaffman and Elizur[45,78] found that differences in child-rearing methods, family functioning style, and social setting influenced the type of problems that became prominent following paternal death.

Circumstances of the Death

The type of death experienced—e.g., anticipated versus unanticipated, in the home versus in the hospital—influences the child's bereavement response. Erna Furman[53] comments that there are no peaceful deaths for parents of young children, and each type of death is associated with particular anxieties; the kinds and sources of anxiety vary with the child and his situation.

It is generally agreed that an anticipated death is easier for children to cope with than sudden loss—just as it is for adults—because forewarning seems to provide an opportunity to prepare at least cognitively. If a parent is ill for a prolonged period of time, however, the child often has to deal with knowledge of a series of surgical and medical interventions that may be interpreted as bodily assaults.[53] If the particular form of a parent's or sibling's terminal illness or injury coincides with and gives reality to developmentally appropriate but otherwise transient concerns, the already existing worries may be intensified and rigidified.

Suicide. As discussed in Chapter 4, suicide is generally considered the most difficult type of death to accept. For children, the suicide of a parent or sibling not only presents immediate difficulties, but is thought by many observers to result in life-long vulnerability to mental health problems.

Pynoos and his colleagues[112,113] have reported on children's immediate reactions to witnessing suicide attempts and homicides. Regardless of what has been told to children, it is clear that they know fundamentally what has transpired and that they promptly institute defensive adaptive measures, including denial in fantasy and reworking of the facts in accord with stage-related concerns.

In a partially controlled study, Shepherd and Barraclough[131] followed 36 children (ages 2–17 years) five to seven years after the suicide of a parent and found greater psychiatric morbidity among the suicide survivors than among a comparison group. They also noted that prebereavement home life was abnormal for these subjects because of the stresses of living with a parent who was mentally ill. In fact, for a few of the children, the suicide was experienced as a relief from a previously "insupportable situation."

In their assessment of 45 disturbed children four years after the suicide of one parent, Cain and Fast[34] found a broad range of psychological symptoms, including psychosomatic disorders, obesity, running away, delinquency, fetishism, lack of bowel control, character problems, and neurosis. Compared with other childhood bereavement cases, there was a much higher incidence of psychosis (24 percent versus 9 percent). Common disturbed reactions among this group included a very intense sense of guilt and distortions of communication. As they often receive the message that they should not know or tell about the suicide, these children frequently are in conflict about learning and knowing in general, with resultant learning disabilities, speech inhibitions, and reality sense disturbances.

Parental suicide also appears to be linked with serious long-term negative consequences. For example, Dorpat,[43] examining the case material of 17 adult psychiatric patients who were seen an average of 16 years after the parent's death, found guilt over the suicide, depression, morbid preoccupation with suicide, self-destructive behavior, absence of grief, and arrests of certain aspects of ego, superego, and libidinal development.

Clinical data amassed by Cain and Fast[35] on adolescents and adults whose parents committed suicide when they were children suggest that some ongoing ideas and processes in these bereaved children can cause difficulty, including direct identification with the parent in his suicidal act, conviction that they too will die by suicide, and fear of their own suicidal impulses. According to the data of Blachley et al.[19] and Farberow and Simon,[47] there is in fact a far higher than chance incidence of prior suicide in the family backgrounds of individuals who later commit suicide.

Summary of Risk Factors in Childhood Bereavement

A review of the clinical and research data suggests that the following factors increase the risk of psychological morbidity following the death of a parent or sibling during childhood years:

- loss occurs at an age below 5 years or during early adolescence,
- loss of mother for girls below age 11 and loss of father for adolescent boys,
- psychological difficulties in the child preceding the death (the more severe the preexisting pathology, the greater the postbereavement risk),
- conflictual relationship with the deceased preceding the death,
- psychologically vulnerable surviving parent who is excessively dependent on the child,
- lack of adequate family or community supports or parent who cannot make use of available support system,

- unstable, inconsistent environment, including multiple shifts in caretakers and disruption of familiar routines (transfer to an institutional setting would be an extreme example),
- experience of parental remarriage if there is a negative relationship between the child and the parent replacement figure,
- lack of prior knowledge about death,
- unanticipated death, and
- experience of parent or sibling suicide or homicide.

INTERVENTION STRATEGIES

Adults often become uneasy when called upon to deal with children on topics of conception, birth, or death. Clinical and research findings suggest that parents often fail to inform their children when a loved one dies, or they do so in an inappropriate or upsetting way, thereby increasing the likelihood of further distressing youngsters who are incapable of seeking out the truth for themselves. Although there are no systematic studies assessing the safety and efficacy of different intervention strategies, psychological theory and clinical experience do suggest an approach.

Anticipating Parental Death

When a parent is terminally ill, Erna Furman[53] recommends maintenance of personal contact between child and parent for as long as the parent is not drastically altered in appearance or in the ability to communicate with feeling. She notes that visits should not become an unbearable burden nor should they force the child to discontinue other activities. Hilgard et al.[70] note that a dying parent can convey to a child an acceptance of death that helps the child to accept its finality.

There is some research evidence that short-term professional ''preventive therapy'' with children of fatally ill parents may also decrease the likelihood of subsequent pathology after a parent dies. In a controlled study of normal, randomly assigned children, ages 10–14, Rosenheim and Ichilov[123] found that brief treatment (10 to 12 weekly home visits) made a significant difference in terms of the anxiety level and social and scholastic adjustment of children who were anticipating parental death. Sessions focused on the child's perception of the parent's illness and his or her reactions to it, the factual life situation at home (present, past, and anticipated future), the child's feelings toward his parents, and his or her self-concept. An opportunity was provided for catharsis while therapists helped supply realistic perspectives about inner and outer realities (e.g., the resources available to the child in the face of loss).

Helping Parents to Help Their Children

The most important preventive intervention may be how parents and others deal with children who have been bereaved. In the interests of helping parents to provide their children with a supportive, understanding environment, this section offers some specific suggestions based on information in the literature and on the best judgment of the committee.

Providing optimal support to grieving children may be difficult, not only because the parents themselves are extremely upset, but also because they may be uncertain of what to expect from a child. Thus, it is important that parents learn about the grieving process in children so they will know what to expect and will not become alarmed about the differences between childhood and adult grieving. Knowing that the child may ask distressing questions, such as when will there be a new parent or sibling to replace the one who was lost, may eliminate surprise and hurt. Such questions do not indicate a shallow attachment to the deceased, but rather the manner in which young children typically respond to loss.

Children may confront strangers with news of the death to test reactions and gauge their own responses. They may play "funeral or "undertaker" games for a few days following the death of a family member in order to master the situation. Children may manifest a superficially milder reaction to the loss because of the strong defenses that protect them from becoming flooded with overwhelming emotions. As noted earlier, troubling emotions or behaviors emerging months or years after the death may be related to the bereavement, because children give up their attachment to the deceased much more slowly than adults usually do.[81] Preparing for and understanding such behaviors and coping responses can help avoid or modify reactions of shocked hurt or anger in parents that could intensify the child's feelings of confusion and guilt.

Providing concrete recollections of the deceased parent or sibling may also be helpful.[53] Photographs and clothing or other possessions of the deceased are meaningful to a child because they represent the deceased person as well as the child's own past relationship with that person.

Talking to Children About a Family Member's Death

Most authors agree that there is preventive value in educating children about death when they are young, long before death is likely to enter their lives in an emotionally threatening way. As Reed[118] points out, children begin asking questions about death at an early age. They are naturally curious about such phenomena and provide adults with opportunities to intervene.

Various educational tools have been suggested. Chaloner,[39] Erna Furman,[54] and Koocher[85] recommend using the death of a child's pet or other naturally occurring teaching moment to introduce the concept. Opportunities such as driving past a cemetery or coming across a dead animal while on a nature walk can also be used to provide awareness and understanding, especially that the deceased animal or person will never return. Moreover, it will provide the child with the reassurance that death is not a topic to be avoided with adults. Other means to help children gain awareness about death include children's books (see Goldreich[60] for a list) and formal death education classes.[92]

When informing a child of a family member's death, a number of variables may be important, including who tells the child, the timing of the information, and the manner in which the child is informed.

In most cases, a family's existing belief system will determine what they do. However, families sometimes contact health care professionals to ask for advice. Professionals need to be cautious in making recommendations under these circumstances. Since there is wide cultural and family variation, it is important for the health care provider to draw upon his or her knowledge of that family and their culture, taking into consideration the family's own wishes and inclinations. The child's level of social, emotional, and cognitive development, the meaning of the event to the child and family, and the child's fantasies about the death should all be kept in mind when determining what is appropriate for a particular child to be told. When possible, decisions should be made within the context of a dialogue with the family.[138]

Use of religious explanations, in particular, is controversial. Some Western observers think that explanations about the deceased going to heaven may be upsetting to children who think and interpret things more concretely than adults.[66,84,116] Others, however, have remarked on the comfort that religious beliefs can provide following bereavement.[97] What is most suitable for a particular child will depend on the factors cited above; what is probably most important is that explanations remain consistent with the family's values and beliefs.

A few basic approaches have been found helpful across most families and cultures. For example, it is generally recommended that a child be told the truth, in simple terms he can understand.[39] ''Children always observe and sense situations which adults wish and believe they did not see. Invariably, they sense the strained and sinister, and if not helped to clarify what they think happened, the adults' silence may increase their fears in fantasy, rather than spare them sorrows.''[110] Telling a child that a parent or sibling is dead and will not be alive again, and assuring him that the deceased no longer feels anything and is no longer suffering are important elements of a discussion. Encouraging questions is often an effective way to elicit concerns or fears that adults would not have thought might be worrying the child.[27]

In the case of sudden death, the surviving parent can acknowledge a child's observations and clarify misperceptions or misinterpretations. Specific facts may be added as the child is able to integrate them.[53] As is true for adults, it is generally agreed that knowledge helps provide a sense of security. In disturbing situations or crises, feelings of helplessness increase with ignorance of the facts.

It is relieving for bereaved children to be told that they will not succumb to the same fate as the deceased, and that they will continue to be cared for. Particularly when dealing with young children, it can be important to reassure a child that the family will remain together and that he or she will be told step by step as each arrangement is planned.[53] It is also helpful for young children to gain an understanding of the difference between the self and the deceased. Telling them that neither they nor other surviving family members will die just because of the other death can help the children differentiate reality from fantasy.

Children's questions about death may reflect an unexpressed need for reassurance and emotional security rather than a desire for an intellectual explanation.[118] For example, it is usually a relief for a bereaved child to hear that he or she was not responsible for the death, if a parent has reason to believe that the child fantasizes culpability. Sensitivity to a child's intent[85] can help him verbalize anxiety, which can then be responded to with understanding. Behind questions about death may be fears that the child will be abandoned or stricken with illness. Under the age of seven, such concerns may be only indirectly communicated.

It may be helpful to ask children for a replay of what they have understood by saying something like, ''Now pretend that one of your friends asks you about this. What would you answer?'' By asking specific questions and letting the child reply, the adult can detect and correct misconceptions quickly.

It may be useful for parents to become aware of potential pitfalls that can emerge following bereavement. For example, parents' capacities to nurture their children may diminish after the death of a family member due to their own grief and loneliness. Because of their own needs during this time, parents may be inclined to turn to their children for emotional support. It may feel gratifying to a child to be able to help a distraught parent, but this responsibility may also be experienced as frightening and overwhelming. Feeling excessive responsibility for a parent can also impede subsequent establishment of autonomy and intimacy with others.

Missing the deceased spouse or child, a parent may look for or notice similarities between the deceased and a surviving child, and even comment on these similarities, implicitly suggesting that the child should function as a replacement for the person who died. The child's sense of personal worth and value may be compromised by this view of being a replacement for someone else, and such perceptions may result in unrealistic life plans.

Krell and Rabkin[87] have identified some family maneuvers that place surviving children at risk following sibling death: indirect or evasive communication about the death due to the parents' belief that it was preventable, and a tendency to accord surviving children special status by overprotecting and shielding them. Hagin and Corwin[67] warn that this need to treasure surviving children can stifle emotional development. Also, holding up the dead child as perfect can have the unintended effect of making the surviving one feel that he can never measure up or that he should have died instead.

Attending the Funeral

Parents frequently express uncertainty about whether children should attend funeral services, fearing that such participation might frighten or otherwise upset them. Most authors who deal with this subject recommend that children be allowed, but not forced, to participate in family mourning and funeral rites if they wish to do so. As with adults, participating in mourning rituals helps children to mark the death and cope with their feelings. Such participation may help children understand the finality of death and aid in dispelling fantasies.[66]

The parent can help prepare the child for the funeral service by explaining in advance how the room will look, where they will be sitting, and what they can expect to see and hear. Arranging to have a relative or close family friend sit with the child and be available to leave with him should the child wish to may be helpful.

It should be noted, however, that there is great diversity in funerals across cultures and some services might be more difficult for a child to handle than others. Erna Furman[53] has observed that even a young child can take in stride some aspects that might otherwise be upsetting as long as the parent(s) feel comfortable with the funeral service. She adds, however, that parents can modify customs to ease the experience for the child. For example, arrangements could be made to shorten the service or to have a closed casket. Children should be told in advance if the casket is to remain open, and may be given the opportunity to look at or touch the deceased one last time if they want. Observers agree that it is unwise to insist, however, that a child touch a corpse.

In general, by anticipating and addressing all the things a child might see, hear, or have concerns about regarding the funeral procedures, adults may be better prepared to discuss the event in an emotionally supportive manner. A cemetery, for example, may be explained as a pretty and quiet place where people can go whenever they want to be near the dead person's body and remember that individual.

Anniversary Reactions: A Normal Long-Term Consequence

As discussed in the preceding chapters on adults, not all long-term consequences of bereavement are pathologic. For example, in a pilot study of bereaved former psychiatric patients, Plotkin[111] found that reactions to birthdays, holidays, and anniversaries of the death were a normal and predictable part of the grieving process. She argues that such late-occurring manifestations of grief should not be confused with pathologic grief, and she advocates using such reactions as healthy opportunities to express feelings about the death.

Johnson and Rosenblatt[76] also distinguish between late-occurring "incomplete" or "pathological" grief and the grief that reemerges in children as a result of maturation and new experience. Sometimes anniversaries or life marker events provide occasions for the emergence of psychopathologic symptoms for the first time in previously well-adjusted youngsters; but more commonly, quite normal manifestations of grief will recur with such developmentally significant events as communion, graduation, pregnancy, or the return to a place an individual previously visited with the deceased parent or sibling. Such feelings may be associated with a conscious realization that the deceased is not present to share the event or they may take place without any understanding of why the distress has surfaced at that time. The most helpful intervention for this type of grief is supportive assurance that sadness under these circumstances is normal and common among those who have lost a significant person.

When to Seek Professional Help

As with adults, the distinction between normal and pathologic grieving in children is not always clear. Following a loss as profound as the death of a parent or sibling, some behaviors and reactions are to be expected that otherwise might be considered pathologic. In normal childhood grieving, it is not unusual to see clinical symptoms of emotional disturbance, some regression, denial, and an inability to function. Children may not report much distress, but their behavior may seem immature for their age.

As discussed in earlier chapters, factors such as intensity and duration are usually used to differentiate the normal from pathologic response, but the limits of these descriptors are difficult to establish. A few clinicians have attempted to delineate some bereavement reactions that signal a need for help. Bowlby's[27] warning signals regarding bereaved children include the presence of persistent anxieties (such as fears of further loss or fear that the self will die), hopes of reunion and a desire to die, persistent blame and guilt, patterns of overactivity with aggressive and destructive outbursts, compulsive care-giving and self-reliance, euphoria with depersonalization and identification symptoms, and accident proneness. Raphael[115] categorizes disturbed behaviors in these groups: suppressed or inhibited bereavement responses, distorted grief or mourning (e.g., grief characterized by extreme guilt or anger), and chronic grief, possibly manifested by acting out.

In discussions at one of the committee's site visits, Kliman added to this list the inability or unwillingness to speak of the deceased parent, exaggerated clinging to the surviving parent, and expression of only positive or only negative feelings about the deceased. A manifest absence of grief, strong resistance to forming new attachments, complete absorption in daydreaming resulting in a prolonged dysfunction in school, or new stealing or other illegal acts may also be a cry for help.[140]

Some clinicians (e.g., Kliman) who take the position that all children who lose a parent through death are ''at risk'' recommend at least some time-limited intervention in all cases, whether or not a child displays the behaviors cited. From this perspective, each child who loses a significant family member would be assessed periodically as a preventive measure.

It is important for parents to be aware of danger signals so that they can know if and when professional help should be sought. Educating parents about normal versus pathologic responses can help them make such decisions.

Conclusions About Interventions

Although there is little scientific evidence regarding the effect of intervention either prior or subsequent to bereavement during childhood, there is general agreement that promptness, honesty, and supportiveness help. Information should be geared to the child's emotional and intellectual level and ample opportunities provided for the child to ask questions about the death. Children need rituals in order to memorialize loved ones just as adults do, and should be allowed to participate in funeral or memorial services to the degree to which they feel comfortable.

Although both short- and long-term distress should be expected and are normal, some professional mental health intervention conceivably may be useful for all bereaved children, or at least when particular patterns of troublesome response become evident.

RECOMMENDATIONS FOR FUTURE RESEARCH

In order to achieve better understanding of the nature of the bereavement process and its potential impact, there is a need for methodologically sound studies in which representative samples of bereaved children are followed for several years and are compared with nonbereaved children. Following are some of the important questions that should be addressed:

• What are the signs and symptoms of pathologic versus normal grief following parental or sibling death?
• What conditions foster or inhibit adaptation?
• What are the preexisting or concurrent risk factors associated with poor outcomes, including major psychiatric disorder?
• How do identified risk factors hold up over the course of the first several years following bereavement?
• What is the relationship between the sex of the deceased parent and the age and sex of surviving children on the course of bereavement reactions?
• How do children who are in various stages of normal cognitive and personality development at the time of bereavement do in comparison with each other and how do they compare with nonbereaved children of the same developmental stage?
• How does early loss exert a detrimental impact on children?
• How do the effects of bereavement and the process of grieving differ for surviving parents and children?

Particular attention should be paid to the design of studies seeking to address questions such as these so that methodological shortcomings do not compromise the conclusions. Grieving children who are not in psychotherapy should be directly observed and assessed. Too much emphasis in the existing literature has been placed on retrospective analysis, memories and extrapolations from adulthood, on parental reports of children's reactions, and on observations of children in treatment who may or may not be representative of grieving children generally. Although clinical case studies will continue to provide useful, in-depth information, prospective, clinically sensitive, longitudinal studies of community samples are also needed in order to further current understanding and resolve controversy about the nature of grieving and the impact of loss on children.

Another series of potentially very important studies would involve the random assignment of bereaved children to a variety of different treatment or control groups to determine whether treatment facilitates adaptation to the extent that certain treatment approaches are indeed successful; other studies should identify the essential process or mechanisms by which children are helped. Identification of the most effective methods of preventive intervention for particular children or groups of children, and at what stage of life and what distance from the loss these interventions should take place, would add significantly to current knowledge.

In sum, it is time to move to modern standards of research in the area of childhood bereavement. Young people who have lost a parent or sibling through death need to be tracked to determine both short- and long-term consequences of bereavement and to identify subgroups most at risk for pathologic developments. Methods of intervention must be subjected to tests of efficacy to determine how best to help children, with new or modified techniques being particularly designed for the pathologically grieving child.

REFERENCES

1. Abrahams, M., and Whitlock, F. Childhood experiences and depression. *British Journal of Psychiatry* 115:883–888, 1969.
2. Alexander, I., and Adlerstein, A. Affective responses to the concept of death in a population of children and early adolescents. *Journal of Genetic Psychology* 93:167–177, 1958.
3. Altschul, S. Denial and ego arrest. *Journal of the American Psychoanalytic Association* 16:301–318, 1968.
4. Altschul, S., and Beiser, H. The effect of parent loss by death in early childhood on the function of parenting. In: *Parenthood: A Psychodynamic Perspective* (Cohen, R.S., Cohler, B.J., and Weissman, S.H., eds.). New York: Guilford Press, 1984.
5. Anthony, S. *The Child's Discovery of Death.* London: Routledge and Kegan Paul, 1940.
6. Archibald, H., Bell, D., Miller, C., and Tuddenham, R. Bereavement in childhood and adult psychiatric disturbance. *Psychosomatic Medicine* 4:343–351, 1962.
7. Arthur, B., and Kemme, M.L. Bereavement in childhood. *Journal of Child Psychology and Psychiatry* 5:37–49, 1964.

8. Balk, D. Effects of sibling death on teenagers. *Journal of School Health* 53:14–18, 1983.

9. Barry, H. Significance of maternal bereavement before the age of eight in psychiatric patients. *Archives of Neurology and Psychiatry* 62:630–637, 1949.

10. Barry, H., and Lindemann, E. Critical ages for maternal bereavement in psychoneuroses. *Psychosomatic Medicine* 22:166–181, 1960.

11. Beck, A.T., Seshi, B., and Tuthill, R. Childhood bereavement and adult depression. *Archives of General Psychiatry* 9:295–302, 1963.

12. Bendiksen, R., and Fulton, R. Death and the child. In: *Death and Identity* (Fulton, R., ed.). Baltimore: Charles Press, 1976.

13. Birtchnell, J. The possible consequences of early parent death. *British Journal of Medical Psychology* 42:1–12, 1969.

14. Birtchnell, J. Early parent death and mental illness. *British Journal of Psychiatry* 116:281–288, 1970.

15. Birtchnell, J. Depression in relation to early and recent parent death. *British Journal of Psychiatry* 116:299–306, 1970.

16. Birtchnell, J. The relationship between attempted suicide, depression, and parent death. *British Journal of Psychiatry* 116:307–313, 1970.

17. Birtchnell, J. Early parent death and psychiatric diagnosis. *Social Psychiatry* 7:202–210, 1972.

18. Birtchnell, J. Women whose mothers died in childhood: an outcome study. *Psychological Medicine* 10:699–713, 1980.

19. Blachley, P., Wisker, W., and Roduner, G. Suicide by physicians. *Bulletin of Suicidology*, December: 1–18, 1968.

20. Black, D. What happens to bereaved children? *Proceedings, Royal Society of Medicine* 69:842–844, 1974.

21. Black, D. The bereaved child. *Journal of Child Psychology and Psychiatry* 19:287–292, 1978.

22. Blinder, B. Sibling death in childhood. *Child Psychiatry and Human Development* 2:169–175, 1972.

23. Bluebond-Langer, M. *The Private Worlds of Dying Children.* Princeton, NJ: Princeton University Press, 1978.

24. Bowlby, J. Grief and mourning in infancy and early childhood. *Psychoanalytic Study of the Child* 15:9–52, 1960.

25. Bowlby, J. Childhood mourning and its implications for psychiatry. *American Journal of Psychiatry* 118:481–498, 1961.

26. Bowlby, J. Pathological mourning and childhood mourning. *Journal of the American Psychoanalytic Association* 11:500–541, 1963.

27. Bowlby, J. *Attachment and Loss. Vol. III: Loss.* New York: Basic Books, 1980.

28. Brown, D. Sex-role development in a changing culture. *Psychological Bulletin* 54:232–242, 1958.

29. Brown, F. Depression and childhood bereavement. *Journal of Mental Science* 107:754–777, 1961.

30. Brown, F. Childhood bereavement and subsequent psychiatric disorder. *British Journal of Psychiatry* 112:1035–1038, 1966.

31. Brown, G., Harris, L., and Copeland, J. Depression and loss. *British Journal of Psychiatry* 130:1–18, 1977.

32. Brown, R., and Epps, P. Childhood bereavement and subsequent crime. *British Journal of Psychiatry* 112:1043–1048, 1966.

33. Buxbaum, E. Pathological grief reactions in children. Paper presented at the 14th International Congress of Pediatrics, Buenos Aires, Argentina, October 1974.
34. Cain, A., and Fast, I. Children's disturbed reactions to parent suicide. *American Journal of Orthopsychiatry* 36:873–880, 1966.
35. Cain, A., and Fast, I. Children's disturbed reactions to parent suicide: distortions of guilt, communication, and identification. In: *Survivors of Suicide* (Cain, A., ed.). Springfield, Ill.: Charles C Thomas, 1972.
36. Cain, A., Fast, I., and Erickson, M. Children's disturbed reactions to the death of a sibling. *American Journal of Orthopsychiatry* 34:741–752, 1964.
37. Call, J., and Wolfenstein, M. Effects on adults of object loss in the first five years. *Journal of the American Psychoanalytic Association* 24:659–668, 1976.
38. Caplan, M., and Douglas, V. Incidence of parental loss in children with depressed mood. *Journal of Child Psychology and Psychiatry* 10:225–232, 1969.
39. Chaloner, L. How to answer questions children ask about death. *Parent's Magazine*, November: 99–102, 1962.
40. Darwin, C. A biographical sketch of an infant. *Mind* 2:285–294, 1877.
41. Dennehy, C. Childhood bereavement and psychiatric illness. *British Journal of Psychiatry* 212:1049–1069, 1966.
42. Deutsch, H. Absence of grief. *Psychoanalytic Quarterly* 6:12–22, 1937.
43. Dorpat, L. Psychological effects of parental suicide on surviving children. In: *Survivors of Suicide* (Cain, A., ed.). Springfield, Ill.: Charles C Thomas, 1972.
44. Dorpat, L., Ripley, H., and Jackson, J. Broken homes and attempted and completed suicides. *Archives of General Psychiatry* 12:213–217, 1965.
45. Elizur, E., and Kaffman, M. Children's bereavement reactions following death of the father: II. *Journal of the American Academy of Child Psychiatry* 21:474–480, 1982.
46. Elizur, E., and Kaffman, M. Factors influencing the severity of childhood bereavement reactions. *American Journal of Orthopsychiatry* 53:668–676, 1983.
47. Farberow, N., and Simon, M. Suicide in Los Angeles and Vienna: an intercultural report. *U.S. Public Health Reports* 84:389–403, 1969.
48. Fast, I., and Cain, A. The step-parent role: potential for disturbances in family functioning. *American Journal of Orthopsychiatry* 36:485–491, 1966.
49. Forrest, A., Fraser, R., and Priest, R. Environmental factors in depressive illness. *British Journal of Psychiatry* 111:243–253, 1965.
50. Freud, A. Discussion of Dr. John Bowlby's paper. *Psychoanalytic Study of the Child* 15:53–63, 1960.
51. Freud, S. *Totem and Taboo* (1913). *The Standard Edition of the Complete Psychological Works of Sigmund Freud*, Vol. 13 (Strachey, J., ed.). London: Hogarth Press and Institute for Psychoanalysis, 1955, pp. 1–161.
52. Freud, S. *Mourning and Melancholia* (1917). *The Standard Edition of the Complete Psychological Works of Sigmund Freud*, Vol. 14 (Strachey, J., ed.). London: Hogarth Press and Institute for Psychoanalysis, 1957, pp. 237–260.
53. Furman, E. *A Child's Parent Dies*. New Haven: Yale University Press, 1974.
54. Furman, E. *Children's Reactions to Object Loss: A Report of The American Psychoanalytic Association*. Washington, D.C.: APA, 1978.
55. Furman, R.A. Death of a six-year-old's mother during his analysis. *Psychoanalytic Study of the Child* 19:377–397, 1964.
56. Furman, R.A. A child's capacity for mourning. In: *The Child in His Family: The Impact of Disease and Death* (Anthony, E.J., and Koupernik, C., eds.). New York: Wiley, 1973.

57. Gay, M., and Tonge, W. The late effects of loss of parents in childhood. *British Journal of Psychiatry* 113:753–759, 1967.
58. Gibney, H. What death means to children. *Parent's Magazine*, March 1965.
59. Glick, I., Weiss, R., and Parkes, C. *The First Year of Bereavement*. New York: Wiley, 1974.
60. Goldreich, G. What is death? The answers in children's books. *Hastings Center Report* 7:10–15, 1977.
61. Granville-Grossman, K. Early bereavement and schizophrenia. *British Journal of Psychiatry* 112:1027–1034, 1966.
62. Greer, S. Parental loss and attempted suicide: a further report. *British Journal of Psychiatry* 112:465–470, 1966.
63. Gregory, I. Studies of parental deprivation in psychiatric patients. *American Journal of Psychiatry* 115:432–442, 1958.
64. Gregory, I. Introspective data following childhood loss of a parent. *Archives of General Psychiatry* 13:99–105, 1965.
65. Gregory, I. Retrospective data concerning childhood loss of a parent. *Archives of General Psychiatry* 15:354–361, 1966.
66. Grollman, E. *Explaining Death to Children*. Boston: Beacon Press, 1967.
67. Hagin, R., and Corwin, C. Bereaved children. *Journal of Clinical Child Psychology* 3:39–41, 1974.
68. Herioch, M., Batson, J., and Baum, J. Psychosocial factors in juvenile rheumatoid arthritis. *Arthritis and Rheumatism* 21:229–233, 1978.
69. Hilgard, J. Depressive and psychotic states as anniversaries of sibling death in childhood. *International Psychiatry Clinics* 6:197–211, 1969.
70. Hilgard, J., Newman, M., and Fisk, J. Strength of adult ego following childhood bereavement. *American Journal of Orthopsychiatry* 30:788–799, 1960.
71. Hill, O. The association of childhood bereavement with suicidal attempt in depressive illness. *British Journal of Psychiatry* 115:301–304, 1969.
72. Hill, O., and Price, J. Childhood bereavement and adult depression. *British Journal of Psychiatry* 113:743–751, 1967.
73. Hopkinson, G., and Reed, G. Bereavement in childhood and depressive psychosis. *British Journal of Psychiatry* 112:459–463, 1966.
74. Jacobson, E. Denial and repression. *Journal of the American Psychoanalytic Association* 5:61–92, 1957.
75. Jacobson, E. The return of the lost parent. In: *Drives, Affects, Behavior* (Schur, M., ed.). New York: International Universities Press, 1965.
76. Johnson, P., and Rosenblatt, P. Grief following childhood loss of a parent. *American Journal of Psychotherapy* 35:419–425, 1981.
77. Kaffman, M., and Elizur, E. Children's bereavement reactions following death of father: the early months of bereavement. *International Journal of Therapy* 1:203–229, 1979.
78. Kaffman, M., and Elizur, E. Bereavement responses of kibbutz and non-kibbutz children following the death of a father. *Journal of Child Psychology and Psychiatry* 24:435–442, 1983.
79. Kane, B. Children's concepts of death. *Journal of Genetic Psychology* 134:141–153, 1979.
80. Kliman, G. Death in the family. In: *Psychological Emergencies of Childhood* (Kliman, G., ed.). New York: Grune and Stratton, 1968.
81. Kliman, G. Facilitation of mourning during childhood. In: *Perspectives on Be-*

reavement (Gerber, I., Wiener, A., Kutscher, A., Battin, D., Arkin, A., and Goldberg, I., eds.). New York: Arno Press, 1979.

82. Kliman, G. Childhood mourning: a taboo within a taboo. In: *Perspectives on Bereavement* (Gerber, I., Wiener, A., Kutscher, A., Battin, D., Arkin, A., and Goldberg, I., eds.). New York: Arno Press, 1979.

83. Kliman, G. Death: some implications in child development and child analysis. *Advances in Thanatology* 4:43–50, 1980.

84. Koocher, G. Childhood, death, and cognitive development. *Developmental Psychology* 9:369–375, 1973.

85. Koocher, G. Why isn't the gerbil moving?: discussing death in the classroom. *Children Today* 4:18–36, 1975.

86. Koocher, G. Children's conceptions of death. In: *New Directions for Child Development: Children's Conceptions of Health, Illness, and Bodily Functions*, No. 14 (Bibare, R., and Walsh, M., eds.). San Francisco: Jossey-Bass, 1981.

87. Krell, R., and Rabkin, L. The effects of sibling death on the surviving child. *Family Process* 18:471–477, 1979.

88. Krupnick, J., and Horowitz, M. Stress response syndromes: recurrent themes. *Archives of General Psychiatry* 38:428–435, 1981.

89. LaGrand, L.E. Loss reactions of college students: a descriptive analysis. *Death Education* 5:235–248, 1981.

90. Leaverton, D., White, C., McCormick, C., Smith, P., and Sheikholislam, B. Parental loss antecedent to childhood diabetes mellitus. *Journal of the American Academy of Psychiatry* 19:678–689, 1980.

91. Levi, L., Fales, C., Stein, M., and Sharp, V. Separation and attempted suicide. *Archives of General Psychiatry* 15:158–164, 1966.

92. Leviton, D., and Forman, E. Death education for children and youth. *Journal of Clinical Child Psychology* 3:8–10, 1974.

93. Lifshitz, M. Long range effects of father's loss. *British Journal of Medical Psychology* 49:189–197, 1976.

94. Lloyd, C. Life events and depressive disorders reviewed: events of predisposing factors. *Archives of General Psychiatry* 37:529–535, 1980.

95. Lonetto, R. *Children's Conceptions of Death*. New York: Springer, 1980.

96. Markusen, E., and Fulton, R. Childhood bereavement and behavior disorders: a critical review. *Omega* 2:107–117, 1971.

97. Martinson, I., Moldow, D., and Henry, W. *Home Care for the Child with Cancer: Final Report of Grant No. CA19490*. Washington, D.C.: U.S. Department of Health and Human Services, National Cancer Institute, 1980.

98. McConville, B., Boag, L., and Purohit, A. Mourning processes in children of varying ages. *Canadian Psychiatric Association Journal* 15:253–255, 1970.

99. Menig-Peterson, C., and McCabe, A. Children talk about death. *Omega* 8:305–317, 1978.

100. Miller, J. Children's reactions to the death of a parent: a review of the psychoanalytic literature. *Journal of the American Psychoanalytic Association* 19:697–719, 1971.

101. Morillo, E., and Gardner, L. Activation of latent Grave's disease in children. *Clinical Pediatrics* 19:160–163, 1980.

102. Munro, A. Parental deprivation in depressive patients. *British Journal of Psychiatry* 112:443–457, 1966.

103. Munro, A., and Griffiths, A. Some psychiatric nonsequelae of childhood bereavement. *British Journal of Psychiatry* 115:305–311, 1969.

104. Nagy, M. The child's theories concerning death. *Journal of Genetic Psychology* 73:3–12, 1948.
105. Neubauer, P. The one-parent child and his Oedipal development. *Psychoanalytic Study of the Child* 15:286–309, 1960.
106. Norton, A. Incidence of neurosis related to maternal age and birth order. *British Journal of Social Medicine* 6:253–258, 1952.
107. Piaget, J. *The Child's Conception of the World*. London: Routledge and Kegan Paul, 1951.
108. Pitcher, E., and Prelinger, E. *Children Tell Stories: An Analysis of Fantasy*. New York: International Universities Press, 1963.
109. Pitt, F., Meyer, J., Brooks, M., and Winokur, G. Adult psychiatric illness assessed for childhood parental loss and psychiatric illness in family members. *American Journal of Psychiatry* 121(12):1–10, 1965.
110. Plank, E.N. *Working with Children in Hospitals*. Chicago: Year Book Medical Publishers, 1971.
111. Plotkin, D. Children's anniversary reactions following the death of a family member. *Canada's Mental Health*, June: 13–15, 1983.
112. Pynoos, R., and Eth, A. Witness to violence: the child interview. Presented at the Annual Meeting of the Academy of Child Psychiatry, Washington, D.C., October 1982.
113. Pynoos, R., Gilmore, K., and Shapiro, T. The response of children to parental suicidal acts. Presented at the Annual Meeting of the Academy of Child Psychiatry, San Francisco, October 1983.
114. Raphael, B. The young child and the death of a parent. In: *The Place of Attachment in Human Behavior*. (Parkes, C.M., and Stevenson-Hinde, J., eds.) New York: Basic Books, 1982.
115. Raphael, B. *The Anatomy of Bereavement*. New York: Basic Books, 1983.
116. Raphael, B., Field, J., and Kvelde, H. Childhood bereavement: a prospective study as a possible prelude to future preventive intervention. In: *Preventive Psychiatry in an Age of Transition* (Anthony, E.J., and Chiland, C., eds.). New York: Wiley, 1980.
117. Raphael, B., Singh, B., and Adler, R. Childhood loss and depression. Paper presented at the meeting of the Section of Child Psychiatry, Royal Australian and New Zealand College of Psychiatrists, Sydney, Australia, April 1980.
118. Reed, E. *Helping Children with the Mystery of Death*. New York: Abingdon Press, 1972.
119. Remus-Araico, J. Some aspects of early-orphaned adults analyses. *Psychoanalytic Quarterly* 34:316–318, 1965.
120. Rochlin, G. The loss complex. *Journal of the American Psychoanalytic Association* 7:299–316, 1959.
121. Rochlin, G. The dread of abandonment: a contribution to the etiology of the loss complex and to depression. *Psychoanalytic Study of the Child* 16:451–470, 1961.
122. Rochlin, G. *Griefs and Discontents*. Boston: Little, Brown, 1965.
123. Rosenheim, E., and Ichilov, Y. Short-term preventive therapy with children of fatally-ill parents. *Israeli Annals of Psychiatry and Related Disciplines* 17:67–73, 1979.
124. Rosenzweig, S., and Bray, D. Sibling deaths in the anamneses of schizophrenic patients. *Archives of Neurology and Psychiatry* 9:71–74, 1943.
125. Roy, A. Vulnerability factors and depression in women. *Psychiatry* 133:106–110, 1978.

126. Rutter, M. *Children of Sick Parents*. London: Oxford University Press, 1966.

127. Schmale, A., and Iker, H. Hopelessness as a predictor of cervical carcinoma. *Social Science and Medicine* 5:95–100, 1971.

128. Seligman, R., Gleser, G., and Rauh, J. The effect of earlier parental loss in adolescence. *Archives of General Psychiatry* 31:475–479, 1974.

129. Sethi, B. Relationship of separation to depression. *Archives of General Psychiatry* 10:486–496, 1964.

130. Shambaugh, B. A study of loss reactions in a 7 year old. *Psychoanalytic Study of the Child* 16:510–522, 1961.

131. Shepherd, D., and Barraclough, B. The aftermath of parental suicide for children. *British Journal of Psychiatry* 129:267–276, 1976.

132. Spinetta, J.J. The dying child's awareness of death: a review. *Psychological Bulletin* 81:256–260, 1974.

133. Spitz, R. *The First Year of Life: A Psychoanalytic Study of Normal and Deviant Development of Object Relations*. New York: International Universities Press, 1965.

134. Stone, M. Depression in borderline adolescents. *American Journal of Psychotherapy* 35:383–399, 1981.

135. Tallmer, M., Formanek, R., and Tallmer, J. Factors influencing children's concepts of death. *Journal of Clinical Child Psychology*. Summer: 17–19, 1974.

136. Tennant, C., Bebbington, P., and Hurry, J. Parental death in childhood and risk of adult depressive disorders: a review. *Psychological Medicine* 10:289–299, 1980.

137. Van Eerdewegh, M., Bieri, M. Parilla, R., and Clayton, P. The bereaved child. *British Journal of Psychiatry* 140:23–29, 1982.

138. Vaughan, V.C. Critical life events: sibling births, separations, and deaths in the family. In: *Developmental-Behavioral Pediatrics* (Levine, M., Carey, W., Crocker, A., and Gross, R., eds.). Philadelphia: W.B. Saunders, 1983.

139. Wahl, C. The fear of death. In: *The Meaning of Death* (Feifel, H., ed.). New York: McGraw Hill, 1959.

140. Watt, A. Helping children to mourn. Parts I and II. *Medical Insight* 15:29–62, 1971.

141. Wilson, I., Alltop, L., and Buffaloe, W. Parental bereavement in childhood: MMPI profiles in a depressed population. *British Journal of Psychiatry* 112:761–764, 1967.

142. Wolfenstein, M. How is mourning possible? *Psychoanalytic Study of the Child* 21:93–123, 1966.

143. Wolfenstein, M. Loss, rage, and repetition. *Psychoanalytic Study of the Child* 24:432–460, 1969.

*Toward a Biology
of Grieving*

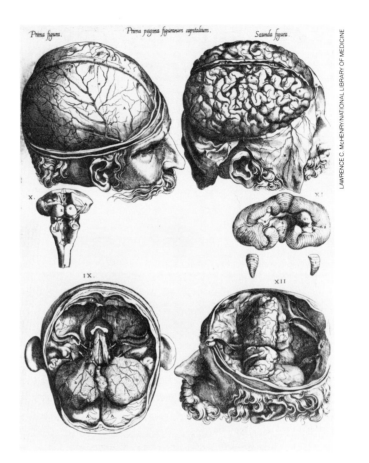

LAWRENCE C. McHENRY/NATIONAL LIBRARY OF MEDICINE

Throughout the ages, people have wondered about the relationship of the brain to emotions and to bodily functions. One of them was Andreas Vesalius, who in 1543 produced the first "modern" concept of the brain, shown above. Although it now is known that the brain regulates many physiologic functions that are commonly disrupted by the stress of bereavement, such as hormones, heart rhythm, and immune responses, the extent to which these disruptions may affect health has not yet been established.

CHAPTER 6

Toward a Biology of Grieving

This chapter reviews the available data on the biologic events that occur during the grieving process and proposes several kinds of pathways through which grief might increase vulnerability to physical illness. The degree to which this vulnerability occurs and results in illness is still open to question.

Research to date has shown that, like many other stressors, grief frequently leads to changes in the endocrine, immune, autonomic nervous, and cardiovascular systems; all of these are fundamentally influenced by brain function and neurotransmitters. However, the significance of these changes is not well understood. They may be primarily adaptive physiologic responses that in some persons become maladaptive and physiologically deleterious.

The notion of a normal adaptive response becoming harmful is not new, especially in the context of the immune system. For instance, there is evidence that chronic active hepatitis is a virally induced or drug-induced autoimmune disease. Craddock[16] suggested other ways

This chapter is based on material prepared by committee members Jules Hirsch, M.D., Myron Hofer, M.D., and Jimmie Holland, M.D., in collaboration with Fredric Solomon, M.D. It draws upon a background paper by Leonard Rosenblum, Ph.D., Director, Primate Behavior Laboratory, Downstate Medical Center, Brooklyn, New York. Additional assistance and background materials were provided by Elizabeth Guilfoyle, medical student, New York University School of Medicine.

the body's natural defenses may cause disease: the appropriate response to endotoxemia is fever and leukocytosis, but if the response is increased it may result in shock, consumption coagulopathy, tissue necrosis, hemorrhage, and death. The complexing of soluble antigen with antibody is a part of the immune response, but deposition of too many immune complexes can lead to severe vascular disease. Likewise, lymphatic hyperplasia is necessary to combat the Epstein-Barr virus, but in severe infectious mononucleosis it can cause serious tissue destruction.

The hypothesis that a normal adaptation to grief can become unregulated and lead to illness is considered further in the section of this chapter on a "psychoneuroimmunoendocrine system." This view is consistent with contemporary stress theory,[17] in which it is postulated that a stressor (x) produces certain transient biological or psychosocial reactions (y) that may (or may not) cumulatively lead to certain health consequences (z). Reactions and consequences may be modified by a number of factors, and the consequences may themselves activate other stressors. In simplified form, the stress model looks like this:

FIGURE 1

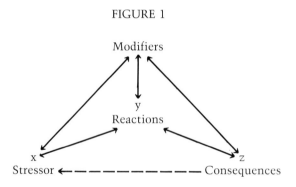

SOURCE: Adapted from Elliott and Eisdorfer.[17]

Epidemiologic studies linking the stress of bereavement with adverse consequences to physical and mental health have been reviewed in Chapter 2; these are x-z correlations, using this model. This chapter reviews the many studies of prompt biological reactions to the stress of bereavement (x-y) and presents conceptualizations and promising leads—but not confirming data—on the implications of these particular physiologic changes for enduring health consequences (x-y-z) in human beings.

ANIMAL MODELS

Finding out more about the involvement of complex biological systems in grief would be greatly facilitated if animal models were available. The history of medical investigation is testimony to the importance of animal research in understanding the pathophysiology of human disease.

Animal models rarely provide precise replicas of human conditions because of species differences. But nature, in evolution, has been conservative, and human beings share many physiological and psychological processes with other species. Thus, a number of the studies discussed in this chapter are based on research with monkeys, dogs, or rats. Social attachments, for example, are widely represented in mammals and in birds, particularly between the young and their social companions, parents, and siblings. Acute behavioral responses of infants to separation from their mothers are quite similar across species, including rat, guinea pig, cat, dog, monkey, and human being. And the few chronic biological responses to early separation that have been studied show striking similarities between monkeys and rats: a similar reduction in rapid eye movement (REM) sleep with insomnia, a lowering of cardiac rate, a thermoregulatory disturbance with decrease of core temperature, and a (very recently) demonstrated decrease in immune competence.[1,26,27,30,46,62,63]

What do these findings indicate about the biology of human grief? Because of the differences between immature and mature organisms, between separation and permanent loss, and between various mammalian species, they can only be suggestive. They confirm that the response to separation has deep evolutionary roots and some biological impact on systems controlling vital processes of sleeping, circulation, thermoregulation, and immune surveillance. These studies require constant innovation in developing methods to detect physiologic changes, methods that may one day be applicable to human beings.

Most important, animal studies provide new conceptual models for approaching an understanding of human bereavement. Examples are given in the section on social relationships as biological regulators and in Chapter 7. In an additional example, a single aspect of grief can be isolated and studied in terms of its biological substrate, as in the work of Weiss[83,84] on learned helplessness. The helplessness of human grief is surely different from the state induced in rats by inescapable shock. Yet an understanding of the simpler case should provide clues about what to measure and how to begin to study the much more complex interrelationship of affects and biological changes that occur in human grief.

BIOLOGIC STUDIES OF BEREAVED HUMAN BEINGS

There have been very few studies employing biologic variables in actively grieving people. The first study of this sort was Lindemann's,[48] in which he concentrated on what he termed the "syndrome" of acute grief. The data he collected from the relatives of victims of the "Coconut Grove" nightclub fire in Boston in the early 1940s, as amplified and extended in the work of Parkes[59] in London in the late 1960s and more recently in studies by Clayton[13] and others (e.g., Bartrop et al.[5]), give a picture of the behavioral and physiologic symptomatology of grief, as outlined in Table 1.

The symptoms described in Table 1 are present to a greater or lesser extent in most bereaved people for a period of weeks or months and in brief reactivation bouts, such as anniversaries, for years. They are the best evidence, thus far, that bereavement involves a physiologic disturbance. Unfortunately, symptoms such as these are not infallible indicators of physiologic change, nor are most of them very specific indicators of which organ or system may be involved. More specific physiologic data have been collected in animal studies of mother–infant separation; and these are summarized in Table 2 (page 165).

In 1944, Lindemann described having made respiratory tracings by polygraph of bereaved people and discovered an unusual pattern that he indicated would be described in detail in a subsequent paper. That paper was never written, and the idea dropped from sight until 1980 when

TABLE 1   Adult Grief Responses (Human Studies)

Behavior	Physiology
Acute episodes: waves of distress, lasting minutes	
Agitation	Tears
Crying	Sighing respiration
Aimless activity–inactivity	Muscular weakness
Preoccupation with image of deceased	
Chronic background disturbance: lasting weeks to months	
Social withdrawal	Decreased or increased body weight
Decreased concentration	Sleep disturbance
Decreased attention	Muscular weakness
Restlessness, anxiety	Cardiovascular changes
Decreased or increased food intake	Endocrine changes
Postures and facial expressions of sadness	Immunologic changes
Illusions or hallucinations	
Depressed mood	

Schiffman and his colleagues,[70] looking for a heritable respiratory defect in relatives of Sudden Infant Death Syndrome (SIDS) victims, found compromised ventilation in recently bereaved parents of children lost to SIDS, suggesting that the chemical regulation of their breathing might be defective. It is unclear from this study whether the alteration in the autonomic regulation of breathing is genetic or acquired, and if acquired whether it is related to the grief state. In order to understand this more fully, Shannon and his colleagues at the Massachusetts General Hospital in Boston are conducting a study to determine the relationship between grieving, depression, and autonomic regulation of breathing and cardiovascular function in recently bereaved parents of SIDS victims, parents whose child died from other causes, depressed patients, and nongrieving/nondepressed parents (D. Shannon, personal communication).

The pituitary–adrenocortical system was studied in the parents of children with leukemia, both before the child's death[86] and in the period of bereavement.[33,34] The researchers found that the operation of psychological defenses played a major role in modifying the extent of activation of this system during the threat of loss. A subject's level of cortisol (a hormone secreted by the adrenal cortex in response to adrenocorticotrophic hormone [ACTH] from the pituitary) could be predicted on the basis of an assessment of defense effectiveness. In follow-up visits six months and two years after the child's death, however, parents no longer maintained the same rank order of cortisol levels as they had prior to the death; cortisol levels varied directly with the extent of active grieving (at the six-month follow-up visit) as judged by an assessment procedure carried out without knowledge of the hormonal data. From these data, it might appear that grief is associated with adrenocortical activation, which continues as long as grief is an ongoing conscious psychological process. However, in those who had been actively grieving at six months and whose grief appeared to have run its course by the two-year return visit, cortisol levels remained high and unchanged. This pioneering study raised as many questions as it answered and gave an early indication of the complications that may arise in this kind of research.

Current psychoendocrine studies at Yale measure plasma levels of pituitary prolactin and growth hormone, as well as cortisol, in recently bereaved subjects during interviews in which the loss experiences were reviewed. Those whose growth hormone output increased during the interview tended to be subjects whose distress had been worsening in the two months between the loss and the interview. Measures of distress during the interview did not correlate in a simple way with pituitary hormone responses, but when one takes into account subtle aspects of the interview situation and the subject's coping mechanisms, interesting correlations begin to emerge.[35,39,41,52] The data suggest a specificity between certain psychological variables and certain hormones; a selective organization of neurohumoral responsiveness seems to be involved in the independent regulation of prolactin, growth hormone, and ACTH.

In the past few years, two studies have addressed the possibility that bereaved individuals have abnormal responses of their cell-mediated immune system. This research was stimulated by suggestions that malignancies may originate more readily among the bereaved. Although, as discussed in Chapter 2, the association is not firmly established on epidemiologic grounds, the clinical observations are frequently intriguing. Researchers in Australia[5] and the United States[71] have found that bereaved persons have an impaired function of T-lymphocytes, the agents of cell-mediated immunity. The lessened T-cell function was not a concomitant of changes in number of circulating T-cells, or of changes in adrenal or thyroid hormones in blood plasma. Neither of these studies was designed to tell whether the reduced T-cell function posed a clinically significant vulnerability of the subjects to disease. These studies require follow-ups that will include investigations of the mounting of specific immune responses. Such research would permit consideration of the relationship of immune function to bereavement and the possible relevance to clinical vulnerability.

PROMISING RESEARCH APPROACHES

Much less is known about the physiology of human bereavement than, for example, about the physiology of exercise or pregnancy. Thus, the most important statement that can be made about the biology of grieving relates to the need for research in this area.

There are at least four areas of knowledge that give useful clues about where to begin: the symptomatology of grief, the epidemiology of bereavement, recent findings in the biology of depression and anxiety disorders, and current knowledge about neuroregulatory mechanisms. In these areas the autonomic, physiologic, biochemical, and endocrinologic systems most likely to be affected by grief and the bereavement process can be identified—regardless of whether the response is viewed as a subcategory of stress response, as a withdrawal of psychobiological regulators, as an adaptive response to a natural event, or as the activation of a neurobiological substrate.

Changes in these systems over time should be studied to reveal the processes of recovery from bereavement as well as the form and duration of the acute disruption. How do children and aging people differ in grief from young and middle-aged adults? What are the special features of the biological responses that are relevant for adverse consequences? In all these areas, the psychological and behavioral responses will have to be related to the biological changes, because there is powerful interplay between these systems in determining the final outcome.

Clues from the Symptomatology of Bereavement

Research should take into account the natural division of symptoms into acute waves of distress, lasting minutes at a time, and chronic disturbance, which can last weeks and months. Acute waves of distress will be reasonably easy to study, because in many people they can be precipitated by an empathetic interviewer and their elicitation is often viewed as helpful to the subject. The symptoms of sighing respiration, dyspnea, substernal tightness, palpitation, weakness, and crying suggest that tests should be made of respiratory control and blood gases, autonomic function (particularly in the cardiovascular system), and energy metabolism (including the rapidly responding hormone systems of the pituitary, thyroid, and adrenal glands). These measures will be most useful if evidence about the subject's inner affective and cognitive state is collected simultaneously and integrated with the physiologic data, so that a comprehensive view of the psychobiological organization of the acute distress ''waves'' will be obtained.

This basic knowledge will be useful in planning clinical studies of patients at risk because of preexisting disease such as asthma, pulmonary emphysema, coronary heart disease, or congestive heart failure. These conditions are most likely to be affected by the physiologic changes of acute distress waves.

The chronic form of disturbance is characterized by symptoms involving a number of different biological systems that are regulated or powerfully influenced by the central nervous system through its autonomic, neuroendocrine, and musculoskeletal outflow channels. Many of the symptoms may be related to the neural regulation of the sleep-wake cycle and related biological rhythms, that is, to disturbance of chronobiological organization. The insomnia, chronic fatigue, restlessness, appetite disturbance, cognitive and perceptual disturbance, and even the illusions and depressive affect may be manifestations of altered integration or patterning of biological rhythms. If this is true, circadian rhythms of body temperature, physical activity, cardiac rate, urinary output, and other vital functions should be examined for evidence of free running (non-24-hour rhythmicity) or internal desynchronization (lack of consistent relationship between physiologic systems).

Clues from the Epidemiology of Bereavement

As documented in Chapter 2, a number of studies suggest that bereavement may enhance vulnerability to neoplastic disease, infection, cardiovascular disease, substance abuse, or depression.

The existence of hormone-sensitive cancers raises the possibility that alterations in hormonal milieu following bereavement may have clinical importance. Estrogen-dependent breast cancers and testosterone-dependent prostatic cancers are some of the best known examples of this sort. Studies are needed of ovarian, testicular, and adrenal hormonal regulation in bereavement, and of the hypothalamic-pituitary stimulating hormones that control these target glands. The potential involvement of the immune system in the recognition and suppression of neoplasia makes it an obvious subject of study during grief. Important interactions are already known among adrenal cortical hormones, autonomic nervous system neurotransmitters, and the immune system.

Susceptibility to bacterial and viral infections has been linked to bereavement in some studies (Chapter 2). This, too, suggests a need for a combined endocrine and immune system investigation. Resistance to infectious agents is known to depend critically on hormonal milieu and on humoral and cell-mediated immune mechanisms. The incidence of pneumonia as a terminal event in the bereaved might also indicate disturbed respiratory regulation during grieving.

The link between disease and bereavement is strongest for the cardiovascular system. Sudden cardiac death, cardiac arrhythmias, myocardial infarction, and congestive heart failure are the most frequently mentioned conditions of that system associated with grief.[72] This presents us with the clue that disturbances in autonomic cardiovascular regulation and in circulating catecholamines may be present in bereavement and may be exaggerated in patients with preexisting cardiovascular disease of the arteriosclerotic or hypertensive variety. Studies have shown that patients with congestive heart failure[12] and with essential hypertension[82] and arrhythmias[60,61] are particularly prone to exacerbation of their condition in response to threatened or actual loss of human relationships. Enough is known about the pathophysiology of these conditions to make quite specific hypotheses as to the probable autonomic and neurohumoral mechanisms involved. In addition, methods to test such hypotheses are currently available.

Vulnerability of the bereaved to substance abuse suggests that they are self-medicating themselves in an effort to alleviate their psychic pain and bodily discomfort. The possibility that sensory and pain thresholds are altered in the bereaved has not been systematically evaluated by modern methods, nor have any of the newer approaches to the study of endogenous, opiate-like peptides and their receptors been employed with this group. Alternatively, substance abuse may be related to depression, a possibility discussed in the next section.

Clues from the Endocrinology and Biochemistry of Depression and Anxiety States

Two well-delineated mental disorders, major depression and panic disorder, may share a common neurobiological substrate with the response to loss in the bereaved. This hypothesis bears testing by looking for the characteristic biochemical, physiologic, and pharmacologic responses of these two patient groups in adults following bereavement uncomplicated by diagnosed psychiatric illness.

Endocrine control during depressive illness and recovery still requires fuller study and documentation. Abnormalities of hypothalamic neurotransmitter systems controlling the pituitary output of ACTH, luteinizing hormone, and prolactin have been found in depressed patients; these findings may also reflect abnormalities in neurotransmitters in other areas of the brain that mediate mood and behavior. Are similar abnormalities found in the bereaved? How are these related to peptide levels in plasma, to immune function, to psychological status?

A characteristic change in sleep-wake state regulation (a shortened latency to the first REM period) has been found in many depressed patients, and reverts to normal with easing of the illness. Might a similar abnormality be found in disturbed sleep following bereavement?

Patients with panic disorder show two biological abnormalities that may have some relevance to the psychobiology of acute grief. They have abnormally wide fluctuations in certain autonomic variables (particularly skin resistance), especially in the prodromal period before a panic attack.[45] And they are extremely susceptible to precipitation of a panic attack by intravenous lactate infusion.[37] This susceptibility appears to be blocked by the tricyclic antidepressant drug, imipramine. The waves of distress, a hallmark of acute grief, bear some resemblance to acute panic attacks; can they be precipitated by lactate infusion and are they heralded by similar patterns of autonomic instability?

The complexity of interactions between the psychologic and the physiologic has been illustrated in a study by Kraemer and McKinney.[42] They used drugs to alter the function of two neurotransmitters that have been implicated in the genesis of depression. With drug doses that failed to produce any detectable effects in juvenile monkeys while they were in their home-peer groups (thus obviating any spurious side effects), increases or decreases in behavior patterns of despair could be produced following peer separation. Thus, only when beset by the significant psychological stress imposed by loss of their peers were these animals responsive to the drug regimen. This complex interaction, in which events at the psychological level affect physiologic processes and where the physiology in turn alters psychological functioning, is a ubiquitous quality of primate psychobiology.

Two neurochemical changes have been found in rhesus monkey infants separated from their mothers and placed in isolation: increases in catecholamine-synthesizing enzymes and in hypothalamic levels of the neurotransmitter serotonin.[8] Suomi and his colleagues[77] subsequently studied rhesus infants raised in peer groups without their mothers until 90 days and then subjected to repetitive peer separations; the tricyclic antidepressant, imipramine, decreased excessive self-clasping and prevented reduction in play behavior characteristically found after such experiences. However, social contact also was reduced and locomotor behavior increased by the drug. Although neurochemical changes clearly occur in infant monkeys separated from social companions, the neurochemical basis for the behavioral changes and the mechanism of their modification by psychoactive drugs are not yet clear.

Clues from Current Knowledge of Neuroregulatory Mechanisms

The neuroregulatory pathways that are known to mediate the conversion of life experiences into changes of bodily function provide many insights into the biology of grief. Whether some or all of these actually are involved in human grief is an empirical question that has received little study. Research on stress physiology has identified many neural and endocrine control systems that are at least a good place to begin investigation. These involve the autonomic neural system, endocrine events, and immune changes related to endocrine and direct neural influences.[17]

Autonomic Neural Effects. Since the time of W. B. Cannon,[9] it has been known that emotional states of rage and fear affect such biological functions as blood flow and cardiac rate by increasing the activity in widely distributed nerve fibers called the autonomic nervous system. This system comprises two main divisions, distinguished by anatomic features, range of distribution, and characteristic neurotransmitter types into sympathetic and parasympathetic divisions. These systems are both afferent and efferent and serve to control and coordinate vital functions of digestion, metabolism, circulation, and respiration. In addition to maintaining what Cannon[10] termed "homeostasis," the autonomic system mobilizes the resources of the body in preparation for "fight or flight."

Autonomic nervous system function has been found to be altered in a variety of ways during an organism's responses to exercise, sex, mental arithmetic, and relaxation and meditation states. Although there have not as yet been any specific and systematic studies of autonomic neural physiology during grief, a number of studies have found autonomic changes to be associated with themes and events associated with rejection, abandonment, and loss. No clear-cut pattern has emerged, however, and the situations and affects were quite disparate.

Patterns of physiologic response following loss have been studied in the biotelemetry research of Reite and his colleagues.[62,63] Using implanted devices to record a number of measures simultaneously in free moving monkeys, they studied the response of pigtail macaques to infant-mother separation. These data show that after initial increases in heart rate and body temperature in the first day after the loss, sharp drops in both measures occurred during the first night, and levels did not return to normal for the next several days. Disturbances in sleep, particularly in REM sleep, emerged in the first evening and disruption of normal sleep patterns continued throughout the 10-day study. Thus, the period of heightened heart rate and temperature roughly coincided with the protest behavior that was observed, while the sleep disturbance and decrease in the levels of these parameters approximated the subsequent despair phase of the response.

One example will illustrate how knowledge of autonomic nervous system physiology could help researchers understand the biology of bereavement. The excess mortality found in several epidemiologic studies during the first six months after bereavement is predominantly caused by cardiovascular events. And studies by Engel[18] and Reich[60,61] have described a number of episodes of sudden death proved or presumed to be due to ventricular fibrillation that occurred in the setting of loss and grief. How could grief stop a heart?

Working with dogs, Lown and his associates[49] have identified a phase during the electrical events of cardiac contraction, lasting only microseconds, when the heart is particularly vulnerable to developing multiple beats and even ventricular fibrillation in response to a weak electrical current. Verrier,[80] working with Lown, then studied the threshold for this "ventricular vulnerable period" as it might be influenced by the emotional state of the experimental animal and by brief episodes of coronary narrowing and reperfusion (as might occur with coronary artery spasm). They discovered that unfamiliarity with the testing chamber and expectation of receiving mild punishment reduced the threshold by 41 percent. They were then able to analyze this effect in terms of the contribution of sympathetic and parasympathetic autonomic influences. Using pharmacologic blocking agents, measurement of plasma norepinephrine and epinephrine, and surgical excision of the stellate ganglia, they found that the reduced threshold was the result of increased sympathetic influences—both along neural pathways and through increased circulating levels of norepinephrine and epinephrine.

These experimental findings do not bear directly on the question of how grief may contribute to cardiac arrhythmias, for they involved a different emotional setting and a different species. But they do suggest how growing knowledge about autonomic mechanisms may help direct the search for biological mechanisms in grief that may predispose individuals to health risks.

Endocrine Events. Psychological events cause many changes in the internal hormonal milieu, principally via the hypothalamic-pituitary axis. The response of the hypothalamic-pituitary-adrenocortical axis to stress has been well documented. Increased urinary and plasma levels of 17-hydroxycorticosteroids (17-OHCS) have been demonstrated in response to movies of emotionally charged material,[21] the stress of army basic training,[66] test-taking, aircraft flight, preoperative period novel situations,[22] hospital admission,[53] athletic events,[78] and other stressful situations.[51]

Secretion of other hormones also is altered by stressful situations. Testosterone decreases during stress.[43] Sowers and colleagues[74] found that physical and psychological stress related to diagnostic procedures and surgery was associated with decreased thyrotropin and thyroxine and with increased prolactin, growth hormone, cortisol, and luteinizing hormone, with no evident effect on follicle stimulating hormone. Stress increases prolactin in the morning when the level is low, and suppresses it in the afternoon when levels are high.[23] Mason[51] found that in monkeys performing a learned avoidance task, there was an increase in catabolic hormones and growth hormone and a decrease in anabolic hormones.

Different emotional responses to stress are reflected in hormonal patterns. Von Euler et al.[21] measured urinary catecholamines in young men shown films of murders, fights, tortures, executions, and cruelty to animals and found that those who were the most emotionally distressed by the films had the most significant endocrine reaction. Psychiatric interviews, field observations, and measurements of 17-OHCS excretion in army recruits showed that low excretors had better defense mechanisms and that high excretors were less successful in dealing with the stress of basic training.[66]

Animal studies have shown that stress, especially uncontrollable or inescapable shock, causes many changes in norepinephrine, epinephrine, and dopamine concentrations in peripheral blood and in different parts of the brainstem, hypothalamus, and limbic system.[68] Although the link between these neuroendocrine substances and the hypothalamic-pituitary axis has not been completely elucidated, a relationship certainly exists. The "helpless-hopeless syndrome" seen in animal studies of inescapable shock situations appears to have special effects on endocrine activity that may have some potential relevance for studies of human stress, including bereavement. In patients entering the psychiatric ward of a general hospital, most of whom had recently suffered a very difficult interpersonal event, Board et al.[7] found that those diagnosed as the most distressed had the highest levels of 17-OHCS and that they tended to be sad, hopeless, and "retarded" rather than agitated. In animal studies, investigators have found that stress-induced increases in plasma and urinary 17-OHCS are highest in situations in which long-established rules have changed and previously effective behavior no longer works to alleviate the stress.[21]

Research on the response of the endocrine system to disruption of attachments has been conducted by Levine and his associates in both the squirrel monkey and the rhesus macaque.[15,47] These studies generally have involved relatively brief and often repeated separation experiences, usually lasting for periods of hours or a few days. This work has shown quite consistently in both species that the sudden loss of the partner causes rapid and often dramatic increases in adrenal function with marked cortisol secretion evident even 30 minutes after separation. In general, the period of highest cortisol concentration is found during the first 24 hours following separation, with a decline thereafter. This period coincides with the initial phase of "protest" in response to loss. In squirrel monkeys, at least, both the mother and infant show these rapid cortisol increases; the mother's return to baseline levels is more rapid than her infant's.[14] The diminution of response after the first day notwithstanding, recent research by this group reveals that increased adrenal activity may be detected as long as two weeks after the separation.[85]

Further research[25,81] illustrates another significant fact that has emerged in physiologic research—the potential for discontinuity between the behavioral and physiologic measures of the loss response. Consider the following: infant monkeys can develop strong attachment bonds toward inanimate surrogate mothers. When infant squirrel monkeys are separated from their surrogate mothers, they show a very dramatic behavioral response of the "protest" variety. If the infant, at separation, is removed to a novel pen, it shows a large increase in blood cortisol—thus, the behavioral measures of stress used here, that is, screaming and agitated activity, are congruent with the physiologic measure. If the infant is left in its home cage and it is the surrogate that is removed, however, the infant still screeches, but its cortisol level remains undisturbed. In rhesus monkeys separated from their biological mothers, elevated cortisol coincided with the protest pattern of the first day, but cortisol levels returned to baseline after 24 hours while various aspects of the initial behavioral response continued for 11 days after separation.[15]

Immune Changes Related to Endocrine Events. It is well known that adrenal cortical activity has the effect of reducing circulating lymphocytes and increasing thymic involution, resulting in diminished immune function.[55,58] Riley and others have conjectured that an increase in adrenal cortical activity induced by stressful manipulation of experimental animals was causally related to an enhanced susceptibility to the growth of malignant tumors.[64,65] Thymic involution and fewer circulating lymphocytes implicate T-cell deficiency as a possible factor in tumor susceptibility; hence Riley and others have shown tumor enhancement. But Newberry[57] and others have found the opposite effect: that some stressors suppress tumor development, which suggests that timing, tumor model, and type of stressor all are factors to be considered.

Immune Changes Related to Psychological Events: Psychoneuroimmune Reactions. Palmblad[58] demonstrated that stress-induced immunosuppression occurs independent of endocrine function. Based on previous findings that the surgical stress of thoracotomy increased the number of lung metastases and tumor growth, Hattori and colleagues[24] administered immunopotentiators (streptococcal preparation and mitogens) to animals with cancer and reduced the number of metastases after thoracotomy, suggesting that tumor spread after surgery was due to immunosuppression.

Coe et al.[15] report that squirrel monkeys separated from their mothers for seven days showed immunosuppression as well as "a marked reduction in their antibody response" when challenged with a benign bacteriophage. However, in keeping with the importance of the environment in affecting response to loss, infants left in their home cage during separation showed less immunologic deficit than those moved to novel settings. In support of hypotheses regarding the role of genetic factors, parallel studies in the rhesus macaque have suggested rather different results. Despite their typically pronounced behavioral response to separation, but perhaps related to their lower adrenal response profiles, the rhesus failed to show immunosuppression after seven days of separation.

The development of virally induced neoplasms in animals and infectious diseases in human beings and animals may be enhanced or diminished depending on the type of stressful situation.[2-4,17] Stress has been shown to affect humoral and cell-mediated immunity and macrophages, with acute stress increasing the immune response and chronic stress decreasing it.[11,75] Stress such as sleep deprivation has caused initial immunosuppression, followed by enhancement of the immune response.[58]

In reviewing the positive and negative effects of stress on immune function in animals, Ader[3] concluded that "in general, high stress scale scores combined with a presumed unsuccessful coping response were correlated with depressed immunologic defenses." The impact of stress on disease depends on "the quality and quantity of stressful stimulation, the quality and quantity of immunogenic stimulation, the myriad host factors upon which stress and immunogenesis are superimposed, the temporal relationship between stress and immunologic stimulation, procedural factors such as the nature of the dependent variable and sampling procedures, and the interaction between any or all of the above."

Human beings also respond to stress with immunologic changes, which probably are determined by a combination of the same variables. Among psychiatry trainees facing their final exam for fellowships, those who were highly stressed psychologically displayed transient increases in T- and B-cells but decreases in plaque formation and response to mitogens prior to the exam. These values returned to normal later. Palmblad[58] cites studies of bereavement and other life changes that have shown depression of both humoral and cell-mediated immunity, correlating most highly with the amount of subjectively perceived stress. Schleifer and his colleagues[71] studied immune function in a group of 15 widowers and found that in vitro lymphocyte response to stimulation by common mitogens was significantly lower in the two months following the deaths of their wives, compared with prebereavement levels. The total numbers of B- and T-cells were unaltered, suggesting alterations in subpopulation ratios or defects in responsivity. After two months, some responses improved but others did not. Bartrop and others[5] also found that T-cell function was significantly decreased after bereavement, without a change in T-cell number. There was no change in B-cell function, nor in adrenocortical, adrenomedullary, or thyroid hormones.

Further evidence of psychoneurologic influence over the immune system is provided by the many studies of behavioral conditioning of immune function.[4] Ader[2] has written a historical account of conditioned immunobiologic responses, in which he notes that studies of such responses originally done in Russia early in this century were based on the belief that immunologic mechanisms were basically physiologic phenomena under complete control of the brain. Repeated experiments have shown that so-called "natural" defense mechanisms (cell-mediated immunity, phagocytosis, etc.) were readily conditionable, with less evidence being provided for conditionability of humoral immunity. Ader points out the variability of results, depending on the antigen used, the conditioned stimulus, and other factors, and states that it is too early to determine the mechanism by which conditioned immunosuppression occurs. There is also evidence that immunosuppression can be hypnotically induced in human beings.[6,73,75]

These findings indicate that immune systems are influenced directly by the central nervous system as well as by hormonal factors. The precise mechanisms are as yet unclear, but it appears that stress of many kinds affects both the endocrine and immune systems and that grieving, considered as a type of stress, would be expected to do so as well.

A cautionary note about interpreting measurements of immune function must be added, however, along with an argument for clinically relevant research involving human subjects. Assessment of T-cell or B-cell functions in vitro is of uncertain meaning in regard to actual vulnerability to infection. When these measures are done in a clinical setting, extreme values generally do indicate immune incompetence. Further evidence is required to demonstrate that the association of grieving with lesser immune changes actually bears a relationship to health.

Studies of bereavement and immune function have primarily investigated mitogen-induced lymphocyte stimulation, which is an in vitro correlate of immunity and provides a general measure of the lymphocyte's ability to synthesize deoxyribonucleic acid and ultimately divide.

Mitogen activation is a useful probe, but it does not involve processes associated with the induction of an immune response. The ability to mount an immune response to an antigen is a primary and specific function of the immune system requiring both antigen recognition and effector processes. One approach, which has yet to be applied systematically, is the direct measure of immune functions in human beings in vivo. For example, by skin testing two agents to which nearly everyone is sensitive ("allergic"), such as candida or trichophyton, it seems possible to establish the nature and intensity of the skin response as a function of psychological state, changing over time. Alterations in measurements of antibodies to cytomegalovirus or herpes virus might also be considered. Another potentially helpful advance would be development of reliable techniques for assessing the incidence of minor cutaneous infections, head colds, and other infections during the grieving process. There are not only urgent needs but also promising opportunities for the direct study of the clinically relevant biology of grieving, including immunity, in the human being.

GRIEF AS AN ADAPTATION IN A "PSYCHONEUROIMMUNOENDOCRINE SYSTEM"

There are abundant data on the effect of psychological events on the endocrine and immune systems and a growing body of information on the endocrine-immune interaction. Probably these interactions are not a one-way street. Thus, a "psychoneuroimmunoendocrine system" can be envisioned. Grief may be viewed as a series of events or reactions in an activated "psychoneuroimmunoendocrine" system that may come to a favorable—or at least neutral—outcome for health or to less favorable and maladaptive consequences.

As shown in Figure 2, the system in simplified form is composed of elements that fluctuate in terms of blood level or activity level. Implicit in the diagram is the existence of effector arms linking each system to another, and also feedback arms. The description in previous sections has already dealt extensively with many of the effectors. There are possibilities for connections with other mechanisms and systems.

This system is hypothesized to be a basic, coordinated mechanism for the response of the organism to stress or arousal and to more chronic events such as loss and bereavement. The activated hypothalamus secretes corticotropin releasing factor, which triggers release of a large peptide synthesized in the pituitary. This peptide, pro-opio-melano-cortin (POMC) contains ACTH, β-endorphin, and other peptides with

FIGURE 2   The Psychoneuroimmunoendocrine System.

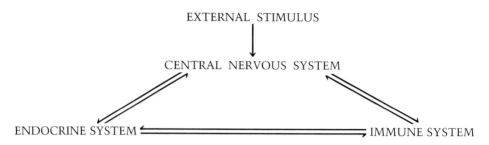

less well understood functions. Some of these peptides or some smaller peptides derived from them are believed to play a role in affective and cognitive function.

There is the possibility that the secretion of one or more products of POMC leads to the activation of various portions of a psychoneuroimmunoendocrine system with separate and important functions. Thus, the effect of adrenal stimulation may be of consequence in the metabolic "preparation" for threat of injury. The catabolic state induced by adrenal activation may provide the organism with an important substrate for energy metabolism. The simultaneous secretion of substances that suppress immune function may serve as a protection by transiently halting the immune response to a flood of antigens appearing from endogenous (proteolysis) or exogenous (injury) effects. The presence of β-endorphin and other brain-related peptides may provide the transient analgesic or even mental alertness required to focus on the external threat and deal with it in the most appropriate way possible.

This integrated system may also be utilized in dealing with chronic arousal such as grief. In this circumstance, the presence of neurohormones that may assist in denial and may therefore permit the metering of recognition of external events in a slow and staged way may be called upon with each new flood of arousing stimuli. The immune or other effects of the system may become increasingly "maladaptive" in the chronic situation. The adverse biological consequences of continued, "inappropriate" need for activation of the system are evident. Perhaps certain genetic characteristics, the use of culturally learned practices, the intervention of key figures in the social network, or other such factors can reduce a person's "need" to utilize this system in the solution of the problem of grief.

The approach outlined above has the merit of suggesting how immunosuppression, for example, might come about as a maladaptive use of a system, functioning on behalf of the need for unusually prolonged

or excessive autopalliation in the face of grief that is particularly difficult to resolve. Such a unified approach, which ties together psychological, endocrine, and immune events, is most attractive but will require
validation by much clinical, cross-disciplinary, long-term observation.

CONCEPTUAL FRAMEWORKS

In the absence of good data, theories abound. And theoretical positions determine what questions are asked and what data are collected as
well as how studies are interpreted. Thus, it is important to have some
insight into the main theoretical outlooks with which clinicians and
investigators approach the subject of the biological nature of grief. The
remainder of this chapter summarizes three current theoretical frameworks. It should be noted that they are not mutually exclusive and may
even be integrated eventually as data are obtained.

Bereavement as a Stressor

As mentioned previously, the current information available on stress
and health has been summarized in an Institute of Medicine report.[17]
The physiologic responses to a range of external events viewed as stressful have identifiable effects on biological systems. The stress imposed
on the bereaved person derives from the internal disequilibrium created
both by loss and the attempt to regain homeostasis and by the external
disruption of the environment following loss of someone close. Grief
could be considered a reaction to stress that is unusual in at least two
respects—its chronicity (the loss of the loved object is forever) and the
absence of an effective repertoire of behaviors to undo the stressor (the
love object cannot be brought back without hallucinations or a denial of
reality).

Rose and his colleagues[66] pointed out that successful mechanisms for
managing stress are not always equivalent to adaptive coping mechanisms. In bereavement, the common immediate response to loss is denial. As discussed in Chapters 3 and 5, this response is not adaptive over
time, but it allows the bereaved to function immediately after the loss.
The longer-term goal is to recognize and accept the loss and to return to
normal functioning. The active, goal-directed behavior so commonly
used successfully in adapting to other stressful situations is useless.

The central task for the bereaved, therefore, is to reconcile themselves to a situation that cannot be changed and over which they have
no control. Studies on both human beings and animals indicate that the
sense of control is an important variable in the psychological and physi-

ologic consequences of stress. Uncontrollable shock in animals has been demonstrated to be more effective than controllable shock in the promotion of gastric ulcerations,[83] immunosuppression,[55] tumor growth,[36,74] and a depression-like syndrome.[84] In animals given uncontrollable shock, Weiss et al.[84] observed similar behavior to the criteria for major depression as defined in the American Psychiatric Association's *Diagnostic and Statistical Manual*. Neuroendocrine changes were also correlated with both. In observing the development of gastric ulceration in rats subjected to inescapable shock, Engel[19] proposed that

> to be without the information and/or the psychological behavioral resources to cope effectively with a particular life circumstance appears to be a highly significant variable. Under such conditions, the organism typically alternates between activity and inactivity, the first reflecting efforts to maintain or reestablish control, the second waiting or giving up. If its efforts succeed, or if circumstances change soon enough, illness may be averted. But the longer such cycles of struggling and inactivity go on, the greater the risk of morbidity. Several human studies indicate that it is the *subjective experience*, rather than the external situation, which is the best predictor of a person's reaction, be it emotional or physical.

There is physiologic evidence indicating that responses to the stresses of bereavement are not the same for all people and that individual responses are situation-specific. In comparing psychological and endocrinologic data on parents before and after loss of their children, Hofer et al.[33] emphasized that the "chronic stress mean" of a person anticipating loss applied only to that situation and could not be applied to other stressful experiences. Schleifer et al.[71] arrived at the same conclusion in studying lymphocyte activity before and after death of a spouse. Mason[51] has shown that hormonal response patterns vary, depending on the stimulus. He described several situations of "stress" (such as acute avoidance, sleep deprivation, and fasting) in which the patterns of cortisol, norepinephrine, and epinephrine are different.

Kuhn and his colleagues[44] also observed different physiologic responses, as measured by ornithine decarboxylase activity, in response to maternal separation and other types of stress in rats. Both Engel[19] and Ader and Cohen[4] noted that the relationship between "stress" and disease in animals depended on both the type of stress and the nature of the disease. Thus, it cannot be assumed that because one physiologic pattern is present in response to one type of stress, it is the prototype for all stress responses. The use of inescapable or uncontrollable punishment in animal studies appears to result in a type of stress similar to the hopelessness-helplessness syndrome described by Engel and Schmale.[20] These studies may be helpful in providing a conceptual framework from which to investigate the biology of grieving, in particular the response to unavoidable stress.

Social Relationships as Biological Regulators

Disruption of Biological Rhythms.   As described earlier in this chapter and in several previous chapters, people typically have a number of symptomatic responses to bereavement. These include physiologic, behavioral, cognitive, and perceptual disturbances as well as a disorganization of ego functioning. Although the links between all these changes are not well understood, it has been hypothesized that social relationships may be an important regulator of these various responses.

Reviewing animal studies and some human studies, Hofer[32] summarized the behavioral and physiologic components of the infant separation response and called attention to the similarities between it and the human adult response to bereavement (Table 2).

In studies on infant rats, there is a clear difference between the acute and chronic phases of the separation response; the phenomena of the slow phase remain even when the acute phase is prevented.[27-31,76] What

TABLE 2   Infant Separation Responses (Animal Studies)

Phase	Behavior	Physiology
Acute		
"Protest" phase lasting minutes or hours	Agitation Vocalization Searching–inactivity	Increased heart rate Increased cortisol Increased catecholamines
Chronic		

Slow developing "despair" phase lasting hours or days	Decreased social interaction, decreased play
	Mouthing, rocking
	Hypo- or hyper-responsiveness
	Decreased or increased food intake
	Postures and facial expressions of sadness
		Decreased body weight
		Sleep disturbance
		Decreased rapid eye movement
		Increased arousals
		Metabolic:
		  decreased core temperature
		  decreased oxygen consumption
		Cardiovascular:
		  decreased cardiac rate
		  decreased resistance
		  increased ectopic beats
		Endocrine:
		  decreased growth hormone
		Immune:
		  decreased T-cell activity

Hofer has suggested is that the slow phase response is actually the sum of many responses to the loss of many separate aspects of the mother–infant interaction. He found that preservation of a single aspect of the mother–infant relationship could prevent a single physiologic change, without affecting any other of the physiologic responses to separation. From analytic studies on infant rats separated from their mothers, a number of "hidden regulators" have been discovered within the mother–infant relationship, which act to maintain the homeostasis of the developing child.

There is evidence of biologically powerful sensorimotor regulators even within adult social relationships, such as the menstrual synchrony that develops in young women who live together,[54] and bereavement may constitute a loss of these regulators as well as an emotional loss. The data (Table 3) from studies of sensory deprivation, jet lag, and work shift changes can be used to emphasize the importance of unseen regulators in human behavior and to illustrate the similarities in the physiologic responses to these varied disturbances of internal equilibrium.

There is an obvious similarity between these responses and the cognitive and perceptual disturbances seen in the chronic grief response, all

TABLE 3   Responses to Disrupted Regulation of Homeostasis (Human Studies)

Symptoms following sensory deprivation:
  Fluctuating concentration and attention
  Restlessness, anxiety
  Difficulty in ordering thoughts
  Decreased food intake
  Illusions and hallucinations
  Decreased body weight
  Sleep disturbance
  Muscular weakness

Symptoms following jet travel across time zones:
  Decreased vigilance, decreased attention span
  Decreased appetite
  Sleep disturbance
  Malaise, fatigue

Symptoms following work shift change:
  Decreased vigilance
  Cognitive impairment
  Insomnia
  Weakness, fatiguability
  Depression, hostility

of which contribute to the feeling of losing control. The similarities in physiologic disturbances resulting from bereavement, sensory deprivation, jet lag, and work shift change have led Hofer[32] to postulate that the regulators' function was to maintain the biological rhythms of the individual. The death of someone with whom a person has lived in close proximity involves the loss of social entraining stimuli for circadian systems, and may therefore disrupt normal biological timing. In fact, there is evidence that social interactions for human beings may be the cues regulating human biological rhythms, rather than light or temperature as in other species.

Hofer[32] suggests that these somatosensory regulators may be the precursors of psychological regulators that take over as the infant matures. He contends that disturbances of physiologic regulation may be involved even in the loss of someone who has been living far away, because internal representations of the person may have served a regulatory function; when these are altered in the psychological process of grieving, their regulatory function may be dissolved. Study of the regulatory aspects of social relationships may eventually lead to some understanding of the mechanisms by which the presence or absence of social support systems modifies physiologic responses to stress and vulnerability to disease.

Rhythms in the Endocrine and Immune Systems. It is well known that cortisol levels in plasma and urine are cyclical. There is evidence that many other hormones and biochemical systems also have cyclical patterns.[56] Catecholamine excretion displays periodicity, for example, and growth hormone secretion, although not itself rhythmic, changes in response to other variables that are in turn rhythmic. The cycles of all hormones are influenced by many environmental variables, and it seems likely that social interactions and their sudden alteration after bereavement may exert major disruptive effects.

The immune system also follows a daily rhythm. Tavadia and colleagues[79] found that the circadian rhythm followed by cortisol secretion is accompanied by changes in the number of lymphocytes and in mitogen-stimulated lymphocyte transformation. Cortisol and lymphocyte transformation were directly correlated, but both varied inversely with absolute numbers of lymphocytes. Maestroni and Pierpaoli[50] suggest that the lymphopenia seen after pinealectomy may be due to the loss of rhythmicity previously regulated by the pineal body. Others[58] have found circadian rhythms involved in immune competence, and Kort and Weijma[38] recently demonstrated that the stress of a chronic light-dark cycle shift in rats resulted in decreased lymphocyte response to a mitogen and decreased immune response as measured by popliteal lymph node assay, but not in a change in adrenocortical activity.

Grief and Depression on a Neurobiological Continuum

As discussed in the section on promising research approaches, the phenomena of bereavement mirror to a considerable extent the symptoms and signs of depressive illness and share some aspects of anxiety states. Because overt depressive illness and, to a lesser extent, severe anxiety states are often precipitated by major losses, it seems reasonable to look for connections between bereavement and these two common psychiatric disorders. Indeed, it is a plausible hypothesis that the three conditions share a common neurobiological substrate.

Klein[37] has made a strong case for this point of view, and his conceptual basis for this involves the temporal contiguity of the protest and despair phases in infantile separation responses as early "Anlagen" of the adult conditions. Klein follows Bowlby's view that these two infantile responses are deeply embedded in phylogenetic history, and hypothesizes that some individuals, even when they are adults, have low thresholds for elicitation. In some, the system may even discharge spontaneously, resulting in classical panic attacks. As Klein points out, patients with panic attacks also have an increased incidence of depressive episodes. But it was the finding that the same drug, the tricyclic antidepressant, imipramine, prevented panic attacks as well as depression that prompted Klein to develop his theory. He supposed that imipramine raised the threshold to both conditions by acting on a common neurochemical substrate.

Other findings tend to link depressive illness with bereavement. Both conditions seem to imperil the resistance of an individual to major physical challenges and have been associated with increased incidence and severity of a number of medical conditions. Second, both conditions result in increased rates of suicide. In addition, there is some limited evidence for similarity in neuroendocrine responses. Thus, in women undergoing psychotherapy for reactive depression, Sachar and his collaborators[69] noted a peak in corticosteroids when patients confronted the fact of the precipitating loss during therapy. The bereavement is often considered more painful than the chronic depression after loss, which may be defensive and help the person to avoid experiencing the loss.

Abnormal endocrine patterns are present in major affective disorders such as depression. Abnormalities in growth hormone, insulin, and thyroid-stimulating hormone are often observed in depression.[67] Depressed individuals tend to have high ACTH and cortisol levels and fail to follow normal diurnal rhythmicity; many severely depressed people fail to depress cortisol levels in response to an exogenous corticosteroid, dexamethasone. However, a new study[40] from Yale of the dexamethasone suppression test in bereaved individuals who met the criteria for a diagnosis of major depression revealed the great majority as having *normal* adrenocortical responses—not those considered typical of depression.[40] On this dimension, then, severe grief reactions would seem to occupy a place on a neurobiologic continuum that is distinct from the one occupied by major depression.

This study notwithstanding, most of the evidence suggests that bereavement may bear more than a superficial resemblance to depressive illness and that it would be appropriate to continue to search in the bereaved for some of the biological phenomena that have been found in depressed patients and in those with panic disorders.

CONCLUSIONS

Very little is known about the biology of the varying states of grief. Clues about promising avenues for research in this field can be gleaned from the symptomatology and epidemiology of bereavement and from current knowledge about several of the body's regulatory systems. Active grieving produces a number of symptoms that suggest involvement of the respiratory, autonomic, and endocrine systems. The epidemiology of bereavement suggests that cardiovascular and immune function may be substantially altered by grief. And there are enough similarities between grief and depression to merit a comparison of neuroendocrine and other biological changes in the two conditions.

Studies are needed on basic neurophysiologic parameters, including cardiovascular, thermal, and central nervous system regulation. In particular, more information is needed on the long-term effects of bereavement: how do physiologic responses change during prolonged grief, both "spontaneously" and in response to specific stimuli and to other significant life events? As more substantial baseline material is collected, possible genetic and experiential precursors should be sought to account for the variability in response encountered so often in studies of both animals and human beings. Considerable expansion of the knowledge of neurochemical changes accompanying the response to loss is required, including further investigation of neuroendocrine functions across a wider array of hormones as well as more studies of the neurotransmitter alterations that may underlie the dramatic and more subtle affective, motivational, and cognitive changes that emerge. In each of these areas, further development of remote, miniaturized blood collection devices (which would permit study of free-moving subjects, as in neurophysiologic research) would provide substantial opportunities to gather significant new data.

The preliminary data now available make it clear that traumatic loss experiences may have a long-term impact on the body's immune system. Expanding the data base on the disease susceptibility of bereaved subjects under controlled conditions and gaining further understanding of the basic immune processes that are affected will improve the chances that appropriate intervention models are developed.

The relationship between the responses to loss and the patterns observed in response to other life stresses should be established more fully. Do the patterns during bereavement parallel those in other situations in which "loss of control" is a prominent element? What types of physical and social environmental factors alter the intensity and time course of human physiologic responses? What is the meaning, in terms of basic processes and the possibilities for effective intervention and treatment strategies, of the fact that events at the behavioral and physiologic level are not always as congruent as might otherwise be expected? Research involving animal models plays a crucial role in generating new hypotheses and methods. But even more urgent is the need for prospective human studies employing the most modern biological and psychological methods and concepts.

REFERENCES

1. Ackerman, S.H., Keller, S.E., Schleifer, S.J., Shindledecker, R.D., Camerino, W.S., Hofer, M.A., Weiner, H., and Stein, M. Effect of premature weaning on lymphocyte stimulation in the rat. (Abstract.) *Psychosomatic Medicine* 45:75, 1983.
2. Ader, A. (Ed.) *Psychoneuroimmunology.* New York: Academic Press, 1981.
3. Ader, R. Stress and illness: immune processes. Paper prepared for the Institute of Medicine, Washington, D.C., 1981.
4. Ader R., and Cohen, N. Behaviorally conditioned immuno-suppression. *Psychosomatic Medicine* 37:333–340, 1975.
5. Bartrop, R., Luckhurst, E., Lazarus, L., Kiloh, L.G., and Perry, R. Depressed lymphocyte function after bereavement. *Lancet* 1:834–836, 1977.
6. Black, S., Humphrey, J.H., and Niven, J.S.F. Inhibition of mantoux reaction by direct suggestion under hypnosis. *British Medical Journal* 5346:1649–1652, 1963.
7. Board, F., Persky, H., and Hamburg, D.A. Psychological stress and endocrine functions: blood levels of adrenocortical and thyroid hormones in acutely disturbed patients. *Psychosomatic Medicine* 18:324–333, 1956.
8. Breese, G.R., Smith, R.D., Mueller, R.A., Howard, J.L., Prangle, A.J., Lipton, M.A., Young, L.D., McKinney, W.T., and Lewis, J.K. Induction of adrenal catecholamine synthesizing enzymes following mother-infant separation. *Nature New Biology* 246:94–96, 1973.

9. Cannon, W.B. *Bodily Changes in Pain, Hunger, Fear and Rage* (2nd edition). New York: Appleton, 1929.

10. Cannon, W.B. Stresses and strains of homeostasis. *American Journal of Medical Science* 189:1–14, 1935.

11. Case, R.M., and Sachar, E.J. Psychoendocrinology. In: *Textbook of Endocrinology* (6th edition) (Williams, R.H., ed.). Philadelphia: W.B. Saunders, 1981.

12. Chambers, W.N., and Reiser, M.F. Emotional stress in the precipitation of congestive heart failure. *Psychosomatic Medicine* 15:38–60, 1953.

13. Clayton, P.J. Mortality and morbidity in the first year of widowhood. *Archives of General Psychiatry* 30:747–750, 1974.

14. Coe, C.L., Mendoza, S.P., Smotherman, W.P., and Levine, S. Mother-infant attachment in the squirrel monkey: adrenal responses to separation. *Behavioral Biology* 22:256–263, 1978.

15. Coe, C.L., Wiener, S.G., and Levine, S. Psychoendocrine responses of mother and infant monkeys to disturbance and separation. In: *Symbiosis in Parent–Offspring Interaction* (Rosenblum, L.A., and Moltz, H., eds.). New York: Plenum, 1983.

16. Craddock, G.C. Corticosteroid-induced lymphopenia, immunosuppression, and body defense. *Annals of Internal Medicine* 88:564–566, 1978.

17. Elliott, G., and Eisdorfer, C. (Eds.) *Stress and Human Health: A Study by the Institute of Medicine*. New York: Springer, 1982.

18. Engel, G. Sudden and rapid death during psychological stress. *Annals of Internal Medicine* 74:771–782, 1971.

19. Engel, G. Memorial Lecture: the psychosomatic approach to individual susceptibility to disease. *Gastroenterology* 67:1085–1093, 1974.

20. Engel, G., and Schmale, A. Conservation-withdrawal: a primary regulatory process for organismic homeostasis. *Physiology, Emotion and Psychosomatic Illness* (Ciba Foundation Symposium No. 8). New York: Elsevier, 1972.

21. von Euler, U.S., Gemzell, C.A., Levi, L., and Strom, G. Cortical and medullary adrenal activity in emotional stress. *Acta Endocrinologica* 30:567–573, 1959.

22. Franksson, C., and Gemzell, C. Adrenocortical activity in preoperative period. *Journal of Clinical Endocrinology and Metabolism* 15:1069–1072, 1955.

23. Gala, R.R., and Haisenleder, D.J. Stress-induced decrease of the afternoon prolactin surge. *Life Science* 31:875–879, 1982.

24. Hattori, T., Hamai, Y., Ikeda, T., Takiyama, W., Hirai, T., and Miyoshi, Y. Inhibitory effects of immunopotentiators on the enhancement of lung metastases induced by operative stress in rats. *Gan* 73:132–135, 1982.

25. Hennessy, M.B., Kaplan, J.N., Mendoza, S.P., Lowe, E.L., and Levine, S. Separation distress and attachment in surrogate-reared squirrel monkeys. *Physiological Behavior* 23:1017–1023, 1979.

26. Hofer, M.A. The role of nutrition in the physiological and behavioral effects of early maternal separation in infant rats. *Psychosomatic Medicine* 35:350–359, 1973.

27. Hofer, M.A. The effects of brief maternal separations on behavior and heart rate of 2 week old rat pups. *Physiological Behavior* 10:423–427, 1973.

28. Hofer, M.A. Survival and recovery of physiologic functions after early maternal separation in infant rats. *Psychosomatic Medicine* 15:475–480, 1975.

29. Hofer, M.A. Studies on how early maternal separation produces behavioral change in young rats. *Psychosomatic Medicine* 37:245–246, 1975.

30. Hofer, M.A. The organization of sleep and wakefulness after maternal separation in young rats. *Developmental Psychobiology* 9:189–206, 1976.

31. Hofer, M.A. On the relationship between attachment and separation processes in

infancy. In: *Emotion: Theory Research and Experience, Vol. 2; Early Development* (Plutchik, R., ed.). New York: Academic Press, 1983.

32. Hofer, M.A. Relationships as regulators: a psychobiological perspective on bereavement. *Psychosomatic Medicine* (in press), 1984.

33. Hofer, M.A., Wolff, C.T., Friedman, S.B., and Mason, J.W. A psychoendocrine study of bereavement. Part I: 17-hydroxycorticosteroid excretion rates of parents following death of their children from leukemia. *Psychosomatic Medicine* 34:481–491, 1972.

34. Hofer, M.A., Wolff, C.T., and Mason, J.W. A psychoendocrine study of bereavement. Part II: observations on the process of mourning in relation to adrenocortical function. *Psychosomatic Medicine* 34:492–504, 1972.

35. Jacobs, S., Mason, J.W., Kosten, T.R., Ostfeld, A.M., Kasl, S.V., Atkins, S.R., Gardner, C.W., and Schreiber, S.J. Bereavement, psychological distress, ego defenses, and adrenocortical function. Paper presented at American Psychosomatic Society Meeting, March 1984.

36. Keller, S.E., Weiss, J.M., Schleifer, S.J., Miller, N.E., and Stein, M. Suppression of immunity by stress: effect of a graded series of stressors on lymphocyte stimulation in the rat. *Science* 213:1397–1400, 1981.

37. Klein, D.F. Anxiety reconceptualized. In: *Anxiety: New Research and Changing Concepts* (Klein, D.F., and Rabkin, J., eds.). New York: Raven Press, 1981.

38. Kort, W.J., and Weijma, J.M. Effect of chronic light-dark shift stress on the immune response of the rat. *Physiological Behavior* 29:1083–1087, 1982.

39. Kosten, T.R., Jacobs, S., and Mason, J.W. Psychological correlates of growth hormone response to stress. (Abstract.) *Psychosomatic Medicine* 45:82, 1983.

40. Kosten, T.R., Jacobs, S., and Mason, J. The dexamethasone suppression test during bereavement. *Journal of Nervous and Mental Diseases* (in press).

41. Kosten, T.R., Jacobs, S., Mason, J., and Wahby, V. Growth hormone response during the stress of bereavement. Paper presented at American Psychosomatic Society Meeting, March 1984.

42. Kraemer, G., and McKinney, W. Interaction of pharmacological agents which alter biogenic amine metabolism and depression. *Journal of Affective Disorders* 1:33–54, 1979.

43. Kreuz, L., Rose, R., and Jennings, J. Suppression of plasma testosterone levels and psychological stress. *Archives of General Psychiatry* 25:479–482, 1972.

44. Kuhn, C.M., Grignolo, A., Johnson, M., and Schanberg, S.M. Heterogeneity in the response pattern of organ systems to stress: mediators and mechanisms. *Psychopharmacological Bulletin* 18:96–99, 1982.

45. Lader, M.H. Palmar skin conductance measures in anxiety and phobic states. *Journal of Psychosomatic Research* 11:271–281, 1967.

46. Laudenslager, M., Reite, M., and Harbeck, M. Suppressed immune response in infant monkeys associated with maternal separation. *Behavioral and Neural Biology* 36:40–48, 1982.

47. Levine, S., and Coe, C.L. Recent advances in psychophysiology: endocrine regulation. In: *Handbook of Psychosomatic Medicine* (Cheren, S., ed.). New York: State University of New York Press (in press).

48. Lindemann, E. The symptomatology and management of acute grief. *American Journal of Psychiatry* 101:141–148, 1944.

49. Lown, B., Venner, R.L., and Corbalan, R. Psychologic stress and threshold for repetitive ventricular response. *Science* 182:834–836, 1973.
50. Maestroni, G.J.M., and Pierpaoli, W. Pharmacologic control of the hormonally mediated immune response. In: *Psychoneuroimmunology* (Ader, A., ed.). New York: Academic Press, 1981.
51. Mason, J.W. Emotion as reflected in patterns of endocrine integration. In: *Emotions—Their Parameters and Measurement* (Levi, L., ed.). New York: Raven Press, 1975.
52. Mason, J.W. Bereavement: endocrine aspects. Paper presented at American Psychosomatic Society Meeting, March 1983.
53. Mason, J.W., Sachar, E.J., Fishman, J.R., Hamburg, D.A., and Handlon, J.H. Corticosteroid responses to hospital admission. *Archives of General Psychiatry*, 13:1–8, 1965.
54. McClintock, M.K. Menstrual synchrony and suppression. *Nature* 229:244–245, 1971.
55. Monjan, A.A. Stress and immunologic competence: studies in animals. In: *Psychoneuroimmunology* (Ader, A., ed.). New York: Academic Press, 1981.
56. Moore-Ede, M.C., Sulzman, F.M., and Fuller, C.A. *The Clocks that Time Us.* Cambridge, MA: Harvard University Press, 1982.
57. Newberry, B.H. Effects of presumably stressful stimulation (PSS) on the development of animal tumors: some issues. In: *Perspectives on Behavioral Medicine* (Weiss, S.M., Herd, J.A., and Fox, B.H., eds.). New York: Academic Press, 1981.
58. Palmblad, J. Stress and immunologic competence: studies in man. In: *Psychoneuroimmunology* (Ader, A., ed.). New York: Academic Press, 1981.
59. Parkes, C.M. *Bereavement: Studies of Grief in Adult Life.* London: Tavistock, 1972.
60. Reich, P. Clinical observations on the psychobiology of life-threatening arrhythmias. In: *Biobehavioral Factors in Sudden Cardiac Death* (Solomon, F., Parron, D.L., and Dews, P.B., eds.). Washington, D.C.: National Academy Press, 1982.
61. Reich, P., DeSilva, R.A., Lown, B., and Murawski, B.J. Acute psychological disturbance preceding life-threatening ventricular arrhythmias. *Journal of the American Medical Association* 246:233–235, 1981.
62. Reite, M., Kaufman, K., Pauley, J.D., and Stynes, A.J. Depression in infant monkeys: physiological correlates. *Psychosomatic Medicine* 36:363–367, 1974.
63. Reite, M., and Short, R.A. Nocturnal sleep in separated monkey infants. *Archives of General Psychiatry* 35:1247–1253, 1973.
64. Riley, V. Psychoneuroendocrine influences on immuno-competence and neoplasia. *Science* 212:1100–1109, 1981.
65. Riley, V., Fitzmaurice, M.A., and Spackman, D.H. Psychoneuroimmunologic factors in neoplasia: studies in animals. In: *Psychoneuroimmunology* (Ader, A., ed.). New York: Academic Press, 1981.
66. Rose, R.M., Poe, R.O., and Mason, J.W. Psychological state and body size as determinants of 17-OHCS excretion. *Archives of Internal Medicine* 121:406–413, 1968.
67. Rose, R.M., and Sachar, E. Psychoendocrinology. In: *Textbook of Endocrinology* (Williams, R.H., ed.). Philadelphia: W.B. Saunders, 1981.
68. Saavedra, J.M. Changes in dopamine, noradrenaline and adrenaline in specific septal and preoptic nuclei after acute immobilization stress. *Neuroendocrinology* 33:396–401, 1982.

69. Sachar, E.J., Mackenzie, J.M., Binstock, W.A., and Mack, J.E. Corticosteroid responses to the psychotherapy of reactive depressions. *Psychosomatic Medicine* 30:23–44, 1968.
70. Schiffman, P.L., Westlake, R.E., Santiago, T.V., and Edelman, N.H. Ventilation control of parents of victims of Sudden Infant Death Syndrome. *New England Journal of Medicine* 302:486–491, 1980.
71. Schleifer, S.J., Keller, S.E., Camerino, M., Thornton, J.C., and Stein, M. Suppression of lymphocyte stimulation following bereavement. *Journal of the American Medical Association* 250:374–399, 1983.
72. Solomon, F., Parron, D.L., and Dews, P.B. (Eds.) *Biobehavioral Factors in Sudden Cardiac Death: Summary of an Institute of Medicine Conference*. Washington, D.C.: National Academy Press, 1982.
73. Solomon, G.F., and Amkraut, A.A. Emotions, stress, and immunity. In: *Frontiers of Radiation in Therapeutic Oncology*, Vol. 7 (Vaeth, J.M., ed.). Baltimore: University Park Press, 1972.
74. Sowers, J.R., Raj, R.P., Hershman, J.M., Carlson, H.E., and McCallum, R.W. The effect of stressful diagnostic studies and surgery on anterior pituitary hormone release in man. *Acta Endocrinologica* 86:25–32, 1977.
75. Starkman, M.N., Schteingart, D.E., and Schork, M.A. Depressed mood and other psychiatric manifestations of Cushing's syndrome: relationship to hormone levels. *Psychosomatic Medicine* 43:3–18, 1981.
76. Stone, E., Bonnet, K., and Hofer, M.A. Survival and development of maternally deprived rats: role of body temperature. *Psychosomatic Medicine* 38:242–249, 1976.
77. Suomi, S.J., Seaman, S.F., Lewis, J.K., Delizio, R.D., and McKinney, W.T., Jr. Effects of imipramine treatment of separation-induced social disorders in rhesus monkeys. *Archives of General Psychiatry* 35:321–327, 1978.
78. Sutton, J.R., and Casey, J.H. The adrenocortical response to competitive athletics in veteran athletes. *Journal of Clinical Endocrinology and Metabolism* 40:135–138, 1975.
79. Tavadia, H.B., Fleming, K.A., Hume, P.D., and Simpson, H.W. Circadian rhythmicity of human plasma cortisol and PHA-induced lymphocyte transformation. *Clinical and Experimental Immunology* 22:190–193, 1975.
80. Verrier, R.L., and Lown, B. Autonomic nervous system and malignant cardiac arrhythmias. In: *Brain, Behavior and Bodily Disease* (Weiner, H., Hofer, M.A., and Stunkard, A.J., eds.). New York: Raven Press, 1981.
81. Vogt, J.L., and Hennessy, M.B. Infant separation in monkeys: studies on social figures other than the mother. In: *Child Nurturance: Studies of Development in Nonhuman Primates* (Fitzgerald, H.E., Mullins, J.A., and Gage, P., eds.). New York: Plenum, 1982.
82. Weiner, H., Singer, M.T., and Reiser, M.F. Cardiovascular responses and their psychological correlates: a study in healthy young adults and patients with peptic ulcer and hypertension. *Psychosomatic Medicine* 24:477–498, 1962.
83. Weiss, J.M. The effects of coping responses on stress. *Journal of Comparative Physiology and Psychology* 65:251–260, 1968.
84. Weiss, J.M., Bailey, W.H., Goodman, P.A., Hoffman, L.J., Ambrose, M.J., Salman, S., and Charry, J.M. A model for neurochemical study of depression. In: *Behavioral Models and the Analysis of Drug Action* (Levy, A., and Spiegelstein, M.Y., eds.). Amsterdam: Elsevier, 1982.

85. Wiener, S., Johnson, D., and Levine, S. Behavioral and physiological response of infant squirrel monkeys following weaning. Paper presented at American Society of Primatologists Meeting, East Lansing, Michigan, 1983.
86. Wolff, C.T., Hofer, M.A., Friedman, S.B., and Mason, J.W. Relationships of psychological defenses and mean urinary 17-hydroxycorticosteroid excretion rates in the parents of children with leukemia. Parts I and II. *Psychosomatic Medicine* 26:576–609, 1964.

Monkeys' Responses to
Separation and Loss

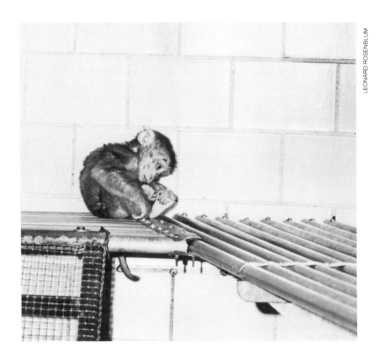

LEONARD ROSENBLUM

This six-month-old monkey who has been separated from its mother exhibits many signs of depression in its posture and behavior. Because of the many parallels with human responses, researchers are studying nonhuman primates to better understand bereavement and how pre- and post-bereavement circumstances affect adjustment to loss.

CHAPTER 7

Monkeys' Responses to Separation and Loss

An infant, having reached an age when independent locomotion is readily accomplished, wanders around a room, eagerly touching and exploring everything he sees. He plays vigorously with two young companions. But when he suddenly discovers that his mother is nowhere in sight, he quickly becomes agitated, moves about the room in rapid, distracted movements, and begins to scream and cry. He no longer approaches the objects in the room, nor does he initiate play with his friends. Indeed, efforts by his friends to initiate play with him result in brief distracted encounters, quickly terminated by the repeated crying and searching of the motherless infant.

Over the next few hours the infant overtly calms somewhat, but any of a variety of stimuli sets off the whole train of emotional responses once again. The time to go to sleep, for example, triggers a striking increase in crying and agitation. In the next day or two, the pattern shifts from one of agitation to one in which the infant gradually withdraws from his environment almost completely, directing much of his activity towards himself. Thumb-sucking, genital manipulation, and self-clasping emerge, as do changes in posture and facial expression. The infant seems lethargic and unresponsive, almost unable to hold his body nor-

This chapter was prepared by Leonard A. Rosenblum, Ph.D., consultant to the study, Professor, Department of Psychiatry, and Director, Primate Behavior Laboratory, State University of New York, Brooklyn, New York.

mally upright; his face appears drawn, and he frequently closes his eyes in apparent, but often not true, sleep. This depressed pattern continues, relatively unabated, for a dishearteningly long time.

The pattern described is not of a human youngster's response to loss, but the reaction of a six-month-old monkey. This description reflects a number of aspects of a phenomenon observed in human beings throughout history and studied in detail in other primates during the past two decades. In both human and nonhuman primates, when a strong emotional bond has been established between two individuals, loss of one has important psychological and emotional consequences for the other. Although researchers have been able to learn much about the factors that influence the course and intensity of bereavement in people, the constraints imposed by a number of ethical and practical matters leave current understanding of the role of many factors relatively uncertain. Working with appropriate animal models, however, while bearing in mind the ethical issues that must still be considered, the environment and experiences can be controlled and the impact of important events can be assessed at preselected times under the rigorous light of experimental scrutiny.

VARIATIONS IN THE RESPONSE TO LOSS

Like people, nonhuman primates are genetically heterogeneous and intelligent enough to be influenced in complex ways by their past experiences and current circumstances. Thus, it is not surprising that their responses to the loss of the mother range across a wide spectrum of behavior. Indeed, a special relevance of the work on nonhuman primates in this domain derives from the fact that the higher primates show a diversity of response, as humans do. By pursuing the sources of this variation, and the forces that intensify or ameliorate the potentially debilitating effects of loss, understanding of the human condition can be advanced.

In monkeys, individual variation in response to the loss of the mother early in life can range from merely several hours of intermittent crying and restlessness to a pattern in which the infant cries and moves incessantly immediately after experiencing the loss and then virtually collapses into an unresponsive heap the next day. Some infants show very strong reactions in the first two to four days but appear to begin recovery quickly; others may still be quite disturbed weeks after the separation. It should be noted, however, that the absence or lessening of behavioral signs of disturbance does not necessarily imply that stressful reactions may not be emerging within several physiologic domains.[4]

Over the last 20 years, the responses of more than a half dozen species of primates to the sudden loss of the mother or other close companions have been studied. The bulk of this work has focused on several Asian macaque species and on the South American squirrel monkey. This range of species has been particularly important because the combination of closely related species and a phylogenetically quite distant one allows an assessment of both the effects of a number of social and environmental conditions and the role of clearly primate, but nonetheless quite diverse, genetic predispositions.

These studies make it clear that although each of these species shows emotional disturbance following a loss, the intensity and duration of the reaction as well as its qualitative form may vary from species to species. The rhesus and pigtail macaques, for example, appear most susceptible to the severest forms of depressive reaction in response to loss of the mother.

One final element in consideration of the potential genetic source of variations in some aspects of the response to separation or loss is the role of individual genetic, or at least prenatal, influences. Recent work by Suomi[43,44] has shown that an infant rhesus' emotional reactivity to an auditory conditioning procedure at three weeks of age significantly predicts subsequent intensity of response to maternal loss. Also, half-siblings (infants with the same father) seem to resemble each other in the intensity of their reactions.

It seems reasonable to conclude from these data that although all primates are emotionally responsive to the experience of loss, there are important congenital contributions (genetic, prenatal, or both) to the form and intensity of that response. This "background" source of variation should be kept in mind when considering the developmental, social, and environmental factors being considered in research results.

PHASES OF REACTION TO LOSS

In general, studies of the response to sudden loss in primates have identified several successive phases through which the infants pass. Before the factors that have been identified as contributing to variation in response are discussed, the behavior that has been observed and the time dimensions along which it proceeds must be considered.

The "Protest" Phase

In almost every study reported in the literature, the initial reaction of an infant to the sudden disappearance of its mother includes frequent, loud, repetitive, rather plaintive calls. This high-pitched, relatively pure wail takes the form of the "coo" vocalization of the separated infant macaque or the ear-piercing, repetitive, relatively pure tones of the lost squirrel monkey baby. Accompanying the vocalizations is rapid activity, often distracted rather than focused.[3,37,38] High outbursts of energy (a factor of no little significance if the youngster is expected to survive for very long on its own) are expended in the immediate aftermath of the loss.

During this "protest" period the infant may briefly interact with either its social or physical environment. Even brief play bouts may be seen. But the form of infant activity is clearly altered. This ubiquitous initial phase of protest appears likely to represent a relatively closed genetic system[18] that leaves only limited room for individual variation, regardless of other environmental or experiential factors.

Most authors agree that the repeated vocalizations and high levels of locomotor activity are designed to effect rapid reunion of the separated infant and its mother or some other member of its group who might offer the protection and care needed for survival. This investment of limited and thus quite precious energy resources by the infant in an effort to regain contact as rapidly as possible may well reflect the fact that, under natural conditions, infants who become separated during the first year or so of life rarely survive (e.g., Rhine et al.[30]). Numerous laboratory observations of animals requiring support during separations attest to the potentially devastating combination of limited physical coping capacity and the trauma of the sudden loss of an important attachment figure.[6]

Despair/Depression Phase

Infants begin to vary considerably in their pattern of response within 24 to 36 hours following the loss of the mother or rearing partner. The most extreme responses have been observed in several laboratory settings (as well as in the field; e.g., van Lawick-Goodall[14]) and in a number of species. These vulnerable subjects, following protests of varying intensity, cease spontaneous locomotion and lose virtually all interest in the world around them. They will neither initiate play nor respond to the efforts of others. Even the presentation of a novel object, normally the stimulus for great excitement and interest in young monkeys, fails to arouse them. While immobile, the infant is unable to maintain the normal alert posture, with head up and eyes open, and is changed into an infant seemingly rolled into a ball, its head lowered to the floor and pressed against its body. Its eyes are closed much of the time, even during the day, when infants never sleep if out of contact with the mother. In addition to the postural collapse, these subjects often begin sustained oral contacts with their fur, limbs, digits, or genitalia.

In most instances, even the most severe cases of this type begin to improve five to ten days after the separation. The infant gradually begins to sit more normally, and the hunched-over posture is increasingly reserved for periods in which the infant is frightened. Its eyes are generally open now and oral contacts with its own body diminish. Finally, following a gradual return of interest in the physical environment, social play responsiveness and then social initiations reappear at increasing levels. By the end of two to four weeks, many infants look overtly like normal infants of their age, although more precise behavioral records indicate that recovery is by no means complete even a month after the loss.

Several important issues must be addressed to appreciate more fully the significance of these depressed patterns as one form of response to loss. First, are these patterns as common in primates as the protest behaviors described earlier? A review of the literature[38] reveals that many studies fail to record any instances of the despair/depression pattern. In general, even in studies in which these extreme reactions do appear, only a portion of the subjects show it at all. Thus, as in humans, the most severe forms of behavioral and emotional debilitation occur in a limited number of subjects. Study of these extremely disturbed individuals could reveal much about the potency of certain factors, perhaps including specific phylogenetic or ontogenetic (developmental) ones, in producing at least certain types of depression. It is at this form of response that efforts at intervention may best be directed.

Before considering the behaviors of these animals further, one should ask if the severe reaction just described could be merely the product of a physiologically disturbed youngster. Perhaps the sudden change in diet is important; infant monkeys generally continue to receive some mother's milk until their next sibling is born, after about a year. Or perhaps the reaction merely reflects the fact that sleep patterns have been abruptly disturbed because its mother, on whose ventrum it has always slept, is no longer available. The pattern described above, this line of cautious concern suggests, is merely the response of a tired young infant whose stomach is upset. In a week or 10 days it will start to feel better and its behavior will improve. This is a significant alternate hypothesis to the one proposed earlier—that the loss of the mother is extremely disturbing psychologically and emotionally for nonhuman primates.

Observations of the presumed depression after loss in primates make clear that the separation pattern is indeed the result of severe emotional response to the loss, and not merely the product of digestive or sleep disturbances. Data presented below indicate that nonhuman primates may well experience a period of detachment from the lost object as a later phase of response to loss.

Detachment Phase

Several studies have been done to assess the actual nature of the most severe forms of depressive response to the loss of mother, as well as to test the applicability of a "detachment phase" to nonhuman primates. In a variety of circumstances during reunions following a prolonged separation from their parents, human infants have been observed either to avoid the parents or to behave in an emotionally detached manner in their presence[7,31] Such behavior seems counterintuitive if not paradoxical. There is a clear suggestion that some alteration in the infant's emotional response to the lost care-giver has emerged during the separation. At the very least, such infants may be seen as having conflicting approach/withdrawal motivations in place of the initially unambiguous drive to move to mother at all costs. Main[16] has suggested, for human infants, that avoidance of the mother under these circumstances may be a part of the particular pattern of sustained mother-infant interaction. She suggests that an infant who is frequently rejected in its attempts to achieve contact with its mother may develop a pattern of avoidance when in proximity to her. Nonetheless, both Main[16] and Bowlby[2] have suggested that the apparent detachment behavior at reunion reflects an effort to cope with the conflict between attachment to and anger at the lost parent.

In laboratory studies of nonhuman primates, at a reunion following the enforced separation of the mother-infant pair, the mother almost always retrieves her infant immediately. Thus the infant has little opportunity to express hesitancy or avoidance if it were so inclined. Nonetheless, in an investigation of separated rhesus infants (8–20 weeks of age), Abrams[1] observed unusual behavior on the part of the infants in 25 percent of reunions: ". . . the mother entered the cage and retrieved the infant as before, but the infant usually screeched as she did so. Ventral contact was established; but after some period of time, from one to five minutes, the infant broke contact and withdrew from the mother. . ." Other instances in which the returning infant actually avoided the mother's initial efforts at retrieval are described as well. These data suggest at least ambivalence on the part of these reunited infants, indicating perhaps an altered emotional response to the previously lost parent.

Studies by Rosenblum[32,33] provide strong evidence in support of the emotional disturbance hypothesis and indications of the detachment phase as well. In one portion of this work, five pigtail infants, 7–8 months of age, were separated from their mothers for a period of 8–10 weeks. The infants, separated two at a time, remained with the rest of the social group in the pens where they had been raised. During the separation the infants showed the normal range of response, from severe depression in two infants and a moderate depressive reaction in a third, to two infants who showed rather minimal reactions after the protest phase. Recovery progressed normally and the depressive phase began to disappear after about 10 days following the loss. Two to three times a week during the separation, the mother of one infant at a time was returned to the home pen for half an hour. For control purposes, both the infant whose mother was returned and the other separated infants were observed in each return trial, thus allowing determination of the specificity of any observed reactions.

Most striking were the reactions of the several infants who had shown strong "depressive" patterns in the days following the loss. Well after these infants had shown relative recovery in the absence of the mother, they showed a virtually complete return of the depressive pattern each time the mother was brought back to the pen. Even nine weeks following loss, one infant that generally looked quite normal, playing socially and actively exploring and playing with its environment, had dramatic reactions to the returned mother.

During these reinvoked depressive episodes, infants would not move toward the cage in which their mother was restrained (for control purposes), although they readily approached the cage when someone else's mother was present. Upon removal of their mother, these infants would almost immediately return to very high levels of activity and play. As a follow-up to this work, the reactions of young infants to color videotapes of their mothers and other social stimuli have recently been studied. In one instance, a 10-month-old pigtail infant that had been terminally separated from its mother three months earlier had an opportunity to produce a taped image of its mother in an operant situation. After several minutes of alternating between the mother's image and that of another female, the infant turned on the image of mother, began to "coo" softly, then closed its eyes and gradually dropped into the collapsed posture typical of the depressive pattern. Holding the lever to maintain the mother's image for the remaining 13 minutes of the trial, the infant stayed in the depressed posture, only occasionally looking up at the image of its mother, cooing briefly, closing its eyes, and dropping its posture once again.

These observations indicate that it is the emotional disturbance in reaction to the loss of mother and the adaptive demands of the separation environment that produce the second-phase effects that have been labeled despair/depression. At the same time, the data suggest that some aspects of the pattern that have been described as reflecting "detachment" in humans may have their counterpart in the reaction of at least some monkey infants to a severe loss experience.

PRESEPARATION INFLUENCES

The Nature of the Attachment Bond

For a strong emotional relationship to be established between an infant and its mother, that relationship must be specific and unambiguous. Indeed, it is a precondition for any consideration of attachment that a particular set of responses be directed selectively toward a specific partner. Despite early anecdotal reports that infant monkeys come to recognize their mother in the first days or week of life, experimental evidence indicates that, as in humans, such recognition matures more slowly and may be affected by a number of factors.

Consider the case of bonnet macaque infants, raised in a complex social group that contains a number of mothers and infants. If offered a controlled choice of responding to their mother or to a complete stranger of the same species, it is not until about 12 weeks of life that significant preferences for the mother are shown.[35] Males, incidentally, appear to be several weeks slower in achieving this capacity than females. If, however, an infant bonnet monkey is reared alone with its mother, without other adults or peers, even as late as six to eight months of age it moves to a complete stranger as readily as it does to its own mother. Some infants reared in this condition failed to select their mothers consistently even as late as a year of age.[39]

In a final study in this series, it was shown that if an infant is reared by its mother in the company of another female–infant pair, the infant at about three months responds selectively to its mother rather than to the familiar female, but may not select her in preference to a stranger until two to three months later. Thus the specificity of an infant's response to its primary care-giver may vary as a function of circumstances. As Spitz[42] initially suggested for human children, individuals will, at the very least, be expected to differ markedly in response to loss in the periods before and after the acquisition of selective, individually focused attachment behavior.

According to Bowlby,[2] the reliability with which the attachment figure is able to respond appropriately to the infant's needs (the degree to which the mother is "available and accessible"[22]) influences the security of the attachment. Thus one speaks of relatively "anxious" or "secure" attachments, with those subjects at the anxious end of the continuum more likely to show severe reactions to loss.

Although some evidence regarding this issue has been provided by efforts to account for variations in response among members of single treatment groups,[10,41] most of the relevant information derives from comparative studies. One striking illustration may be seen in detailed comparisons of the bonnet and pigtail macaques.[34,37]

The pigtails, studied in the laboratory in social units of unrelated individuals, form rather hostile groups in which animals rarely sit or sleep close together. The infants are zealously guarded by their mothers and in the early months rarely have contact with other adults. The mothers, in the early weeks, not only prevent others from contacting their baby, but initially restrain the efforts of their infants to leave. Even as the infant grows more competent, the pigtail mother retrieves it frequently as it attempts to run and play about the pen. As the time for rebreeding approaches (when the infant is four to five months old), the pigtail mother begins active, often punitive weaning and removal of the infant from her body. Such rejections last for varying periods of time. It is not until the infant reaches eight or nine months of age that this "punitive deterrence" abates.

In comparison, bonnet macaques rapidly form close, gregarious groups in which members often intertwine while resting and sleeping in close contact. When infants are born this adult pattern remains undisturbed, and from the first day of life onward the infants are the frequent object of communication and contact by many others in the group. As the bonnet infant matures, the mother, although protective when necessary, is typically passive to its comings and goings, neither preventing nor actively encouraging its departure.

In terms of the concepts described above, as a result of the inconsistency of maternal response and the limitations on their range of social and environmental experience early in life, the pigtails might be expected to develop more anxious "attachments" than their bonnet counterparts, and should therefore show the more severe responses to loss. This has indeed been the case. In numerous studies[12,29,32] pigtails have often shown very severe depression following loss, while bonnets rarely show the most extreme forms of negative response.[13,24,37] Bonnet infants often pass through the loss period relatively unscathed, whether they are "adopted" by others or not.[32]

Further support for the influence of the security provided by the attachment bond has been obtained in other recent research on bonnet macaques.[38] In an effort to determine the effects of maternal "employment" on mother-infant relations and infant development, "working" bonnet mothers were required to spend a portion of their day searching for food, which was hidden within specially constructed "foraging devices." Control mothers, living in identical pens, had their food provided for them without any work required. During the course of early development, the infants of the foraging mothers appeared to be functioning more independently than the infants in the no-work group. They were apart from their mothers more and for longer periods. Although weaned somewhat more than the infants in the other group, the forager infants were not dramatically or consistently rejected by their mothers, at least during laboratory observations. However, the normal equanimity of bonnets was quite disturbed in the work group. More overt hostility and less gregarious behavior were observed. The group situation was clearly more tense.

Nonetheless, when pairs were separated it was the infants of the foraging mothers that showed the most severe reactions (including depression) and were the slowest to recover even nominally normal functioning. It seems reasonable to suggest that the mothers required to spend a portion of their day preoccupied with their search for food were often not as available to their infants as the control mothers were. Indeed the records showed that the foraging mothers generally were engaged in active foraging when their infants were out of contact. The requirement that the mother share time between the infant's care and other survival needs, coupled with the decreased friendliness of the social group, may well have left the infants less secure in their attachment to their mothers and less able to learn the skill and approaches necessary to cope with the requirements of the surrounding environment.[26]

In recent research in which bonnet mothers and infants lived in environments where the work requirements (of foraging) changed repeatedly over time, the social group became increasingly aggressive. Mother bonnets became unusually rejecting of their infants as they became more distressed themselves. The infants, forced to spend periods of time apart from the mothers, showed increasing disturbance, in some cases culminating in the repeated expression of the full depressive pattern. In some ways this debilitating response duplicated the reactions of the pigtails to the repeated returns of the "lost" and rejecting mother. As in the case of their reinvoked depressions, these apparent "loss patterns" in the presence of a psychologically unavailable figure alert researchers to the continuity of emotional responses between a pre-loss and loss period.

It appears from these comparative data that in nonhuman primates, and presumably in humans beings, many of the types of behavior that are clearly recognized as emotional responses to loss may appear in various degrees and configurations as part of the ongoing pattern of interaction prior to the final loss experience.[47]

Artificial Mother Surrogates

Although it has been clear since the early work of Harlow that monkeys can form very strong emotional attachments to artificial mother surrogates that embody certain specific stimulus characteristics, new evidence makes clear that these attachments differ from those formed toward biological mothers. Although a surrogate may offer emotional support during rearing, the loss of this object does not impair the functioning of a young infant to the same degree that loss of a biological mother does. This important difference in the response to loss has now been demonstrated in rhesus,[20] pigtail,[28] and squirrel[19] monkeys.

What is there about the relationship of infant and surrogate, as compared to infant and mother, that results in less severe response to loss? Two factors seem relevant. First, the security of the relationship depends in part on the reliability and consistency of the responses of the caretaker. Second, the nature of the infant's experience with the non-maternal environment depends, at least in part, on the affective state of the infant during encounters with the outside environment.

In the case of the surrogate mother, there can be no questions of consistency or availability. Thus, there is the possibility of a rather secure attachment being formed. Moreover, within the confines of the relatively simple environments in which surrogate-rearing usually occurs, the infant is free to explore and contact its environment whenever it feels comfortable doing so. It may return to the consistently available surrogate when its level of arousal or fear becomes too great and may return once again when it feels comfortable. From a variety of perspectives, an individual's opportunities to learn how to deal effectively with the requirements of its environment will be affected by the individual's emotional status at the time of potential learning. The more complex the situation, the more significant the role of the emotional state. Thus it seems reasonable to suggest that the relatively securely attached surrogate infants, having had the most opportunity to learn the nature of their cage environment to best advantage, may be expected to fare better than infants raised by biological caretakers, at least when tested "at home."

Response of Older Subjects to Loss

Nonhuman primate research on the effects of a disruption of social bonds in subjects older than about one year of age has not progressed as far as the work on early infant–mother separation. It does appear clear, however, that nonhuman primates show some evidence of emotional disturbance after the loss of a close partner at virtually all ages tested. For example, monkeys raised in so-called "nuclear families" have been shown to be markedly disturbed following separation from their family units at three, four, and even five years of age, which is well after puberty.[21] Similarly, three-year-old, peer-reared rhesus monkeys have shown very marked depressive behavior after repeated separations from their lifetime partners.[23] Finally, there are suggestions of depression in adult female pigtails after the loss of a close associate,[27] and transient emotional changes do occur in mothers after loss of their infants, although in general these responses are often rather limited.

EFFECTS OF THE SEPARATION ENVIRONMENT

The primary focus of most of the early work on separation has been the effects of the "loss" per se. In certain respects, too little attention was paid to how the nature of the separation environment might have influenced the individual's capacity to deal effectively with the loss. Consequently, at times there has been a confounding of the loss experience with simultaneous alterations in the social or physical environment. It has now been clearly established that the circumstances in which the grieving individual must function markedly influence the response to loss.

Social Environment

A number of studies of bonnet macaques,[37,38] squirrel monkeys,[4,36] pigtails,[32] and langurs[5,6] have indicated that when an infant is able to receive substitute caretaking from some other member of the group, the overt disturbance of behavior following loss of the mother is markedly reduced or even eliminated almost completely. This ameliorative effect of substitute care-giving in nonhuman primates fits well with the general experience with human infants under comparable circumstances.[2]

In general, there is an indication that the impetus to "adoption" often lies with the infant,[6] and that this capacity to move to others and to transfer filial responses to a foster care-giver may be a crucial coping skill for dealing effectively with the loss experience. The target of the transfer of attachment behavior does not seem to be rigidly fixed, as infants have been shown to shift to other females, adult males, juvenile siblings, other peers, other species,[17] and artificial surrogates after the loss of mother.

If they occur immediately after the separation, these transfers of attachment may preclude both the initial protest behaviors as well as the subsequent despair patterns. Initial vocalizations in squirrel monkeys are virtually eliminated when separation occurs in the presence of an "aunt" (already a partial caretaker of the infant) who immediately accepts the infant. Even the sensitive indicator of infant affect—social play—may show insignificant changes during separation if the infant has been adopted. As these foster relationships continue past a week or two, the new attachments may become so strong that the infant will fail to return to the biological mother when she is returned to the group.

The nature of the infant's familiarity with the other animals appears to be important even if an actual "adoption" does not occur. In one case, for example, a bonnet infant separated from its mother and all other members of its own species but left with several pigtails with whom it had been living showed a marked depressive response to separation. As noted earlier, bonnets left in more supportive groups of their own species generally show minimal disruption of behavior following loss of the mother. Similarly, there is an indication in rhesus monkeys that infants left with familiar peers are less emotionally disturbed following separation than those left with unfamiliar peers.[45]

Physical Environment

Current data make it clear that when separation is confounded with the transfer to a novel environment, the pattern of response is altered. Unfamiliar environments appear to increase and prolong initial protest reactions of the infant and either delay or ameliorate subsequent despair behavior.[8,9] Similarly, when surrogate-reared squirrel monkeys are separated from the surrogate, only when they are simultaneously placed into a novel environment do they show marked emotional distress (reflected particularly in their hormonal stress response[46]).

There is now reason to believe that the requirements of the environment, if appropriately tailored to the capacities of the infant, may actually facilitate recovery following loss of the mother. In a recent study of pigtail macaque infants,[25] subjects were reared by their mothers in a no-work environment. In a series of separations from their mothers, however, these infants either were required to spend several hours a day digging for their food in a layer of sawdust on the floor or were provided their food freely. During the separations in which work was required, infants showed diminished symptoms of emotional distress and depression. Most important, this easing of disturbance occurred not only during the actual foraging activity, but also carried over to the remaining part of the day as well.

It is not simply a matter of "work" per se, or work effort exclusively, that might prove beneficial under these circumstances. It may be that any focused activity that the infant is motivated to engage in and that it can perform successfully would serve as well or better than the foraging task.

Suggestions from the Environmental Data

Available information suggests ways to lessen the intensity of the inevitable emotional response to loss and to increase an individual's capacity to overcome problems and return to effective functioning. It is clear from the data on nonhuman primates that the more familiar a subject is with the setting confronted following a loss and the more supportive the individuals within it are, the less severe the sustained emotional response will be and the more rapid the recovery. Furthermore, individuals confronted with a readily accomplishable and rewarding task may show fewer behavioral difficulties after a loss. In a broad sense, both the "coping" skills brought to the loss experience that are specific to the characteristics of the surrounding environment, and the individual's past successful experiences coping with a variety of situations prior to separation, markedly affect the severity of a bereavement.[15]

RESEARCH RECOMMENDATIONS

Much of the current evidence argues against earlier views[11,40] that the nominal "phases" of protest, despair, and detachment are "phases of a single process"[2] inevitably tied to one another as a result of evolution. The patterns of behavior, characterized more by an intersubject and intersituational variability than by consistency, are perhaps best studied from the "coping" perspective on separation phenomena that has been developed by Levine and his associates.[4] In this view, it is the infant's active efforts to cope with the imposed loss, both in terms of behavioral and physiologic responses, that are seen in each phase of the loss pattern. These efforts are shaped largely by the social and physical circumstances during the loss period, not by a prior evolutionary history of adaptation to loss per se. This view also stresses the importance of prior experience with the attachment figure and the prior environment, which are seen as affecting the capacity of the subject to cope with or strategically adapt to suddenly altered conditions. These environmental features, as well as the contingent, interactive qualities of past experience, may reveal the factors controlling the severity and extent of a bereavement and the types of intervention that can ameliorate the potentially disastrous effects of the loss.

Although research on the response to loss of significant partners has shown considerable progress during the past two decades, in many areas researchers have just begun to examine a number of important issues. Pursuit of these topics in further animal studies is sure to enhance researchers' growing understanding of the bereavement process in human beings and help them to distinguish among the numerous interacting factors that are often confusingly interwoven at the human level.

The data base on response to loss throughout life and on continuities or changes in the patterns of response in different groups should be expanded. Moreover, data on the effects of early loss upon emotional response to subsequent social disruptions are extremely limited and must be increased through longitudinal studies. Again, the advantages of the nonhuman primate models here are obvious, as the pace of maturation allows for examination of these continuities and discontinuities across a life span of manageable length.

A wider variety of social partnerships needs to be studied in the context of the loss experience. How do sibling, peer-peer, peer-adult, and adult-adult relationships parallel or differ from the infant-mother bonds that have been the subject of extensive study? How are these differences reflected in patterns of behavior after loss of the specific partner?

Given current thinking about the effect of the availability and contingent responsivity of a partner on the initial bonding and subsequent response to loss, more detailed observations prior to loss are needed. This might help account for at least some of the notable variation in the form and extent of the capacities needed to handle the trauma of loss.

It is now clear that in a number of ways the social and physical environment in which adaptation to loss must occur significantly influences the bereavement reaction. Further studies can investigate the factors that promote or retard the support of other individuals for the grieving subject, as well as the environmental factors that may facilitate recovery or exacerbate the negative responses of various individuals. What features engage the subject productively? What features overwhelm the already disturbed individual?

That these same questions arise in discussions of the human experience points to the importance of following current leads under the controlled conditions obtainable in animal research.

REFERENCES

1. Abrams, P. Age and the effects of separation on infant rhesus monkeys. Paper presented at APPA meeting, Mexico City, 1969.
2. Bowlby, J. *Separation: Anxiety and Anger.* New York: Basic Books, 1973.
3. Coe, C.L., and Levine, S. Normal responses to mother-infant separation in nonhuman primates. In: *Anxiety: New Research and Changing Concepts* (Klein, D.F., and Rabkin, J., eds.). New York: Raven Press, 1981.
4. Coe, C.L., Rosenberg, L.T., and Levine, S. Endocrine and immune responses to maternal loss in nonhuman primates. Paper presented at American Psychological Association meeting Anaheim, California, 1983.
5. Dolhinow, P. An experimental study of mother loss in the Indian Langur monkey (*Presbytis entellus*). Folia Primatologica 33:77–128, 1980.
6. Dolhinow, P. Langur monkey mother loss: profile analysis with multivariate analysis of variance for separation subjects and controls. *Folia Primatologica* 40:181–196, 1983.
7. Heinicke, C., and Westheimer, I. *Brief Separations.* New York: International Universities Press, 1965.
8. Hinde, R., and Davies, L. Removing infant rhesus from mother for 13 days as compared with removing mother from infant. *Journal of Child Psychology and Psychiatry* 13:227–237, 1972.
9. Hinde, R., and McGinnis, L. Some factors influencing the effects of temporary mother-infant separation: some experiments with rhesus monkeys. *Psychological Medicine* 7:197–212, 1977.
10. Hinde, R., and Spenser-Booth, Y. Effects of brief separations from mothers on rhesus monkeys. *Science* 173:111–118, 1971.
11. Kaufman, I.C. Developmental considerations of anxiety and depression: psychobiological studies in monkeys. In: *Psychoanalysis and Contemporary Science* (Shapiro, T., ed.). New York: International Universities Press, 1977.
12. Kaufman, I.C., and Rosenblum, L.A. The reaction to separation in infant monkeys: anaclitic depression and conservation-withdrawal. *Psychosomatic Medicine* 29: 648–675, 1967.
13. Kaufman, I.C., and Stynes, A.J. Depression can be induced in a bonnet macaque infant. *Psychosomatic Medicine* 40:71–75, 1979.
14. van Lawick-Goodall, J. *In the Shadow of Man.* New York: Houghton-Mifflin, 1971.
15. Levine, S. A psychobiological approach to the ontogeny of coping. In: *Stress, Coping and Development in Children* (Garmezy, N., and Rutter, M., eds.). New York: McGraw-Hill, 1982.
16. Main, M. Analysis of a peculiar form of reunion behavior in some day care children: its history and sequelae in children who are home-reared. In: *Social Development*

in Children: Day Care Programs and Research (Webb, R., ed.). Baltimore: Johns Hopkins Press, 1977.

17. Mason, W., and Kenney, M. Redirection of filial attachments in rhesus monkeys: dogs as mother surrogates. *Science* 183:1209–1211, 1974.

18. Mayr, E. Behavior programs and evolutionary strategies. *American Scientist* 62:650–659, 1974.

19. Mendoza, S., Smotherman, W., Miner, M., Kaplan, J., and Levine, S. Pituitary adrenal response to separation in mother and infant monkeys. *Developmental Psychobiology* 11:169–175, 1978.

20. Meyer, J., Novak, M., Bowman, R., and Harlow, H. Behavioral and hormonal effects of attachment object separation in surrogate-peer reared and mother-reared infant rhesus monkeys. *Developmental Psychobiology* 8:425–435, 1975.

21. Mineka, S. Depression and helplessness in primates. In: *Child Nurturance: Studies of Development in Nonhuman Primates* (Fitzgerald, H.E., Mullins, F.A., and Gage, P., eds.). New York: Plenum, 1982.

22. Mineka, S., and Suomi, S.J. Social separation in monkeys. *Psychological Bulletin* 85:1376–1400, 1978.

23. Mineka, S., Suomi, S.J., and DeLizio, R. Multiple peer separation in adolescent monkeys: an opponent process interpretation. *Journal of Experimental Psychology* 110:56–85, 1981.

24. Paully, G., and Rosenblum, L.A. Variability of environmental characteristics and mother-infant relations. *Child Development* 55:305–314, 1984.

25. Plimpton, E. Environmental variables and the response to maternal loss. Unpublished doctoral dissertation: State University of New York—Downstate Medical Center, 1981.

26. Plimpton, E., and Rosenblum, L.A. Ecological and temporal dimensions of maternal loss in nonhuman primates. In: *The Psychology of Separation Through the Life-Span* (Bloom-Feshbach, J., and Bloom-Feshbach, S., eds.). San Francisco: Jossey-Bass (in press).

27. Rasmussen, K., and Reite, M. Loss-induced depression in an adult macaque monkey. *American Journal of Psychiatry* 139:679–681, 1982.

28. Reite, M., Short, R., and Seiler, C. Psychological correlates of maternal separation in surrogate-reared infants: a study in altered attachment bonds. *Developmental Psychobiology* 11:427–435, 1978.

29. Reite, M., Short, R., Seiler, C., and Pauley, J.P. Attachment, loss and depression. *Journal of Child Psychology and Psychiatry* 22:141–169, 1981.

30. Rhine, R., Norton, G., Roetgen, W., and Klein, H. The brief survival of free-ranging baboon infants (*Papio cynocephalus*) after separation from their mothers. *International Journal of Primatology* 1:401–409, 1981.

31. Robertson, J. Young children in brief separation: a fresh look. *Psychoanalytic Study of the Child* 26:264–315, 1971.

32. Rosenblum, L.A. Infant attachment in monkeys. In: *The Origins of Human Social Relations* (Schaeffer, R., ed). New York: Academic Press, 1971.

33. Rosenblum, L.A. Affective maturation and the mother-infant relationship. In: *The Development of Affect* (Lewis, M., and Rosenblum, L.A., eds.). New York: Plenum, 1978.

34. Rosenblum, L.A. The influence of the social and physical environment on mother-infant relations. *Annali dell Istituto Superiore di Sanita* 18:215–222, 1982.

35. Rosenblum, L.A., and Alpert, S. Fear of strangers and the specificity of attachment

in monkeys. In: *The Origins of Fear* (Lewis, M., and Rosenblum, L.A., eds.). New York: Wiley, 1974.

36. Rosenblum, L.A., and Cooper, R.W. (Eds.). *The Squirrel Monkey*. New York: Academic Press, 1968.

37. Rosenblum, L.A., and Kaufman, I.C. Variations in infant development and response to maternal loss in monkeys. *American Journal of Orthopsychiatry* 38:418–426, 1968.

38. Rosenblum, L.A., and Plimpton, E. Adaption to separation: the infant's efforts to cope with an altered environment. In: *The Uncommon Child* (Lewis, M., and Rosenblum, L.A., eds.). New York: Plenum, 1981.

39. Rosenblum, L.A., and Smiley, J. Therapeutic effects of an imposed foraging task in disturbed monkeys. *British Journal of Child Psychology and Psychiatry* (in press), 1984.

40. Solomon, R., and Corbitt, J. An opponent process theory of motivation: I. temporal dynamics of affect. *Psychological Review* 81:119–145, 1974.

41. Spenser-Booth, Y., and Hinde, R. Effects of six-days separation from mother on 18- to 32-week-old rhesus monkeys. *Animal Behaviour* 19:174–191, 1971.

42. Spitz, R.A., Anaclitic depression. *Psychoanalytic Study of the Child* 2:313–347, 1946.

43. Suomi, S.J. Genetic, maternal and environmental influences on social development in rhesus monkeys. In: *Primate Behavior and Social Biology* (Chiarelli, A.B., and Correuccino, R.S., eds.). Berlin: Springer, 1981.

44. Suomi, S.J. Social development in rhesus monkeys: consideration of individual differences. In: *The Behavior of Human Infants* (Oliverio, A., and Zappella, M., eds.). New York: Plenum, 1983.

45. Suomi, S.J., Collins, M.L., and Harlow, H.F. Effects of permanent separation from mother on infant monkeys. *Developmental Psychology* 9:376–384, 1973.

46. Vogt, J.L., and Hennessy, M.B. Infant separation in monkeys: studies on social figures other than the mother. In: *Child Nurturance: Studies of Development in Non-human Primates* (Fitzgerald, H.E., Mullins, J.A., and Gage, P., eds.). New York: Plenum, 1982.

47. Weintraub, M., and Lewis, M. The determinants of children's responses to separation. *Monographs of the Society for Research in Child Development* 42:172, 1977.

Sociocultural Influences

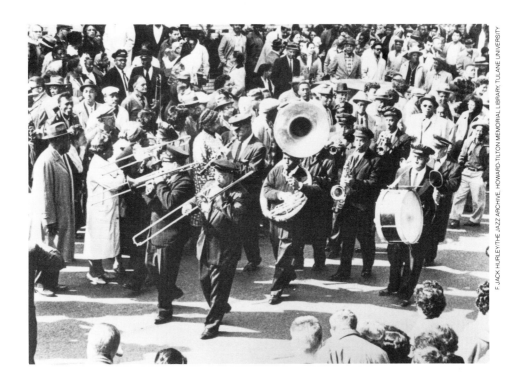

F. JACK HURLEY/THE JAZZ ARCHIVE, HOWARD-TILTON MEMORIAL LIBRARY, TULANE UNIVERSITY

Every culture has rituals to mark the deaths of its members and to assist survivors. These outward expressions of mourning may be solemn or joyous, depending on the group's beliefs about death. Pictured here is the Young Tuxedo Brass Band of New Orleans playing outside the funeral home for the crowd that mingles around the casket in the background.

CHAPTER 8

Sociocultural Influences

Bereavement is less akin to the acute experimental stress created in a laboratory (such as a film that makes viewers uncomfortable) than it is to the stress of immigrants' uprooting and acculturation. It ushers in altered social roles, a new set of interactions with individuals and social institutions, and a search for meaning.

Moreover, bereavement can be a source of distress not solely for one individual, or even a social network, but also for an entire community. Death poses a challenge or threat (at least symbolically) to the moral order and systems of ultimate meaning (religion) in society, one responded to by the institutions that maintain and authorize social reality. Hence, bereavement is a social and cultural as well as a psychobiologic phenomenon.

THE SOCIETAL CONTEXT

The social organization of bereavement practices, as well as the social reaction to death and dying, has changed in response to epidemiologic and demographic transitions. The shifts in age-specific mortality patterns and cause of death that accompanied industrialization, urbanization, and economic development altered the relationship between death and the social structures that surround it.

In preindustrial societies mortality rates were high, concentrated in the early years of life, and subject to great fluctuations due to epidemics and famines. Life expectancy ranged between 20 and 30 years. Preindus-

This chapter is based on material prepared by committee members Arthur Kleinman, M.D., Berton Kaplan, Ph.D., and Robert Weiss, Ph.D., drawing on background information prepared by committee member William Wendt, S.T.D., and consultant Maurice Eisenbruch, M.D.

199

trial societies were also organized differently, with great emphasis on kinship, joint households, and religion. Communities were small and close-knit, with each individual and kinship unit tightly integrated into a community's economic and political sphere. The death of an individual in such a social structure affected not only the surviving kin but often the entire community.[4]

Because death in such a society represented a serious loss to the community's identity and continuity, bereavement and mourning practices were highly ritualized. Funeral ceremonies lasted months—sometimes years—and the entire community participated in these ceremonial occasions. Mourning rituals in a preindustrial society reinforced and reaffirmed the group sentiments, common bonds, and social solidarity threatened by death.[9]

The contrast between that picture and modern societies is striking. Mortality rates in Western countries are now low and controlled, and degenerative diseases dominate as the major cause of death. Infant and child mortality has declined significantly while proportional mortality over age 50 has risen as life expectancy has increased.

The rise and rule of rational bureaucratic efficiency in modern society are clearly evident in what Blauner[4] calls the "bureaucratization of modern death control." Until recently, care of the dying, as well as death itself, took place in the home. Today modern bureaucratic institutions have, for the most part, not only removed death from the home, but have also effectively concealed many aspects of death and dying from patients and their families. One consequence is that survivors are less well equipped to deal with the aftermath of death.

Despite this standardization of the event of death, mourning practices in Western countries, especially in the United States, remain highly individualistic and variable. The norms and institutionalized conventions that govern these practices are less readily apparent when people live in large heterogeneous communities, in relative isolation from extended families, than in more homogeneous communities of persons who share the same ethnic and religious beliefs. A bereaved person may be unsure about how long and how much to grieve because grief is no longer shared and ritualized by the community. The mourning process in America today is supposed to be brief and private. According to Blauner,[4] "the individualization and deritualization of bereavement" lead to difficulties in adjustment because of ambiguity about the phases of, and behavior appropriate to, grieving and mourning. The lack of social prescriptions concerning mourning and bereavement may result in serious adjustment and recovery problems for the recently bereaved.

Over the years, there have been great changes in the social phasing of mourning in America. Until fairly recently, people in mourning were expected to wear dark clothes, often black, and to sequester themselves; to attend a movie a month or two after a spouse's death would be shocking. Now many feel that the opposite is true and that displaying grief in a public fashion is in bad taste. Private life is now more and more separated from public view.

All these salient characteristics of contemporary Western society, and others—such as the decline of kinship and religion, the nuclearization and high mobility of the family, a diminished sense of community, and the disengagement of the elderly—have important implications for recovery from bereavement and grief.

Although there are a variety of different cultural and religious prescriptions for mourning in the United States, social institutions today tend to be more uniform in the views they embody. These macroinstitutions—the law, the work place, funeral homes, and the medical care system—place explicit constraints on individuals' bereavement behaviors. And the attitudes underlying these institutional requirements may place implicit constraints on behavior.

Laws governing the disposal of dead bodies are designed to ensure the health of the community, yet public health legislation may be at odds with particular religious beliefs about when and how bodies should be disposed of. Because of such laws, for example, funeral homes, rather than the homes of the bereaved, have become the site of wakes.

This body of legislation has resulted in the development of specialists whose function it is to carry out the law. As recently as 100 years ago, undertakers were usually furniture makers and carpenters who built and sold coffins.[17] In the past few decades, the role of funeral directors has changed dramatically. Not only do they provide coffins, but they are trained in the technical skills of mortuary science and, most recently, as funeral "counselors." Students entering this profession must be interested in working with living people and receive some training in the psychology of grief and grief management.[31] This evolution from carpentry to mortuary science to human service profession reflects not only changes in public health laws, but also an increasing reliance on external supports as extended family and community networks have diminished in importance.

Another major change that has resulted in increased involvement of macrosocial institutions in death and bereavement relates to where people die. Most deaths now occur in hospitals or nursing homes. Thus, what happens prior to and immediately following death is likely to be governed by institutional requirements and norms of the health professions, an issue discussed in detail in Chapter 9.

Employers, through leave policies, explicitly define a legitimate period of acute mourning when people are relieved of their work obligations without penalty. Such policies, which are uniformly restrictive, may inadvertently do a disservice to the bereaved who expect themselves to be able to perform adequately after only a few days but who find they are unable to concentrate and function well.

The federal government's policy, for example, is simply that a person may use annual leave in the event of a death in the family. However, government employees may take up to three days' bereavement leave to attend the funeral of a family member who was in the military. It appears from this policy that the government believes military personnel are likely to be away from home when they die, but that others will be at home. And yet a person's elderly parents or grown children are just as likely to live far away.

Other employers, such as the National Academy of Sciences, permit a three-day leave with pay in the event of the death of an immediate family member. Additional time, if needed, may be taken as annual leave or leave without pay. As discussed at length in Chapters 2 and 3, the bereaved are unlikely to be able to function after only a few days. Thus, these leave policies are unrealistic in terms of human nature.

In contrast, at least one Japanese automaker, Toyota, has no set leave allowance and treats a death in the family as an illness that has befallen the worker. Bereavement leave is left up to the work group, with tasks being covered by the survivor's co-workers and with the understanding that the bereaved person will take as much time as needed. Similarly, public utilities in Tokyo allow two weeks' leave for a death in the immediate family.

A number of publications in recent years have criticized the so-called American way of death.[2,32,42] At this point, however, there is strikingly little information on the impact of funeral and leave practices on the bereavement process. For example, does cremation versus burial make any difference? What about the attitudes inherent in the allocation of leave time? It would seem appropriate to consider the effects of these practices on recovery.

Social Support

The concept of social support has a rich and varied set of meanings. Insofar as it suggests a stable and reliable interpersonal scaffolding that sustains an individual's morale, well-being, or functioning, the term "social support" is misleading. In reality the social ties individuals maintain not only serve to sustain their functioning but are themselves affected by that functioning. Kaplan states: "A large number of environmental and individual characteristics interact to produce a person's social support system at any one point in time [and] the nature of all these determinants changes with sequential role changes and other life events as an individual proceeds through the life cycle."[20]

In its broadest sense, social support refers to optimum personal and social integration[10] and may include the following elements:

- supportive religious and other social rituals
- supportive values and beliefs by which individuals and families are comforted
- supportive shared norms that provide "meaning"
- social networks that supply supportive needs
- the fit between the role(s) of the bereaved and the meeting of acute dependency needs at death and recovery time
- the availability and supply of nurturant others
- the availability of support that "protects" the self
- the function of self-supports in terms of the ability to seek and get support
- the availability of supportive others who "permit" or elicit emotional release
- structural supports such as community, work, and the like.[21]

Four aspects of social support—enhancing self-esteem and a feeling of being loved, problem-solving, networking, and providing relationship resources for meeting life cycle transitions—are thought to modify the effects of traumatic loss and to facilitate recovery from bereavement.[7,18,21] As discussed in Chapter 3, social relationships are an important determinant of self-esteem. They may enhance individual well-being by providing "information leading the subject to believe that he is cared for and loved . . . esteemed and valued . . . [and] that he belongs to a network of communication and mutual obligations."[7] Social support also is viewed as an important factor in the coping process, because relationships provide information and problem-solving skills an individual can draw on to solve basic tasks and devise strategies for meeting life cycle transitions.[3,16,18]

In addition, as a person's life situation changes, different constellations of support may be better able to meet his needs than others; a support network that may be optimally helpful at one point in time may be dysfunctional at another time. For example, during the early phase of grief, a small, dense network is most helpful. Later on, however, such a network "may entrap the individual within a limited set of normative expectations, information, and social contacts, rather than fulfill his need to make a transition to new social roles."[44]

Thus, it is believed that social support may exert a number of important modifier effects predicting who will and who will not do well following bereavement.[6,8] As discussed in several earlier chapters, perceived social support seems to be important in deciding the course of grief and the likelihood that the individual will return to effective functioning.[35,36,43] The hypothesized link between social support and outcome has not yet been adequately tested. The perception of support has usually been measured in gross terms by a few questions about the availability of others to be with and talk to but what these supports actually are like has not been specified in detail. Nor have particular groups of people who are likely to be lacking in social support been singled out for study. For example, certain types of professionals, immigrants, and migrant workers are all geographically mobile by the nature of their jobs. When a family member dies, the only "community" that might be available for support is that of new friends and co-workers. It is not known whether this kind of social isolation automatically places such individuals at risk following bereavement.

THE CULTURAL BACKDROP

Culture exerts a significant influence on the way loss is perceived and experienced. Culture authorizes categories and norms for labeling the consequences of loss, priorities for ranking loss among other stressful life events, expectations about social support and coping styles, sanctioned idioms for articulating personal and family distress, and shared ways of regarding and responding to a death. The meaning of bereavement or other stressful life events may vary across groups with respect to who died and who is grieving.[13,26]

Cultural influences on bereavement interact with economic and other social influences that may amplify or dampen cultural effects. As intracultural diversity among members of a culture is often as great as intercultural differences, individual persons respond to loss differently, sometimes even differently from ways specified by group norms. Quite obviously, social class, economic and even sociopolitical factors will contribute (to greater and lesser extents) to negotiations of group norms guiding how bereavement ideally should be experienced and handled in particular local contexts. And there are only a limited number of ways that bereavement experiences can be socially organized.[40] Hence, there is both substantial continuity and significant variation in the bereavement experience across cultures, ethnic groups, and social classes.

The distress that death produces in a person (and group) will be articulated in more or less distinctive idioms—in one group, a particular pattern of somatization (the manifestation of emotional distress in physical symptoms); in another, through particular religious concerns; in still another, in particular social, moral, kinship, and other symbolic terms.[33] Responses to the distress will vary according to whom the group or individual regards as the locus of responsibility for coping (the individual, nuclear family, extended family, friends, co-workers, etc.); what coping styles are applied; which institutional resources are viewed as most relevant as appropriate sources of help; and how those resources are tapped and their responses assessed.[24] It is not just that different sources of support may be brought to bear but that there are distinctive cultural notions of what constitutes authorized support, how it is to be elicited, who can elicit it, and how it is to be evaluated.

With respect to cross-cultural variations in specific health consequences of bereavement, there is so little systematic research on this topic that it is only possible to speculate on what contingencies health care providers and prevention experts ought to consider. The consequences of the stress of bereavement may vary because of the genetic predisposition of particular groups, relative vulnerability of members of the culture owing to cultural and psychological processes in development, relative stressfulness of particular kinds of loss in particular cultures, differential efficacy of cultural resources, and varying categories for assessing outcome. Where there are no postbereavement expectations or categories of illness, none will be labeled as illness, even if the survivor has a poor outcome following bereavement.[38,41] Another label, such as religious or moral, will be applied.

Therefore, pathologic consequences of grieving, not surprisingly, are differentially evaluated and labeled. The contemporary Western practice of systematically looking for the health consequences of bereavement is so unusual in cross-cultural perspective (in spite of the fact that most ethnopsychological systems are aware of the more untoward outcomes) that it can be regarded as a result of Westernization.

The development of bodily complaints following bereavement (somatization), while common in the general population, appears to be even more common among ethnic minorities, especially those whose members belong predominantly to the working class and who possess relatively lower levels of education.[22] Culturally approved somatization of bereavement among ethnic group members may be particularly difficult for health providers to identify and respond to effectively.[39] It may lead to misdiagnosis; costly, potentially dangerous, and unnecessary tests; delay in appropriate referral; or multiple prescriptions of potentially toxic pharmaceutical agents—all of which are likely to be inappropriate and potentially harmful.[25]

In America's widely pluralistic society, within the same ethnic group can be found extremes of secular and sacred, traditional and modern orientation that in part reflect levels of education and Westernization. The tendency of ethnic minorities undergoing acculturation and social mobility to alter beliefs and behaviors, coupled with the wide range of intra-ethnic diversity, should caution against stereotyping behaviors in an attempt to be culturally sensitive. In addition, because it is very difficult to predict in advance whether members of a given ethnic group have maintained traditional values, modified them, or replaced them entirely with those of the dominant culture, elicitation of bereavement beliefs and norms is essential if health care providers are to determine whether such practices are relevant in a particular episode of bereavement.

Uprooting, migration, and acculturation may leave first generation members of an American minority group few traditional resources for carrying out culturally expected bereavement practices and yet not make it appropriate for them to use mainstream bereavement practices.[1,12,19] For Southeast Asian refugees, for example, funeral homes are not an expected means of dealing with death, and bereavement counseling by health professionals is unprecedented. For certain more traditional ethnic groups, kinship networks play a bigger role in all aspects of the bereavement experience than professional agencies, which may be seen as alien and intrusive.

Thus, marginality in relation to mainstream culture may result in keeping traditional practices of an adaptive kind intact or may result in barriers (economic, linguistic, cultural) to access, knowledge, and the necessary skills for dealing with the secular bureaucracies that loom larger and larger on the American bereavement scene. The most marginal people are impoverished refugee and ethnic members who are moving away from traditional resources and support systems and who have not yet arrived at assimilation of, or even access to, the mainstream cultural orientations and institutions. Impressionistic observations of the Southeast Asian refugees suggest potentially negative health consequences of the loss of indigenous cultural support systems. The effects of marginality on the bereavement process should be systematically investigated.

Somatization is not the only culturally authorized idiom of distress through which grief is articulated. Religious and moral idioms among traditionally oriented ethnic group members are at least as prevalent, and probably more so.[19,25,33] It is not known, however, whether these public manifestations of distress differ with respect to the personal health consequences of the stress of bereavement. Are some more protective of the bereaved and others less so? This is a subject worth investigating among ethnic group members and also in the mainstream population.

Idioms of distress are at least as significant for the help-seeking pathways they authorize as for the psychophysiologic processes they activate or inhibit.[30] Somatic idioms lead mourners to clinics and patienthood, while religious and moral idioms lead to quite different sources of help.[24,38,41] It is intriguing to recognize that the chief contemporary professional sources of help—funeral home directors and staff—have not been systematically assessed to determine effect on outcome. Do satisfaction, compliance, and health consequences vary not only with individual traits of the bereaved, but also with the traits, functions, and competence of "bereavement professionals"? Do bereaved members of ethnic groups have better outcomes when helped by bereavement professionals of the same ethnicity, or by professionals of different ethnicity who have been systematically trained to deal with cross-cultural problems? These are questions for which there are as yet no answers.

A list of other potential problems could be cited based on the ethnographic and clinical literatures, but in the absence of empirical research data it is best merely to point up the likelihood that cultural and ethnic aspects of bereavement, abetted by the economic and social class problems that frequently accompany ethnicity, are likely to place minority ethnic group members, especially refugees and recent immigrants, at greater risk for negative health consequences. Because both poverty and migration are associated with higher mortality and morbidity rates,[1,12] it will be difficult to detect the actual cultural contribution of ethnicity, but it is worth considering recent migration or refugee status, along with low socioeconomic status or unemployment, as placing ethnic group members at greater risk for negative health consequences of bereavement.

With respect to the mainstream middle class population, historians, social critics, and behavioral scientists have maintained that the culture of individualism, the social arrangement of close nuclear families and loose social networks, and the weakening of traditional sacred and secular rituals for responding to bereavement have all placed the bereaved under greater strain with less traditional support.[28,29] Yet no research demonstrates an increase in the scope or severity of negative health consequences from bereavement in the West at present. Comparisons of bereavement outcomes across social class and cultural lines are important precisely for this reason: as natural experiments on the impact of different social circumstances on the bereavement process and its effects.

Finally, a cultural approach to bereavement should make researchers and clinicians sensitive to their own potential bias and barriers. The mental health and medical fields tend to discount the normative and the social dimensions of experience and to provide too superficial an understanding of a profoundly existential experience. Bereavement cannot be understood without taking these aspects into account. Hence, from the cultural perspective it is important to understand the distinctive ways families and networks shape bereavement, and to search for potential cultural conflicts with professional models that are also the product of a culture: the professional subculture.

Mourning Rituals

Although the cultural forms of mourning rituals and practices vary greatly, their structure is similar. Ethnography discloses in all societies an obdurate human grain that runs through the bewildering variety of cultural forms: grieving everywhere must be *experienced*. Mourning rituals involve changes in self-concept and transition to a new stage of personal identity. Viewed in a cultural perspective, they provide for the sanctioned public articulation of private distress; the reordering of disrupted social relationships; the reassertion of threatened core cultural codes of meaning that address existential human questions; the remoralization of those demoralized and made desperate by loss; and both the reincorporation of the bereaved into the social fabric and reaffirmation of their solidarity with the group.[37,40]

Bereavement rituals order the disruptions of normal social roles so that the transitions are celebrated and thereby legitimized. The bereaved, whose transitional position in the society poses a threat to the social and moral order as much as to their own inner world, are symbolically and pragmatically escorted through these threatening stages.[15] In the vivid mythology of one Native American group, the widow, who must wear sack cloth during the bereavement period, throws off her rags at the end of mourning to display a dress in the colors of the rainbow. She is enacting her people's creation myth, which centers on the birth of the butterfly, and in the authorized symbolism of that myth her society announces she is once more available as a marriage partner and is expected to return to a normal social role.

Anthropologic findings suggest that the personal experience of grief, like the public articulation of mourning, may be quite distinctive in different social settings.[11] Puerto Rican bereaved women are expected to express their sorrow dramatically through displays of seizure-like attacks and uncontrollable emotions. Various Southeast Asian-American groups participate in public displays of wailing and open expression of sad emotion, but in private are expected to be contained and stoical, demonstrating their endurance and forebearance in the face of life's tragedies. Traditionally oriented Greek and Portuguese widows are expected to enact a lifetime role of grieving in which they demonstrate loyalty to the memory of the dead. In contrast, grief among middle class, college-educated Americans is increasingly regarded as an acute transitory stage, to be gotten through as quickly as possible with successful outcome measured in terms of developing new relations and giving up ties to the dead. Compare this with the no longer practiced but still deeply respected Hindu and Balinese traditions of ritual suicide of the wife on the funeral pyre of her dead husband as a sign of loyalty to the lasting commitments of marriage.[14]

The dominant institution in earlier times, and still one of great significance in the management of death and the rituals surrounding it, is formal religion. Among Western religions, key ritual activities for dealing with the dead have included washing the body, anointing, watching over the body, the recitation or singing of prayers, and wakes. Traditionally, these rituals assure survivors that life has gone out of the body, show respect and love for a person dear to their lives, and turn over to a transcendent reality the lives of the dead through meditation and prayer.[5,27] One of the few religious rituals that has survived in Western society in the twentieth century is the funeral. Some assert that the decline of other long-established rituals has contributed to the lack of socially acceptable guidelines to deal with dying, death, bereavement, and grief. This predicament may be worsened by mobility, as described earlier, and the resultant breakdown of neighborhoods as religious or ethnically distinct communities.

The social institutions available to recent refugees and immigrants, for example, may not be the same as those traditionally made available for bereavement. Puerto Ricans and other Hispanics in many American cities may find that churches lack Spanish-speaking clergy who can be effective in organizing expected religious rituals, like the long wake of many traditional Hispanic populations, and also that funeral homes and health care facilities neither understand nor tolerate traditional Hispanic dramatic enactments of grief. The absence or weakening of institutional resources such as traditional healers and religious experts may lead to increased negative consequences of bereavement.

Anthropologists of religion have observed that rituals are frequently very adaptive both for affected individuals and for their groups. Unlike contemporary Western culture, where rationalization, secularization, and demystification undercut this traditional work of culture, in more traditional societies and ethnic groups spiritual suffering is regarded as central to grieving and is seen not as an individual but as a group problem. Rather than being viewed as an illness, it is an occasion to assume a religious perspective on the world. The suffering is then worked through in a process involving religious rites which create an image of the deceased as an immortal and recast social relations of the living so they are no longer dependent on the deceased.[23,34]

CONCLUSIONS AND RECOMMENDATIONS

Considering the heterogeneity of American society, health and mental health professionals should use great caution in interpreting the bereavement experience of refugees, immigrants, and traditionally oriented ethnic group members as deviant because of the possibility that the norms for these groups may differ from their own and from those of the mainstream culture. Bereavement specialists should make an effort to be aware of and accommodating to alternative cultural practices for handling bereavement, and should be instructed in cultural differences in the bereavement process in an attempt to reduce the potential for cross-cultural miscommunication and iatrogenic effects.

The pluralistic cultural context of bereavement, its secularization, and the concern with therapeutic means among the relevant professions, make it understandable that individuals and families in the United States often feel uncertain about how to proceed in the bereavement process. This is an issue that should be addressed by the relevant religions and mortuary, mental health, health, and governmental agencies with respect to public education about existing knowledge and choices.

Research is needed on the various grieving experiences of ethnic group members to determine cultural norms of grieving and to lay the groundwork for determining pathology. High priority should also be given to research on the potentially greater risk for negative health consequences of bereavement among refugees, recent immigrants, and ethnic group members who experience social marginality and economic deprivation. In planning and conducting research in such communities, group members should be involved in the research process to determine risks and to plan culturally appropriate preventive and therapeutic interventions.

REFERENCES

1. Ahmed, P.I., and Coelho, G. (eds.). *Uprooting and Migration.* New York: Plenum, 1981.

2. Becker, E. *The Denial of Death*. New York: Free Press, 1973.
3. Billings, A.G., and Moos, R.H. The role of coping responses and social resources in attenuating the stress of life events. *Journal of Behavioral Medicine* 4:139–157, 1981.
4. Blauner, R. Death and social structure. *Psychiatry* 29:378–394, 1966.
5. Bowman, L. *The American Funeral*. New York: Landmark, 1973.
6. Broadhead, W.E., Kaplan, B., James, S.A., Wagner, E.H., Schoenback, V.J., Grimson, R., Heyden, S., Tibblin, G., and Gehlback, S.H. The epidemiological evidence for a relationship between social support and health. *American Journal of Epidemiology* 117:521–537, 1983.
7. Cobb, S. Social support as a moderator of life stress. *Psychosomatic Medicine* 38:300–314, 1976.
8. Dean, A., and Lin, N. The stress-buffering role of social support. *Journal of Nervous and Mental Disease* 165:403–417, 1977.
9. Durkheim, E. *The Elementary Forms of Religious Life* (1915). Glencoe, Ill.: Free Press, 1947.
10. Durkheim, E. *Suicide* (1899). Glencoe, Ill.: Free Press, 1951.
11. Eisenbruch, M. Cross cultural aspects of bereavement and its health consequences. Paper prepared for the Institute of Medicine, Washington, D.C., 1983.
12. Eitinger, L., and Schwarz, D. (Eds.). *Strangers in the World*. Bern, Switzerland: Huber, 1981.
13. Geertz, C. *The Interpretation of Culture*. New York: Basic Books, 1973.
14. Geertz, C. *Local Knowledge*. New York: Basic Books, 1983.
15. van Gennep, A. *The Rites of Passage* (1906). Chicago: University of Chicago Press, 1960.
16. Gore, S. *The Influence of Social Support in Ameliorating the Consequences of Job Loss*. Unpublished dissertation. Ann Arbor: University of Michigan, 1973.
17. Haberstein, R.W., and Lamers, W.M. Early american funeral undertaking. In: *The Individual, Society and Death* (Berg, D.W., and Daugherty, G.G., eds.). Baltimore: Waverly Press, 1972.
18. Hamburg, D., Adams, J.E., and Brodie, H.K.H. Coping behavior in stressful circumstances. In: *Further Explorations in Social Psychiatry* (Kaplan, B.H., Wilson, R.N., and Leighton, A.H., eds.). New York: Basic Books, 1976.
19. Harwood, A. (Ed.) *Ethnicity and Medical Care*. Cambridge: Harvard University Press, 1981.
20. Kaplan, B.H. Toward further research on family and health. In: *Family and Health: An Epidemiological Approach* (Kaplan, B.H., and Cassell, J.C., eds.). Chapel Hill: Institute for Research in Social Science, University of North Carolina, 1975.
21. Kaplan, B.H., Cassell, J.C., and Gore, S. Social support and health. *Medical Care* 15:47–57, 1977.
22. Katon, W., Kleinman, A., and Rosen, G. Depression and somatization. *American Journal of Medicine* 71:127–135, 241–246, 1982.
23. Keyes, C.F. The interpretive basis of depression. In: *Culture and Depression* (Kleinman, A. and Good, B.J., eds.). Berkeley: University of California Press, forthcoming.
24. Kleinman, A. *Patients and Healers in the Context of Culture*. Berkeley: University of California Press, 1980.
25. Kleinman, A. Neurasthenia and depression. *Culture, Medicine and Psychiatry* 6:117–190, 1982.
26. Kleinman, A., and Lin, T.Y. (Eds.) *Normal and Abnormal Behavior in Chinese Culture*. Dordrecht, The Netherlands: Reidel, 1981.

27. Lamm, M. *The Jewish Way in Death and Mourning*. London: Jonathan David, 1969.
28. Lasch, C. *Haven in a Heartless World: The Family Besieged*. New York: Basic Books, 1977.
29. Lifton, R.J. *The Broken Connection*. New York: Simon and Schuster, 1979.
30. Lin, T.Y., Tardiff, K., Donetz, G., and Goresky, W. Ethnicity and patterns of help seeking. *Culture, Medicine and Psychiatry* 2:3–13, 1978.
31. Martin, E.A. *Psychology of Funeral Service*. Grand Junction, Colo.: Colorado Printing, 1977.
32. Mitford, J. *The American Way of Death*. New York: Simon and Schuster, 1963.
33. Nickter, M. Idioms of distress. *Culture, Medicine and Psychiatry* 5:379–408, 1981.
34. Obeyesekere, G. Depression, Buddhism, and the work of culture in Sri Lanka. In: *Culture and Depression* (Kleinman, A., and Good, B.J., eds.). Berkeley: University of California Press, forthcoming.
35. Parkes, C.M., and Weiss, R.S. *Recovery from Bereavement*. New York: Basic Books, 1983.
36. Raphael, B. *The Anatomy of Bereavement*. New York: Basic Books, 1983.
37. Reid, J. A time to live, a time to grieve: patterns and processes of mourning among the Yolngu of Australia. *Culture, Medicine and Psychiatry* 3:319–346, 1979.
38. Rosaldo, M. *Knowledge and Passion*. Cambridge: Cambridge University Press, 1981.
39. Rosen, G., Kleinman, A., and Katon, W. Somatization in primary care. *Journal of Family Practice* 14:493–510, 1982.
40. Rosenblatt, P.C., Walsh, R.P., and Jackson, D.A. *Grief and Mourning in Cross-Cultural Perspective*. Washington, D.C.: HRAF Press, 1977.
41. Schieffelin, E.L. *The Sorrow of the Lonely and the Burning of the Dancers*. New York: St. Martins Press, 1976.
42. Stannard, D.E. *Death in America*. Philadelphia: University of Pennsylvania Press, 1974.
43. Vachon, M.L.S., Sheldon, A.R., Lancee, W., Lyall, W.A., Rogers, J., and Freeman, S.J.J. Correlates of enduring distress patterns following bereavement: social network, life situation and personality. *Psychological Medicine* 12:783–788, 1982.
44. Walker, K.N., MacBride, A., and Vachon, M.L.S. Social support networks and the crisis of bereavement. *Social Science and Medicine* 11:35–41, 1977.

Roles of Health Professionals and Institutions

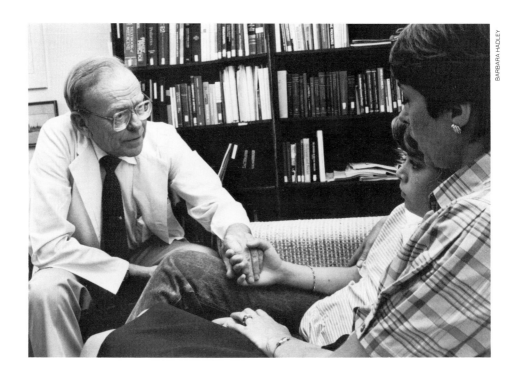

BARBARA HADLEY

Health care professionals have an obligation to family members of terminally ill or recently deceased patients. To carry out this role responsibly, they should be able to communicate about sensitive issues, to understand the nature of normal and abnormal bereavement reactions, and to be knowledgeable about community resources to which the bereaved can be referred for specialized help if needed.

CHAPTER 9

Roles of Health Professionals and Institutions

Although grief is not an illness, health professionals and health care institutions have important roles to play in caring for the bereaved, both before and after the death of a patient. One hundred years ago, most people were born and died at home; now most are born and die in a hospital. The widespread perception of hospitals as bureaucratic, impersonal institutions gives people the impression that the psychosocial needs of dying people in hospitals are often underserved, that families are provided no regular help in understanding and coping with death, and that the capacity for compassion has been lost in a technologically oriented, strange world.[15,42]

A recent editorial in the *British Medical Journal*[10] pointed out that the failure of care-givers to respond to families' needs for reassurance and information has been fostered by increasing fears of malpractice actions as well as by physicians' inabilities to deal with their own failures. However, several concrete, helpful suggestions were made:

> First, . . . medical students and young doctors must be taught how to give help and comfort to the relatives of patients who have died. . . . Secondly, consultants and general practitioners should recognize and accept an obligation to talk to the relatives

This chapter is based on material prepared by Morris Green, M.D., chairman of the study committee, from background papers by committee members Eric Cassell, M.D., Jimmie Holland, M.D., Ida Martinson, R.N., Ph.D., Jack Medalie, M.D., and Joan Mullaney, D.S.W., and by Catherine Low of Memorial Sloan-Kettering Cancer Center, New York.

whenever there is an unexpected death.... An interview should be offered—not every relative has the courage or the social skills required to ask for one—and its prime purpose should be to give comfort and answer questions. ... Finally, [we] must not let lawyers set our priorities.... Most relatives simply want to know what happened.

That Americans want such issues to receive more attention is evidenced by the grass-roots development of the primary care and hospice movements and by the establishment of numerous support groups to assist the bereaved (discussed further in Chapter 10). In no small part, these have come about because of the shortcomings of traditional medical settings in meeting emotional needs. With the increased emphasis on patients' perceptions of illness and death, quality of life, and medical ethics, more hospitals are beginning to acknowledge a responsibility for providing emotional support that traditionally rested with families and chaplains. However, the nature of an institution's responsibility to survivors, once the immediate concerns surrounding a death have been dealt with, is unclear.

In recent years there have been striking improvements in the care of dying people and their families. Yet family care following bereavement is still generally meager.[23] (The terms "family" and "relatives" are used in this discussion in their broadest senses, to describe the people most affected by an individual's death, although it is worth noting that these individuals are not necessarily related to the patient through birth or marriage.) Limitations in the attention paid to the bereaved by health care professionals appear to derive from three factors: (1) their inadequate training about the nature of bereavement and their own personal feelings toward death; (2) the failure of health care institutions to acknowledge their responsibility for bereavement follow-up, the stress that caring for dying and bereaved persons puts on their staff, and the need for sufficient staff time for these activities; and (3) the financial constraints imposed by the current structure of third-party reimbursement arrangements.

Despite currently inadequate therapeutic guidelines, however, it is necessary for health professionals to formulate some approach to the bereaved because, whether they are trained or untrained, those who interact with a bereaved person will have an impact—negative or positive—on that individual. This chapter offers practical guidance on professional and organizational practices based on humane considerations, professional norms, and the experiences and informed judgment of the committee.

The contributions of individual health professionals to the bereaved depend on the organizational setting in which they work; the religious, psychosocial, and cultural characteristics of the bereaved; the individual characteristics, interest, competence, accessibility, and availability of the professional; and the nature of his or her relationship with the bereaved. Although the exact nature of the assistance given following death varies, several professional tasks following bereavement can be identified:

- information and education, with sensitivity to what people seem to want to know
  - emotional support
  - clinical recognition of abnormal bereavement reactions
  - management and appropriate referral to mental health resources
  - legitimization of the occurrence of death, so that the bereaved are assured that all therapeutically appropriate measures were attempted.

ROLES DURING THE DYING PERIOD

More than 80 percent of the deaths in the United States occur with at least several weeks' warning,[43] and in most cases health care professionals will have been involved.[26] Whether death occurs at home or in an institution, there is a period during which health professionals have multiple opportunities to help the soon-to-be-bereaved.[13,29] Staff members' professional competence and the sincerity and consideration they show toward a patient and his or her family can help the bereaved cope with their grief when the patient dies.[33] By ensuring that the patient and family are made as comfortable as possible during this generally difficult time, staff members establish themselves as people who will help the survivors.

Families usually turn to both physicians and nurses for information about the illness and its management and for assurances that "everything has been done." Because of the many professionals actively involved in the care of gravely ill patients, relationships with any one health professional—doctor, nurse, or social worker—are often poorly defined. In the committee's view, it is important that there be one identifiable health professional who the family knows is responsible for overseeing care and to whom they can turn for support and information. Even in the complex teams of health professionals that care for patients in some institutions, that person most often is a physician. The family should know that person's name, and the rest of the team should be aware of who has that central role. In addition, the primary care physician who cared for the patient prior to admission to the hospital should remain informed about the patient's status and responsive to the family's need for reassurance and information.

Although physicians usually direct patient care activities, in some settings (especially at home and in nursing homes) families may relate most closely and comfortably to a nurse. For this reason the primary nurse should be present when relatives are told that an illness seems to be in its final stage or when the nature of a medical or surgical problem is discussed. The nurse is then fully knowledgeable when the family later asks questions or if it becomes evident that they did not hear or understand the implications of what a physician said. Clear explanations of the cause of the death may prevent misconceptions and self-blame by the bereaved.

Although an institution's responsibility to provide the family with information on the patient's condition is clear, doing so has often proved difficult because the general public is so unfamiliar—and health professionals are so very familiar—with hospital routines and the intricacies of medicine. People are often afraid to question a physician, fearing their confusion or uncertainty will be interpreted as lack of trust. Often, too, they may need help in identifying and formulating their questions. Although these problems are frequently cited in the literature, few detailed solutions have been proposed, suggesting that this is an area in need of much attention.

One project that addresses this problem is the Surgical Nurse Counseling Program[46] at the Memorial Sloan-Kettering Cancer Center in New York. Nurse-counselors visit patients the afternoon before surgery to find out what information each patient wants transmitted to relatives during the surgery. Providing a direct link to the operating room and the surgeons through their rounds of the operating rooms, the nurses carry progress reports to those in the waiting room. Since they are seen as sympathetic and supportive, the nurses also often become aware of misconceptions and fears that may distort a family's understanding of the illness and the surgery. By clarifying the situation and answering questions as they arise, they can help relatives understand what the physician has already told them.

It is increasingly accepted that the care received by a dying patient should facilitate the resolution of relations between patients and those close to them. For this to occur, several goals must be pursued. The first is to allow a smooth and emotionally complete separation at the time of death. Communications between patients and those close to them should be facilitated so that both patient and family know, as much as possible and desirable, the diagnosis and when death is to be anticipated. In the increasingly rare situations where, because of the patient, the family, or the circumstances, precise communication is not possible, the need for reconciliation or other emotional tasks can be conveyed metaphorically.

The physical setting also influences the opportunities to be close to the dying patient. Consequently, increased length and convenience of visiting hours, open access of family to the patient's bedside, and reduced intrusiveness of medical procedures and hospital bureaucratic concerns can all increase the ability of the family to visit the patient. Although health professionals do not directly control many of these matters, they may have considerable influence in easing access to the patient.

The vital fact that must be remembered is that the well-being of the family and others close to a dying person is part of health professionals' responsibility in terminal illness. Naturally, there are limits to that responsibility, and problems arise when the needs of the family and those of the patient conflict. It is generally held that in such cases the primary responsibility of care-givers is to the patient. Here, as in other circumstances, compromise and open discussion often allow conflicts to be resolved. Physicians and nurses will help family members say goodbye in a smooth and fulfilling way when they understand that the family must be permitted to spend as much time as possible at a bedside and that saying goodbye is important for each person.

Unfortunately, the needs of the family are sometimes viewed as obstacles to the essential activity of caring for a patient's disease. Although a family's needs may, on occasion, intrude in the care of a dying patient, physicians, nurses, and social workers must set new goals that include the well-being of the surviving family. Where the outcome is uncertain, as in high-risk myocardial infarction, conflicting responsibilities may be more difficult to resolve. When a realistic chance at meaningful survival exists, current attitudes give the patient's welfare highest ultimate priority.

In addition to facilitating a smooth separation from a dying patient, health care workers should, as much as possible, help relieve survivors of the guilt that often accompanies bereavement. Although the source of this guilt is unclear, its presence is ubiquitous. Nurses and physicians have the opportunity to lessen the reality-basis of survivors' guilt. The newly bereaved should leave a deathbed with the faith that they and the medical staff have done the right thing for the person who died. Health professionals should help diminish the occasions for survivors to blame themselves or the medical and hospital staff. To accomplish this, family members must be kept informed as care progresses and be permitted to take part in decision making whenever possible. They should understand the reasons for important medical actions and realize that the physicians and nurses care as much about the relief of suffering as they do. A family should not be overprotected with undue optimism or false hopes. Rather, to the degree possible, the family should be made aware of forthcoming risks and complications.

Family rivalries often surface and intensify at the bedside of a dying parent. It is impossible for the hospital staff to resolve at the deathbed problems that may have occupied the family for years. It is feasible, however, to insist that everyone be notified, that every family member have a chance to visit and say goodbye, and that appropriate family members partake in, or have access to, the decision-making process when possible. Great diplomacy may be required in such situations.

While facilitating separation and removing as many grounds for future guilt as possible, care-givers must take care not to overburden family members. Compared with obligations to a dying person, which may be perceived as boundless, family members may see their own needs as selfish. Health professionals should encourage families to place reasonable limits on what they expect of themselves and on the degree to which they are exposed to painful sights, smells, and sounds. Because people vary in their ability to tolerate the physical unpleasantness of dying, there can be no hard and fast rules. It is best to err on the side of protection, but to be as flexible as possible about the behavior of individual family members. The custom, followed in many hospice units, of giving visitors one day off a week is a wise one and might guide care-givers in their advice to the family. Parents whose child is dying may not wish to take a day off, but even in this case the aim should be to avoid a family member being so worn out in advance that the person has no reserves left to cope with the death itself.

PRACTICES AROUND THE TIME OF DEATH

Death occurs in many different ways and places, with varying consequences for those left to grieve. Patients die after long illnesses and many hospitalizations or after multiple problems develop with old age. Some die in the operating room, in the recovery room, or on the ward following surgery. The special care or intensive care unit, coronary care unit, and the emergency room are sites of maximal available technology for critical patient care, yet usually have minimal "technology" for emotional support.

It is particularly important that relatives have the opportunity to be present at the actual time of death.[11] They usually feel that they ought to be there. If desired, family members should be able to spend some time privately in the room after the patient dies. If no relatives are present at the time of death, it is imperative that they be informed promptly by someone who cared for the patient (and who knows the family), and that the body not be moved to the morgue until after the family has had the opportunity to see the deceased.

Guidance provided at the time of death may help prepare the bereaved for the often lengthy grieving process, for possible emotional reactions, and for physical symptoms they may experience in the subsequent months. Being forewarned may lessen anxiety if such reactions do occur.[24,38] In addition, by offering the family the opportunity for a later appointment to discuss questions that might come to mind, health professionals make it clear that they are not indifferent to relatives' feelings, that they are available for support, and that they are sensitive to the fact that the shock of death may preclude people's ability to express all their questions and uncertainties immediately.

Although health care institutions have been thought of as insufficiently responsive to patients' and families' needs around death and bereavement, administrative personnel are beginning to acknowledge their responsibility in these areas. To provide support for both family and staff, some hospitals and many hospices conduct periodic nondenominational memorial services to which both the family members and the hospital personnel who care for a patient are invited. Social workers are available in many hospitals and nursing homes to discuss legal, financial, or household problems and funeral arrangements with families. These services may facilitate the process of bereavement, especially in the case of individuals who are, or who perceive themselves to be, socially isolated. Referral to a specialized support group after the death (discussed further in Chapter 10) may also be welcomed by some. Studies indicate that recovery from bereavement may be enhanced when health professionals at a hospital encourage the use of informal and formal support available through family, friends, and the community.[9,17,20,30,41]

The Special Problems of Sudden Death

Although knowledge that someone close is going to die may not measurably lessen the impact of the final loss, sudden deaths and deaths due to suicide, homicide, accident, or war can be especially shocking. If death is anticipated, relatives can be given factual information and can be prepared to some extent for the reactions likely to follow. If a patient dies suddenly, however, it is important to be alert to the needs of the stunned family on a more immediate basis, because it may be most difficult at this time for the bereaved to collect their thoughts and ask questions.

Hospitals are increasingly trying to provide support for parents whose infant dies soon after birth or with Sudden Infant Death Syndrome.[4,35,36] The parental feelings of guilt and responsibility that inevitably follow may be countered, in part, by authoritative medical information. The literature also emphasizes the importance of permitting the parents, if they desire, to see or hold a stillborn infant or a baby who dies shortly after birth.[9,17,20,40]

There are two instances in which caution is required. With some cultural or religious groups, a baby who is born dead or who does not live for at least a few days is not officially accepted into the faith. Individuals in these groups may not want to see the baby. In cases of babies born with devastating congenital malformations, such as anencephaly or cyclops abnormality, parents should not be forced to see the infant. In these situations, no clear-cut advice is possible, but parents' desires can be elicited by careful discussion. Talking with the hospital staff who cared for the baby before death is particularly important in confirming for parents that their baby really did exist, especially when other family members or friends may suggest that it would be better for everyone if the pregnancy and birth were simply forgotten.

Institutions can also structure the response to sudden death so that health care professionals do not become unduly stressed. A protocol used in the emergency room at the Children's Hospital National Medical Center in Washington, D.C., serves to alleviate confusion and lessen the emotional distress of both the staff and family. Since it may be assumed that when a child is brought to an emergency room either dead or dying, the family in crisis cannot be expected to take care of itself, some members of the staff take responsibility for informing and supporting the parents while others attend to the child.[8] The clear delineation of responsibilities for patient care, coordination, and parental support helps alleviate staff stress and confusion.

Although many sudden deaths take place in institutions, many do not. In the case of natural disasters and accidents, for example, health care professionals and institutions may become involved, but often it is the police or criminal homicide detectives who make the initial contact with families of the deceased. In the case of war casualties families are notified by the military and typically have no contact with the health care system. The way families are notified and early efforts to support the family in its grief may have significant consequences for the subsequent course of bereavement.[6] Soldiers who survive but have witnessed others' deaths in combat may need support not only from individuals but from the broader community in order to be reassured of the value of the combat. This has been an especially thorny public and personal issue for veterans of the Vietnam war.[7]

The role of community-oriented health professionals in stimulating "the development of . . . natural supportive links among members of a population exposed to acute or long-term stress" is described by Caplan[6] in the aftermath of the Yom Kippur war in Israel and by Raphael[27] following a major train wreck in Australia.

Raphael[27] describes a psychiatric intervention that was implemented in Sydney, Australia, after a bridge collapsed and crushed several railroad cars. As rescue workers were mobilized and hospitals prepared to accept the wounded, the Disaster Committee of the Australian and New Zealand College of Psychiatrists formed a team to facilitate bereavement counseling. Some members went to the city morgue to assist families in identifying the bodies, many of which were grossly disfigured. Attempts were made to learn what social support was available to each family, provide for further contact with and referral to local support groups, and arrange for material aid. Other members of the team established communication between the hospitals and persons who knew or feared that a family member had been in the accident.

Rescue work lasted two days, but follow-up psychiatric support and referral services continued for several months. Although these services were designed primarily to aid family and friends through the emotional and practical stresses of bereavement, the impact on the rescue workers at the site, the hospital staff, and the psychiatric support teams was acknowledged at a debriefing meeting held to share the stress of the long hours, the large numbers of people dealt with, the intense level of commitment, and the unusually large number of dead and mutilated bodies.

Autopsy Requests

Probably the most controversial and sensitive postdeath issue for health care institutions is the request for autopsy. The task traditionally has been assigned to the house officers with the expectation that they should make a great effort to obtain as many autopsies as possible. Perhaps as a result of the recognition that consideration for the feelings of the grieving family is crucial, an increased sensitivity in discussing this issue with families has developed. It is uniformly recommended that the responsible attending physician should make the request, unless the resident has developed an especially close and supportive relationship with the family.

When a patient dies in a hospital, the autopsy cost is covered under the third-party agreement that covers hospital costs. No such insurance is available for out-of-hospital deaths, however; thus, the family will usually have to pay the cost of an autopsy that they were unenthusiastic about in the first place. This situation probably will lead to even fewer autopsies than at present.

The many studies that document the anxiety experienced by doctors when they request autopsies underline the need to help young physicians deal with their own complex feelings about this procedure.[3,14,16] Although a family's reservations about giving permission must be acknowledged and respected, the positive aspects of an autopsy both for the family and for the advancement of medical science should be noted. For some relatives, knowledge of the precise cause or causes of death appears to help them accept the loss and assuage guilt feelings that might arise. In the case of neonatal deaths, autopsies may offer the possibility of identifying genetic or hereditary factors that could be important if another pregnancy occurs.

Requests for organ donations may also be made at this time, and, like autopsies, may serve to make families feel better. Knowing that the organs of the deceased may preserve the vision or the life of others has the potential of giving some meaning to a death.

If permission for an autopsy is granted it is important to follow through with the family when results become available, to discuss findings and answer any questions they might have.[3,16,28] This expectation of follow-up suggests that the institution has a responsibility to maintain contact with the bereaved for some time; it may also explain why physicians seek to avoid making an autopsy request, with the accompanying necessity of reviewing and remembering what they may have experienced as a "failure" on their part.

CONTINUING RESPONSIBILITIES OF HEALTH PROFESSIONALS AND INSTITUTIONS

Although medical institutions are not commonly expected to have a continuing responsibility to family members once a patient has died, the fact that there may be no one else to fulfill that function has prompted a range of experiments with institutional bereavement programs. The committee believes that health care professionals should not withdraw from this process but rather should remain involved. Because of their familiarity with death and dying, their experience with each particular dying patient, and their opportunity for a special closeness with the family, the hospital staff is in a unique position to alleviate, to some extent, the social isolation and personal distress the bereaved may experience.[8,17,30,41]

Practical support or counseling provided after a death should be responsive to the expressed concerns and needs of the bereaved. It is important to avoid inappropriate remarks such as "He's better off this way," or "If we had seen him sooner, we could have saved him."

When the bereaved find themselves experiencing the death and its aftereffects differently from what they had expected or think is normal they may become isolated from their friends and remaining family and feel threatened. Social workers, nurses, and physicians can be a powerful force in resolving some of the difficulties that may arise when survivors' experiences cannot be explained by culturally acceptable categories of reality. Based on their clinical experience care-givers can assess experiences, provide appropriate assurance that reactions are within normal bounds, or detect those that are truly abnormal.

Staff members pursuing research in relation to the deceased or the bereaved can also be helpful to families, both through the relationship that develops and, perhaps, by pointing out that the deceased and the survivors who participate in the research are able to make a contribution to scientific knowledge. Research, therefore, may have psychologic as well as scientific functions.

Although interactions between a family and health professionals are likely to decrease in intensity or to end shortly after bereavement, each group of health professionals has special skills to offer in caring for the bereaved.

Current nursing education provides a solid conceptual groundwork of knowledge about bereavement, grief, and mourning. Nurses are trained to use this knowledge in support of the bereaved in a preventive and health-promoting manner, as well as to assist them in the process of grieving for their losses and in achieving the most constructive resolution possible. They often are able to make and promote appropriate referrals or suggest other interventions.

The social work role is to maintain and enhance family solidarity at a time of crisis. Social workers regularly encourage communication among the family members most directly involved, refer people for services, and provide indirect service by fostering the establishment of support groups. The social worker may provide valuable help in locating relatives, making burial plans, notifying next of kin, and referring the bereaved to public welfare, visiting nurse, homemaker service, and other community agencies. In addition, specially trained social workers are often available for counseling and psychotherapy to help the bereaved restore personal and family equilibrium when appropriate; this function may also be performed by psychologists and psychiatrists.

After the death of a patient and the return of the family to their homes, the physician's role frequently ends with the performance of some bureaucratic procedure such as filling out the death certificate and writing a condolence letter. That is the usual scenario, particularly for institutionally based care-givers. If the family members have also been patients of the physician who cared for the patient during the terminal illness, it may not be uncommon for one or more of them to call or visit the doctor after the death. They may want to go over details of the illness, just as they did prior to the death, to make sure that they behaved correctly or perhaps to discuss something they think they should have done differently or about which they feel guilty. It is usual and necessary that the bereaved tell their story.

It has been pointed out that the physician may not be the best person to tell this story to, because he or she was directly involved, knows many of the details, and may also be grieving.[21] This difficulty can be overcome if the physician listens patiently and does not interrupt except for comments or questions designed to keep the person talking. Time constraints have also tended to limit many practitioners' patience for such interactions. Furthermore, physicians customarily direct their interviews. Since they are unaccustomed to more unstructured discussion, they may need to be specially trained to carry out such discussions comfortably and effectively. And finally, receptive listening may be difficult if the doctor feels defensive or guilty about the death.[10] It may have taken more days than it should to get the patient admitted to the hospital; there may have been delays in the start of treatment or diagnostic studies; medication errors may have occurred; there may have been pain or other symptoms inadequately relieved; and all of these problems may be ascribed to the physicians by themselves, if not by others. The physician has also suffered a loss and has the need to tell someone. Thus, for the physician to listen to the family member's recitation without interjecting comments is not a simple matter. It takes training and discipline. Physicians occasionally are certain that the family blames them for the death, although they have no concrete evidence beyond their own feelings of guilt. In such circumstances, it takes an effort of will to reach out to the family through telephone calls or letters.

The committee believes, nevertheless, that such continued contacts and telephone calls are important. They provide a concrete demonstration of concern, present further opportunities for families to raise questions, and enable a quick assessment of how the survivors are coping. Such calls may give the health professional hints of difficulties in the bereavement process or the presence of gross dysfunction. Such suspicions should be followed up by inviting the bereaved person to come in and discuss matters related to the bereavement. Except under special circumstances, referral to mental health practitioners or facilities should not be made by telephone or solely on the basis of a telephone call unless the referral is requested by the bereaved person.

Part of the continuing responsibilities of health professionals stems from recent changes in the delivery of health care. Very ill patients are increasingly being transferred to regional facilities for care. When such a patient dies, the family is often left to return home to a community that does not know what happened. It has been suggested[47] and is considered important by the committee that under such circumstances the physicians who cared for the patient in the tertiary hospital should notify the doctor in the patient's home community about the death, including details of final treatment and the nature of the death. It should be remembered that most patients had a primary care physician who remains responsible to the survivors for their health and perhaps, in their eyes, for what happened to the patient who died. This is because the primary care physician will often have been responsible for the initial diagnosis and for making arrangements for transfer to the tertiary facility. The essential point is that medical care and responsibility do not cease with the death of the patient; their focus shifts to the survivors.

In some communities, it will be appropriate to notify the public health nursing agency or visiting nurse association so that follow-up care of the bereaved can be initiated. Social workers at the tertiary care institution are usually able to provide referral to social agencies in the home community when that is necessary. Often the most effective way of assuring the continued care of the family is to ask them whom they wish contacted.

Primary care physicians (internists, family practitioners, pediatricians, and obstetricians/gynecologists) who did not take care of the deceased nonetheless play an important role for the bereaved who are their regular patients. Responsible history-taking by these practitioners should routinely include questions about recent major life changes, including bereavement. Such questions validate patients' feelings and will help to elicit their perceptions about their own or other family members' adjustment, concerns, and questions. The discussion provides an opportunity to educate the survivors about the nature of the bereavement process and to monitor their progress. Effective monitoring requires that physicians understand normal and abnormal bereavement responses and be able to make appropriate referrals as needed.[37]

As discussed in earlier chapters, although there is substantial individual and cultural variation in response to bereavement, there are a number of red flags that should signal primary care physicians and community-based nurses that a bereaved individual is having enough difficulty to warrant intervention by a mental health professional. When a pattern of increased illness in a previously well person is noted, even with no other evidence of a failure to return to full engagement in living, there may be a problem related to the process of bereavement. Increased smoking, excessive alcohol consumption, and difficulty maintaining social relationships are all possible signals of unhealthy bereavement reactions. As discussed in Chapter 8, some ethnic groups appear to be more likely than others to somatize. However, persistent somatic complaints and enduring depressive symptoms usually signal a need for help. In bereaved children, the need for help may be expressed through repeated aggressive or hostile behavior, a drop in school performance, continued regressive behavior, and somatic complaints.

When a physician or other care-giver attends a patient whose terminal illness has been long, complex, or unusually dramatic, the relationship with the family may become particularly intense. The doctor, seen in the hospital regularly or visiting or calling the home frequently, becomes a temporary family member. For the about-to-be-bereaved, the physician may be seen as a particularly strong and emotionally giving individual at a time when the family members' emotions are in turmoil and they are more aware of their own weaknesses than of their strengths. Following the death, if the doctor merely "walks out," another loss has been sustained. To remain close to the family, however, may require walking an emotional tightrope, a situation for which physicians are rarely trained.

One helpful step that health care professionals can take is to make sure the bereaved know, without question, that the professional is available for advice and help should they ever need it—and that the nature of the "need" is a personal matter that differs from individual to individual. As discussed in Chapter 3, some people may have delayed grief reactions and only feel the need for assistance many months after the loss. Whenever these reactions occur, the bereaved should not feel it necessary to have physical symptoms in order to call or visit.

Inherent in most reimbursement schemes is a strong disincentive to the kind of follow-up activities described here as being desirable. Once a patient has died, there usually is no third-party mechanism to pay for members of the person's family to consult with a health professional. Thus, in addition to the discomfort many health professionals feel in talking with the bereaved, there is the added discomfort of having to charge for this service, knowing that the cost will have to be borne out of pocket. The only alternative physicians have is to donate their time, a practice that may be constrained in some institutional settings.

One model that has been adopted by facilities serving many terminally ill patients is to fold the costs of such follow-up services into institutional overhead or daily bed-rate charges. This practice includes recognition that such services are considered a routine part of adequate patient care.

ENHANCING THE WORK OF HEALTH PROFESSIONALS

There are two broad areas in which more changes are needed to enhance and encourage the work of health professionals with the bereaved: the support that institutions give for such work and the education and training that health professionals receive.

Institutional Support

Health care institutions are increasingly recognizing that they cannot expect to provide adequate emotional support for the patient, much less for the family, unless the issues of staff stress, including personal reactions to death and bereavement and the inevitable problems of staff relationships, are acknowledged and allowances made for them in the administration's expectations. Working with dying patients and those who grieve for them presents a challenge that requires special training, adequate support systems, and a considerable amount of professional and personal maturity.[32,34,48] As Raphael's study[27] suggests, any initiative on the part of an institution to take more responsibility in aiding the bereaved must begin with an acknowledgment of the effects of death and dying on its own staff.

The choice of staff and volunteers is particularly important in high-stress areas such as emergency rooms, intensive care units, and hospices.[12] Problems for patients, family members, and personnel themselves have been observed when care-givers are psychologically unstable, uncomfortable with issues of death and grief, and unable to recognize their own limits and make referrals when their competencies are exceeded.[18,39] These issues are discussed in Chapter 10 in relation to the screening and selection of lay volunteers to work in hospice bereavement intervention programs.

Although clinicians need to recognize the boundaries of their tolerance for working with dying patients and the bereaved, stress can escalate quickly in critical care environments. Some mechanism for continually monitoring the staff's emotional response to their work should be in effect.[5,19,45] Signs of potential difficulty include an "I can't empathize any more" attitude, or over-involvement as evidenced by a "nobody can do it but me" attitude. Unusual irritability, insomnia, anorexia, overeating, temper tantrums, argumentativeness, suspiciousness, and over-attachment or hostility to a patient or family are other signs of trouble. Personal stresses such as loss, illness, or serious family conflicts, when added to work-related stress, can cause emotional fatigue. Monitoring staff for evidence of fatigue and suggesting time off, a vacation, or a temporary pullback may avoid major problems.

Apart from drug and alcohol abuse and overt mental illness, which clearly require immediate intervention, most of the problems that arise respond well to staff discussions and sharing. Regular meetings of those who work in highly stressful units should be held to discuss cases, problems, and issues. Even with experienced staff, group meetings have educational value. People can be reminded, for example, that "just listening" to a patient or colleague is an active, professional activity that may help that individual identify and deal with personal feelings or disturbing misunderstandings.

Perhaps the most frequent problem to surface in staff meetings is the unrealistic level of self-expectation common among highly skilled individuals.[39,44] The inevitable failure to live up to these self-imposed expectations often leads professionals to withdraw so that their colleagues will not observe their "failures." This withdrawal results in isolation and severely limits staff members' ability to respond adequately to their patients. Seeing the hostile or demanding behavior of the relative of a patient as part of the bereavement process rather than as a personal attack may relieve the professional of the sense of failure and isolation. The use of multidisciplinary teams with clear role definition and coordinated, shared responsibilities may also reduce individual isolation and thus lessen staff stress.

It is often reassuring in group sessions to hear that colleagues have similar feelings of inadequacy. Indeed, Beszterczey,[5] in reporting his experience as a psychiatrist responsible for both patient and staff care on a palliative care unit, suggests that changing expectations to gain a more appropriate view of the situation demonstrates a successful adjustment to highly stressful patient-care responsibilities. He notes that this may produce an increase in self-confidence that frees professional staff to experience the satisfaction of being able to attend to "the nuances of psychological support." A sense of esprit in the group also helps each member faced with a trying situation. Staff effectiveness and comfort may also be enhanced by the liaison psychiatry consultation service to help with specific cases or with staff feelings.

By encouraging and structuring support for its staff, an institution demonstrates that it is aware of and concerned about the stress inherent in working with dying patients and their families. Coordinated staff activities with clear role responsibilities, regular meetings to discuss problems and staff reactions to them, and adequate back-up from liaison psychiatry are all ways to build a supportive atmosphere for staff.

Education of Health Professionals

Recognizing that the ability to care for grieving people depends heavily on such personal factors as conscious and unconscious reactions, personality structure, family experiences, and styles of coping, the committee also believes that this capacity can be enhanced through professional education. In the same way that information helps the bereaved to understand what is happening and what to expect, concrete knowledge about bereavement assists health care providers.[2,22] Similarly, health professionals who have an opportunity to explore their own feelings regarding death prior to having to help others cope with it are more likely to provide effective and compassionate care.[1,45] Thus, health professionals should be prepared to deal with the realities of their role in bereavement through training that gives them both the necessary knowledge base and the clinical skills, adapted to the personal characteristics of both the clinician and the bereaved. These can be taught.

Relatively little time in the training of physicians is devoted to the affective aspects of the physician-patient relationship or to the personal reactions of medical students and residents to illness, death, and bereavement. Knowledge of how the individual clinician deals with anxiety, depression, grief, anger, guilt, and frustration should be a part of each practitioner's educational experience. Such awareness facilitates that physician's ability to provide effective and compassionate care. The attention paid to death and dying as part of life cycle education in family practice residency programs is to be commended as a step in the right direction.

Current social work education stresses topics relevant to these concerns. A social worker in the health field ordinarily prepares in the clinical track that emphasizes interpersonal skills in individual and group interviewing and with the goal of restoring, enhancing, or maintaining social functioning.[25] Social work curricula always include course work on dying and death using content about the physical, emotional, and social problems faced at various points in the life cycle. Schools of nursing as well as graduate nursing programs emphasize many of the concepts and skills that are necessary in settings of illness and death. The concepts of loss, grief, crisis, dying, death, and bereavement are basic to nursing curricula. So, too, are the acquisition of communication and interpersonal skills required to apply that knowledge. This training should prepare the nurse, whether hospital- or community-based, to participate in the follow-up and care of the bereaved.

The values inherent in the acute-care, crisis intervention model of care most often found in hospitals may provide a disincentive for even the best-trained health professional to exercise those skills that are most appropriate to meet the needs of the bereaved. Because of this, health and social service professionals including physicians, social workers, nurses, psychologists, and clergy may need additional training to acquire the specific knowledge and skills necessary to work with the bereaved.[31]

In summary, the education of health care professionals should specifically enhance the development of skills in an effort to attain the following goals:

- *Attentive listening.* This skill offers substantial support because it provides the bereaved an opportunity to grasp what is happening and express those concerns that may trouble or threaten to overwhelm them.
- *Continuing relationship with the bereaved.* By having a professional with whom they can form a close alliance, families may be helped to realize their potential for coping with this universal human experience.
- *Empathy with the bereaved.* Even though the bereaved's concerns and questions may not be specifically medical, they can often best be dealt with by health professionals.
- *Personal coping strategies.* Health professionals must be prepared to deal with the discomfort precipitated by upsetting events in the lives of their patients.
- *Observational skills.* The health professional should be alert to behavioral as well as physical clues to grief reactions that interfere with the bereaved person's return to full function.
- *Appropriate referrals.* The health professional should be prepared to make appropriate referrals to a mental health resource. This requires knowledge about community resources to which the bereaved can be referred and an appreciation of the particular skills of other health providers. Such supportive professional linkages—which recognize and

value the contribution of other health professionals—reduce feelings of total responsibility for the bereaved and permit appropriate professional involvement.

CONCLUSIONS AND RECOMMENDATIONS

The well-being of the family and those close to a dying or recently deceased person is part of the health professionals' responsibility. The committee believes that health care providers and institutions are professionally and morally obligated to assist the bereaved by offering support and information and by being sensitive to and knowledgeable about grief's impact. The outcome of specific practices in lessening distress or preventing pathologic grief should be studied. Currently, such practices are based largely on what seems most humane and compassionate.

To aid this support process, health professionals need training that provides them with an appropriate knowledge base and specific clinical skills. In the committee's view, it is important that these specific skills rest on the broad and solid foundations that health and mental health education and preparation for the ministry provide in order to have the proper context for understanding the impact of bereavement. Thus, the committee cannot endorse the development or certification of a new profession for ''grief counseling'' that is separate from existing health and social services.

The primary tasks for health professionals in the care of the bereaved include providing information and explanations about the medical factors that caused the death as well as legitimization of it by assuring the bereaved that everything therapeutically reasonable was attempted. The symptoms and signs that may be associated with bereavement should be anticipated, including the lengthy nature of the grieving process and the likelihood of differences in the ways grief is expressed in various ethnic groups and even by members of the same family.

Primary health professionals should monitor the process of bereavement. Visits to physicians for either illness care or health supervision provide an obvious opportunity to inquire about major life events, such as the death of a close relative or friend, during the past year or two and about the patient's adaptation to such events. Physicians, nurses, and social workers must be alert to the ''red flags'' for children and adults discussed in this report that signal the need for mental health intervention.

Clinicians should recognize the boundaries of their own professional competency and personal tolerance for the care of bereaved individuals. By helping to mobilize the bereaved person's support network of family, friends, and community and by being knowledgeable about mental health resources available to assist those whose grief is extreme, health professionals may responsibly limit their own involvement.

Health care institutions have an obligation to provide for the comfort of the family of seriously ill patients and to limit avoidable stress. Relatives should be permitted to be close to and spend as much time as is reasonable with a dying patient, including the chance to be present at the time of death. If they are not present, it is imperative that they be informed promptly of the death.

The hospital's responsibility to aid the bereaved includes an acknowledgment of the stressful effects of death and dying on hospital staff and of the impact management and organizational practices can have on staff functioning in such settings. Avoidable bureaucratic stress needs to be minimized and the staff's emotional response to their work monitored, especially in settings where deaths are likely to be sudden or frequent.

REFERENCES

1. Artiss, K.L., and Levine, A.S. Doctor-patient relation in severe illness. *New England Journal of Medicine* 288:1210–1213, 1973.
2. Barton, D., and Crowder, M. The use of role playing techniques as an instructional aid in teaching about death, dying and bereavement. *Omega* 6:243–250, 1975.
3. Bergen, L.R. Requesting the autopsy: a pediatric perspective. *Clinical Pediatrics* 17:445–452, 1978.
4. Bergman, A.B. Psychological aspects of sudden unexpected death in infants and children. *Pediatric Clinics of North America* 21:115–121, 1974.
5. Beszterczey, A. Staff stress on a newly developed palliative care service: the psychiatrist's role. *Canadian Psychiatric Association Journal* 22:347–353, 1977.
6. Caplan, G. Organization of support systems for civilian populations. In: *Support Systems and Mutual Help* (Caplan, G., and Killilea, M., eds.). New York: Grune and Stratton, 1976.
7. Card, J. *Lives After Vietnam: The Personal Impact of Military Service.* Lexington, Mass.: Lexington Books, 1983.
8. Cohen, G. D.O.A. Preliminary report on an emergency room protocol. *Clinical Proceedings* 35:159–165, 1979.
9. Cohen, L., Zilkha, S., Middleton, J., and O'Donohue, N. Perinatal mortality: assisting parental affirmation. *American Journal of Orthopsychiatry* 48:727–731, 1978.
10. Editorial. Honesty after death. *British Medical Journal* 287:1906, 1984.
11. Engel, G.L. Grief and grieving. *American Journal of Nursing* 64:93–98, 1964.
12. Frader, J.E. Difficulties in providing intensive care. *Pediatrics* 64:10–16, 1979.
13. Friedman, S., Chodoff, P., Mason, J., and Hamburg, D.A. Behavioral observations on parents anticipating the death of a child. *Pediatrics* 32:610–625, 1963.
14. Gardner, R., Peskin, L., and Katz, J. The physician, the autopsy request and the consent rate. *Journal of Medical Education* 48:636–644, 1973.
15. Glaser, B., and Strauss, A. *Awareness of Dying.* Chicago: Aldine Publishing, 1968.

16. Katz, J., and Gardner, R. The intern's dilemma: the request for autopsy consent. *Psychiatry in Medicine* 3:197–203, 1972.

17. Keller, K., Best, E., Chesborough, S., Donnelly, W., and Green, W. Perinatal mortality counseling program for families who experience stillbirth. *Death Education* 5:29–35, 1981.

18. Koocher, G.P. Adjustment and coping strategies among the caretakers of cancer patients. *Social Work in Health Care* 5:145–150, 1979.

19. Kopel, R. Death on every weekend. *Suicide and Life Threatening Behavior* 7:110–119, 1977.

20. Krein, N. Sudden infant death syndrome: acute loss and grief reactions. *Clinical Pediatrics* 18:414–423, 1979.

21. Lattanzi, M., and Coffelt, D. *Bereavement Care Manual.* Boulder, Colo.: Boulder County Hospice, 1979.

22. Linn, M.W., Linn, G.S., and Stein, S. Impact on nursing home staff of training about death and dying. *Journal of the American Medical Association* 250:2332–2335, 1983.

23. Lohmann, R. Dying and the social responsibility of institutions. *Social Casework* 58:538–545, 1977.

24. Macon, L.B. Help for bereaved parents. *Social Casework: The Journal of Contemporary Social Work* 60:558–565, 1979.

25. Mullaney, J., and Fox, R. Clinical nurse specialist and social worker. In: *Rehabilitation Services and the Social Work Role: Challenge for Change* (Browne, J., Kirlin, B., and Watt, F., eds.). Baltimore: Williams & Wilkins, 1981.

26. President's Commission for the Study of Ethical Problems in Medicine and Biomedical and Behavioral Research. *Deciding to Forego Life-Sustaining Treatment.* Washington, D.C.: U.S. Government Printing Office, 1983.

27. Raphael, B. A primary prevention action programme: psychiatric involvement following major rail disaster. *Omega* 10:211–226, 1979.

28. Reynolds, R. Autopsies—benefit to the family. *American Journal of Clinical Pathology* 69:220–222, 1978.

29. Richmond, J., and Waisman, H. Psychological aspects of management of children with malignant diseases. *American Journal of Diseases of Children* 89:42–47, 1955.

30. Rogers, J., Sheldon, A., Barwick, C., Letorfsky, K., and Lancee, W. Help for families of suicide survivors support program. *Canadian Journal of Psychiatry* 27:444–448, 1982.

31. Roskin, M. Integrating primary prevention into social work practice. *Social Work* 25:192–197, 1980.

32. Rothenberg, M. Reactions of those who treat children with cancer. *Pediatrics* 40:507–510, 1967.

33. Sahler, O.J.A. (ed.). *The Child and Death.* St. Louis: C.V. Mosby, 1978.

34. Schowalter, J. Death and the pediatric house officer. *Journal of Pediatrics* 76:706–710, 1970.

35. Schreiner, R.L. The death of a newborn. In: *Ambulatory Pediatrics III* (Green, M., and Haggerty, R.J., eds.). Philadelphia: W.B. Saunders, 1984.

36. Schreiner, R.L., Gresham, E.L., and Green, M. Physician's responsibility to parents after death of an infant. *American Journal of Diseases of Children* 133:723–726, 1979.

37. Secundy, M. Bereavement: the role of the family physician. *Journal of the National Medical Association* 67:649–651, 1977.

38. Silverman, P.R. Transitions and models of intervention. *Annals of the Academy of Political and Social Science* 464:174–188, 1982.
39. Spikes, J. Physicians' reactions to death. *Continuing Education* 10:54–64, 1979.
40. Stringham, J., Riley, J.H., and Ross. A. Silent birth: mourning a stillborn baby. *Social Work* 27:322–327, 1982.
41. Stubblefield, K. A preventive program for bereaved families. *Social Work in Health Care* 2:379–389, 1977.
42. Sudnow, D. *Passing On*. Englewood Cliffs, N.J.: Prentice Hall, 1967.
43. United States Department of Health, Education and Welfare. *Facts of Life and Death*. Washington, D.C.: U.S. Government Printing Office, 1978.
44. Vachon, M.L.S. On the suffering of caregivers in the care of the critically ill and dying. In: *Death, Suffering and Well-Being* (Levine, C., ed.). New York: Plenum, 1983.
45. Vachon, M.L.S., Lyall, W.A.L., and Freeman, S.J.J. Measurement and management of stress in health professionals working with advanced cancer patients. *Death Education* 1:365–375, 1978.
46. Watson, S., and Hickey, P. A support system for families of surgical cancer patients. *American Journal of Nursing* (in press), 1984.
47. Wessel, M.A. Primary care bereavement after tertiary care death. Paper presented at Palliative Care Conference on Bereavement: New Horizons, Philadelphia, September 1983.
48. White, L. The self image of the physician and the care of dying patients. *Annals of the New York Academy of Sciences* 164:822, 1969.

Bereavement Intervention Programs

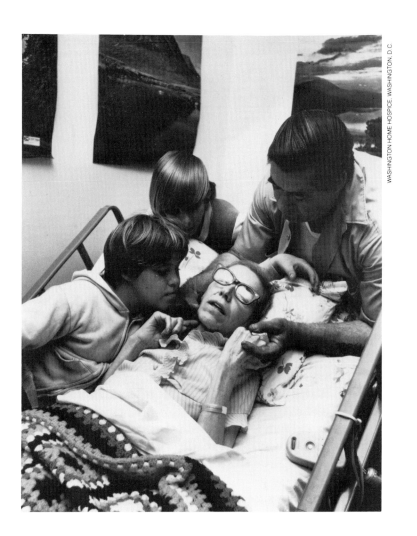

WASHINGTON HOME HOSPICE, WASHINGTON, D.C.

Hospices, many mutual support programs, and some hospitals offer support to families facing the loss of one of their members. They encourage all the members of the family, including children, to remain involved with the dying person. After the death and during the period of bereavement, new needs for support and counseling often appear.

CHAPTER 10

Bereavement Intervention Programs

The previous chapter dealt with the roles and responsibilities of health professionals in relation to the bereaved in the broad context of health care. In this chapter, the more formal bereavement programs and approaches are discussed. Many of the techniques used by mental health professionals and experienced lay care-givers to assist the bereaved are similar to those advocated in Chapter 9 as appropriate for health professionals generally. All are designed to facilitate the grieving process and to have a positive effect on outcomes.

There has recently been a tremendous increase in efforts to assist the bereaved in a variety of ways. Several explanations of this growth can be postulated. First, as discussed throughout this volume, bereavement has been recognized as a powerful, sometimes pathogenic event, both psychologically and physically. This is exemplified by emotional distress, physical symptoms, and loss of social functions in many people and by the excessive mortality, morbidity, and use of health services of some individuals. Second, there has been a growing recognition that the normal bereavement process may take at least a year for most people and often longer. Third, our society has undergone many changes that

This chapter is based on material prepared by Marian Osterweis, Ph.D., study director, from background papers by committee members Marie Killilea and David Greer, M.D., and Phyllis Silverman, Ph.D., consultant. Committee member Gerald Klerman, M.D. prepared the section on medications.

239

have an impact on the circumstances of death and the course of bereavement. As discussed in Chapter 8, for example, geographic mobility has a profound influence on the availability of social support from kin and close friends. Growing concern about limited financial resources has sparked greater public policy interest in preventive measures. And finally, as noted in Chapter 9, some professional care-givers may be ill-equipped, both emotionally and in terms of specific skills, to deal comfortably with the bereaved.

Although most persons recover capacities that had been diminished and adapt to bereavement, the intensity, magnitude, and consequences of grief have attracted the attention of a variety of institutional and individual care-givers. Some programs are designed to facilitate the normal bereavement process while others are intended to help people who are having, or who are at high risk of having, special problems or pathologic reactions to bereavement. Some are directed to the bereaved generally; others focus on people who have particular bereavement circumstances in common. Programs may be designed to help individuals, families, or groups of similarly bereaved people. Increasingly, these programs are based in institutional settings such as hospitals, health maintenance organizations, and community mental health centers. They may be implemented by experienced laypeople, who typically have been bereaved themselves, or by professionals from medicine, nursing, social work, psychology, or the ministry, who may or may not have special training to work with grief reactions.

Many different theoretical perspectives guide the training of grief workers and provide the framework for the actual programs. But whether they are formal or informal, naturally occurring or deliberate, run by peers or by professionals, the goals of all bereavement interventions include the facilitation of the grieving process and, implicitly or explicitly, the prevention or alleviation of the detrimental consequences of bereavement. The many different approaches of current programs and the overlap among the professions preclude a discrete classification of these interventions. In this chapter, four major approaches to helping the bereaved are discussed: mutual support, hospices, psychotherapy, and medication use. Bereaved persons may avail themselves of one or more of these interventions sequentially or simultaneously.

THE MUTUAL SUPPORT APPROACH

Mutual support or self-help groups are associations of people who share the same problem, predicament, or life situation and who unite for the purpose of mutual aid. This element of commonality is solely what determines inclusion in the group.[14] All decisions about content, organization, and external relationships are made by the participants.[43]

Mutual support groups provide their members with:

- person-to-person exchange based on identification and reciprocity
- access to a body of specialized information
- an opportunity to share coping techniques based on realistic expectations for optimal functioning
- an increased sense of personal worth, by focusing on how similar members are to others confronting the same situation
- reinforcement for positive change and maintenance of effort toward change through feedback on performance
- an arena for advocacy and social change
- an opportunity for education, not only of other persons with similar problems, but also professionals and the public
- an opportunity to help others by giving concrete aid and providing a role model
- help for the helpers who themselves are aided by assisting others[36] and by activism toward shared goals.[16,50]

Mutual help groups have been organized as alternative care-giving systems, as adjuncts to the professional care-giving system, and as strategic independent elements in interdependent networks of formal and informal care-giving systems in communities.[7,17]

In recent years there has been an increase in the number of independent mutual support groups and of voluntary associations with support groups concerned with acute and chronic life-threatening illnesses. A few deal with a single issue, such as the "National Committee on Treatment of Intractable Pain," which advocates legislation to permit the use of heroin in control of terminal cancer pain. Most groups are concerned with specific categories of persons, such as parents of children with cystic fibrosis, families of relatives with Huntington's disease, or parents of premature infants. A few, like "Make Today Count" and "Candlelighters," are concerned with the overall needs of adults and children as they face the uncertainty associated with a variety of diseases, especially cancer. Such organizations offer support, education, and practical advice to their members during the course of an illness. It is unclear whether and how these groups offer systematic help with bereavement when death actually occurs, but there is informal support given among a smaller network of individual members.

Postbereavement mutual support groups fall into two categories: (1) those that help people deal with personal grief, with the problems resulting from bereavement, and with the reorganization of their lives around the new status of being a single person (e.g., "THEOS" and the various widow-to-widow programs); and (2) those that attempt to help survivors cope with a grief made particularly difficult by the circumstances of the death, e.g., suicide, homicide, or the death of a child. Some groups (e.g., "Compassionate Friends" or "Seasons") focus primarily on support; others (e.g., "Parents of Murdered Children," "Military Widows," "Vietnam Veterans," "Mothers Against Drunk Driving," "Sudden Infant Death Syndrome"), in addition to giving support, are committed to advocacy and social and political action to remedy the circumstances that caused the death of a family member or adversely affect the lives of survivors. The modalities of communication in both kinds of groups include one-to-one outreach, group meetings, peer counseling by telephone or by mail, and periodic conferences for members and professionals.

Almost all groups have developed literature—based on their own experiences and sometimes in collaboration with professionals—to educate others in similar circumstances, the general public, and health professionals. Many organizations have periodic newsletters with information on, for example, the types of services and benefits offered members; the grief process and its impact on marriage and family, including guidance for sibling grief; suggestions for the behavior of friends, relatives, and health professionals; community resources; reference lists and resource materials dealing with the latest scientific findings on causes and treatments; personal experiences of survivors; and public policy issues.

According to Parkes,[32] the assumption that underlies mutual support bereavement groups is that "the person best qualified to understand and help with the problems of a bereaved person is another bereaved person." The organization that best exemplifies this approach is the Widow-to-Widow program.

The Widow-to-Widow Model

The original Widow-to-Widow Program was a demonstration–research project conducted by Phyllis Silverman under the direction of Gerald Caplan at the Laboratory of Community Psychiatry at Harvard University from 1964 to 1974. Extensive library research, observation, and interviews with widowed persons and community agencies were done in order to learn about the bereavement process, existing services, and widows' perceptions of themselves. This background research revealed several important findings that provided the rationale for the structure and content of the program. Existing services at that time were generally limited to traditional counseling by mental health practitioners. Relatively few widows sought out these services because they did not view their upset and practical problems as "mental illness." When they did seek such help it was typically several years after the bereavement, and grief was rarely identified as the presenting problem, although delayed grief reactions might be uncovered during therapy.[42]

It also became apparent that the bereavement process was not over in a few weeks or months but that it extended over a period of years; that guilt and anger were not identified by widows as the critical issues needing attention, although these were the common therapeutic foci; and that bereavement was best thought of not as a "crisis" but as a "transition." The death of a spouse initiated a critical life transition, marked by a sudden change in social status (from wife to widow) and requiring major changes in self-concept, roles, and tasks. With these observations in mind, Silverman considered how best to assist people in this transition and when to intervene.[43,44]

Because it is not always possible to identify in advance which *individuals* are at risk and because people seemed reluctant to ask for help, it was decided that the intervention should be based on a public health approach rather than a clinical model. Thus, the program was designed for the entire *population* at risk and used an outreach rather than a self-referral approach.[46]

The next question had to do with the timing of intervention. Immediately following bereavement widows are likely to be numb and to act reflexively. Clergy, funeral directors, family, and friends are there to help with the specific tasks of the funeral and mourning rituals. Only somewhat later, during the phase Silverman[43] calls "recoil," does the meaning of the loss begin to become real. But by then family and friends have often gone home, expecting that the widow is over the worst and can manage on her own.

This period of recoil seemed the ideal time to offer help to widows with practical problems, management of extreme and profound feelings, and a general reordering of their lives. Thus, it was decided: (1) that help should not be offered until at least three to six weeks after the bereavement; (2) that in order to be accepted by the entire population at risk, it should be offered by another widow in the neighborhood who could serve as a role model during this critical transition; and (3) that help should be offered initially on a one-to-one basis because the recently bereaved were not often ready for group interactions for several months. Mutual support groups were useful later.

The goals of the program centered around change, not around "recovery." It was discovered in talking to widows that they never "recovered" in the sense of returning to all prebereavement baselines, but that a successful outcome depended on their ability to adapt and alter their images and roles to fit their new status. Although emotional support from a person who has also been through the experience was considered important, the women's more fundamental need was to learn how to change. Thus, in addition to emotional support, the intervention provided specific information about various practical concerns and about bereavement, as well as helping the widows develop alternate coping strategies.[44]

The original program was funded by the National Institute of Mental Health and the national and Massachusetts associations of funeral directors. It was designed by Silverman, who convened a forum in which the widow aides could pool their experiences as widows reaching out to new widows, discuss coping mechanisms, and develop strategies for program development. Silverman provided sanction, legitimization, and technical assistance when appropriate. Over time, the widow aides became very knowledgeable about such issues as insurance, finances, employment opportunities, housing, and community health and social services. As the program developed, social and educational group activities were started by the widow aides.

The initial program, which was conducted in a heterogeneous community in Boston from 1967 to 1970, was limited to widows under age 60. In 1971, it was replicated with elderly Jewish women.[47] There are now programs all over the United States, Canada, and the United Kingdom. In 1973, the American Association of Retired Persons (AARP), in conjunction with the National Retired Teachers Association, established the Widowed Persons' Service. Using materials and consultants from the Widow-to-Widow Program, the AARP began a national effort to develop mutual help programs in communities throughout the country. There are now more than 135 local AARP programs. Groups under different auspices, such as Community Contact for the Widowed of Toronto,[37] are also modeled after the original Widow-to-Widow Program.

It should be noted, however, that there is substantial variation in the application of the original model. Some programs offer only group support while others also provide one-to-one outreach. Some groups have no professional involvement while others have a substantial amount. Professionals may act as occasional consultants, provide routine backup support for the volunteers, train volunteers, or run support groups.

It is also interesting to note that there are very few mutual support groups for widowers or other groups of bereaved men. The reasons for this are not entirely clear. On several site visits it was suggested that men do not readily avail themselves of such services, preferring to deal with their problems alone, and that men are more likely than women to be able to become distracted by their work after bereavement.

Efficacy of the Mutual Support Approach

Many program descriptions include impressionistic, anecdotal data about the perceived usefulness of the support given by one-to-one or group encounters with others who have been through a similar experience. Such reports, although not objective, often provide important insights into the bereavement experience and what some people have found useful. For example, these reports almost uniformly suggest that the discomforts of bereavement extend over many years. Indeed, the respondents to a newspaper notice asking for widows to join a study had been widowed on the average almost five years and only one-third of those replying had been widowed less than two years.[1] In addition, information about the bereavement process and the opportunity to interact with others in similar circumstances appear from these reports to help by reassuring the newly bereaved that they are not ''going crazy'' and by providing a forum for the bereaved to talk openly about their feelings with others who are not uncomfortable listening.

This kind of impressionistic data, useful in some ways, also has its limits. In particular, it provides few clues about the relative benefits of different intervention strategies. Ideally, those helping the bereaved would like to know which programs work best for whom under which circumstances. The diversity of program goals, structure, content, and methods renders comparative evaluations difficult.

There also appear to be some barriers to evaluation that are inherent in the programs themselves. The mutual support programs tend to be run by laypeople in community settings. They are unlikely to have people associated with them who are skilled in research, and the organizers have often been reluctant to be scrutinized by professional evaluators. For these and perhaps other reasons, such as underdeveloped research methodologies appropriate to collaborative research, there is a paucity of research on the impact of mutual support groups. The four studies that have been done are summarized in Table 1.

Two of these studies were large surveys of participants in mutual support groups to determine whether intensity of involvement (meeting attendance and leadership roles) with the group was related to bereavement outcome. Lieberman and Borman[24] surveyed current and former members of 71 different chapters of THEOS, a mutual support group for widows and widowers with chapters throughout the United States and Canada. They found that a number of outcomes (psychosocial, behav-

TABLE 1 Summary of Intervention Research on Mutual Support for the Bereaved

Study Author and Year of Publication	Type of Intervention	Study Population	Type of Evaluation	Measures Used	Results
Barrett, 1978[1]	Three different types of format: self-help groups (specific problems of widowhood), "confidant" groups (development of friendships between pairs of widows), and consciousness-raising groups (women's roles in society). Met for 2 hours/week for 7 weeks. Groups led by 2 doctoral students in clinical psychology.	70 urban widows who responded to a newspaper ad randomly assigned to one of three treatment groups (E) or a "waiting list" control group (C). Average length of bereavement was 5 years.	Pretest, post-test (at 7 weeks), and follow-up (at 13–15 weeks).	Personality, attitude, and behavioral measures; physical, emotional, and social functioning indices.	1. At post-test, all E and C subjects had higher self-esteem, more intense grief, and more negative attitudes toward remarriage. 2. At follow-up the most positive life changes occurred in consciousness-raising group, least positive in self-help.
Vachon et al., 1980[51]	Newly bereaved widows paired with trained widow helpers for 1:1 support and practical assistance followed by group mutual support. No predetermined number of meetings or length of intervention.	162 widows, median age 52, 81% of whose husbands had died of a chronic illness in 7 Toronto hospitals were randomly allocated to intervention vs. no intervention.	Controlled prospective study with assessments at 1, 6, 12, and 24 months postbereavement.	Goldberg General Health Questionnaire, other self-administered questionnaire, and structured interview.	1. No differences between treatment group (E) and control group (C) at 1 month. 2. At 6 months, E better on intrapersonal adaptation. 3. At 12 months, E better on interpersonal adaptation.

246

Reference	Intervention	Sample	Method	Outcomes	Results
					4. At 24 months, overall differences between E and C and high-risk E widows more likely to have become low risk. 5. Perceived social support is key predictor.
Lieberman and Borman, 1981[24]	Post-bereavement mutual support group, THEOS, for widows and widowers.	Current and former members of 71 THEOS groups in U.S. and Canada and people who had declined joining these groups. 721 responded to first questionnaire, 502 to second; 93% were widows; 80% under age 60.	Mail surveys 1 year apart.	Depression, self-esteem, anxiety, somatic symptoms, psychotropic drug use, coping, and well-being.	More intense the involvement with the group, the better the outcomes, especially for depression and self-esteem.
Videka-Sherman, 1982[53]	Compassionate Friends, mutual support group for bereaved parents with chapters throughout U.S. and Canada.	Members and nonmembers of 18 chapters. Paper reports on 194 parents who lost a child in previous 18 months. 70% were mothers, average age 41.	Mail surveys 1 year apart.	Psychosocial adjustment, depression, self-reported personal growth.	1. No significant differences in depression scores by level of involvement in group. 2. Self-reported personal growth varied directly with intensity of involvement in group.

ioral, and physiologic) varied directly with intensity of involvement with the group.

A similar hypothesis was tested by Videka-Sherman,[53] who surveyed members of Compassionate Friends, a mutual support group for bereaved parents with chapters throughout the United States and Canada. Self-reported personal growth varied directly with involvement, as predicted, but no significant differences were found on measures of depression by level of involvement.

Only one study has compared different mutual support approaches. Barrett[1] randomly allocated widows to three different types of mutual support groups and a nonintervention control group. Each support group concentrated on a specific aspect of widowhood. The "self-help" group met for two hours each week for seven weeks and focused on specific, practical problems of widowhood; the "confidant" group focused on the development of new friendships between pairs of widows; and the "consciousness raising" group focused on women's roles in society. Unlike the "pure" widow-to-widow approach, in this study nonwidowed professionals (doctoral students in clinical psychology) led the sessions. At follow-up (seven weeks after the groups stopped meeting), the most positive changes occurred in the consciousness-raising group and the fewest positive changes occurred in the self-help group. This finding lends support to Silverman's thesis[44] that widowhood is best thought of as a life transition, rather than a crisis, and that in order to make that transition successfully widows need to overcome obstacles to changing their self-image so they can learn new roles. Since no additional follow-up was done, however, it is not known whether the group differences persisted over time.

Vachon and her colleagues[51] have conducted the only rigorous study of the efficacy of Silverman's original widow-to-widow model. Women whose husbands had died at age 67 or younger in one of seven participating hospitals in Toronto were contacted by a widow helper who offered one-to-one support, practical help, and eventually small group meetings as well. Of the 185 widows eligible for the study, 162 (88 percent) agreed to participate and were randomly allocated to the intervention or nonintervention group. The program had no predetermined limits on the amount or duration of contact. Personal interviews were conducted with widows in both groups by project staff at 1, 6, 12, and 24 months after the bereavement. The Goldberg General Health Questionnaire (a well-validated psychiatric screening instrument) was administered, along with another self-administered instrument designed to examine demographic and situational variables, social support, and physical symptoms. A structured interview was conducted to elicit more sensitive data regarding the husband's death and other stressors. As summarized in Table 1, the psychologic adaptation of the experimental group members to their new circumstances was better than the control group's at 6 months; at 12 months, interpersonal adaptation was better; and by 24 months the experimental group was better than the control group on all measures. High-risk subjects who were in the experimental group were significantly more likely to have shifted to low risk by 24 months than were highly distressed widows who were in the control group. The best predictor of bereavement adjustment was perceived social support.

Further analyses[52] revealed that deficits in social support and health and financial problems were correlated with enduring high distress at 24 months after bereavement. Personality traits compatible with successful socialization in an appropriate "widow role" were found to differentiate the women with enduring low distress. Emotional stability and maturity (ego strength), conservatism, and superego strength (conscientious and moralistic) were among the traits that distinguished the low-distress group.

HOSPICES

The rapid proliferation of hospices in this country since 1975 has been driven by a powerful grass-roots movement to provide an alternative to overly aggressive hospital care on the one hand and inadequate nursing home care for the terminally ill on the other. In 1979, the General Accounting Office reported to Congress that there were 59 operating hospices and 73 others being planned. In 1981, the American Hospital Association estimated that there were approximately 800 hospices; by early 1983, this figure was revised to 1,200.

The term hospice refers not to an institution but rather to a philosophy of care for the terminally ill and their families that emphasizes:

- control and palliation of symptoms rather than cure of disease
- care given at home or in as home-like an environment as possible
- patient autonomy regarding decisions about care
- attention to emotional, social, and spiritual needs as well as to requirements for physical care.

Because the patient and his family are considered to be the unit of care, hospices aspire to provide support to families both before and after death.[29]

This philosophy, which was adopted from the British,[39,40] has been translated into a variety of programs in this country. Hospice care is delivered in both inpatient and home care settings in a number of different administrative and organizational models. Some are freestanding while others are hospital-based. Many hospices offer only home care, whereas some offer only inpatient care and others offer both. Some hospices provide all their own services, while others represent loose affiliations of a number of pre-existing service providers (e.g., visiting nurses, homemaker services) or contract for services as needed.[31] Despite the fact that patients with many different types of diseases could be appropriately cared for, the vast majority of patients in hospice programs have some form of cancer, and these programs have tended to favor the middle class.

Hospice services are provided by multidisciplinary teams usually composed of physicians, nurses, social workers, chaplains, psychiatrists, physical therapists, and volunteers. Professional bereavement counselors, especially nurses, may also be involved in bereavement care.

In most hospice programs, lay volunteers, who often have themselves been bereaved, perform a substantial proportion of the bereavement work. Most hospices screen lay volunteers very carefully. Screening procedures were discussed at length at three of the committee's site visits. There appears to be a consensus that people whose own bereavement occurred less than a year ago are not ready to assist in these programs and should not be permitted to work directly with other bereaved individuals. Second, people who have their own personal agendas (e.g., religious proselytizing, use of others to work through their own problems, need for companionship) are considered inappropriate because of the special vulnerability of the newly bereaved. Sense of commitment, good listening and communication skills, sensitivity, compassion, sense of humor, and awareness of personal limitations were all mentioned as desirable characteristics for lay volunteers who wish to work with the bereaved. Screening is usually done by the coordinator of volunteer or bereavement services in a face-to-face interview. Applicants may also be required to complete a questionnaire that asks about their bereavement history, personal history generally, current lifestyle, beliefs, and attitudes.

Once accepted as a volunteer, some training is usually provided. This may include education about the bereavement process, hospice philosophy, and community resources; development of communication skills; and role playing. Training may be as brief as a few hours or as long as 30 hours, done either very intensively in a couple of days or spread out. Following didactic training sessions, volunteers may be very closely supervised for some period of time. Regular meetings with all bereavement volunteers usually provide a forum for ongoing evaluation of their work.

Most hospice programs assign a bereavement worker to each family when a patient begins treatment. This person assists the patient and family during the terminal illness and follows up with the family after the death. At some hospices, however, a different pattern is followed. The staff of the Boulder County Hospice, for example, believes that the best person to do follow-up bereavement care with families is someone who has *not* been directly involved with care of the dying patient. Support for the bereaved requires very different skills than active care of dying patients. Initially, nurses served in both these roles. But it seemed that bereavement support became a low priority, with patient care remaining the nurses' first concern. Second, it was found that following bereavement, families needed to tell their story over and over again. This need could be met more effectively by having a new person available to listen rather than one who had been intimately involved around the time of death, who might have his or her own version of events. Thus Boulder County Hospice has two rather separate sets of care-givers available—one for patient and family care before the death, the other for follow-up family support after the death.[22]

Although all hospices offer some type of bereavement intervention to families, at least in preparation for the death, they vary greatly in the breadth and magnitude of services offered. During the predeath phase, the interventions are likely to be informal rather than formal, with a focus on information and education, support, and validation by the care-givers who are tending to the patient's needs and assisting the family. Because hospice care is most often given in the patient's home by the family, support of those responsible in this endeavor may take on a significance that is absent in other care settings. The entire ethos of hospice care is also likely to lend support through its implicit acceptance of death and willingness to discuss and plan for it.

Hospices have certain opportunities to assist families prior to the patient's death that are intrinsic to their basic functioning. These include ongoing possibilities for support and education of the family, as well as for observation of family functioning in order to plan for effective follow-up. Like hospitals, however, once the patient has died, hospices must organize their services in a different way in order to support families effectively.

Although about 70 percent of hospices[6] offer services for about a year following bereavement, these efforts are often modest. Such services may include home visits, phone calls, letters, social gatherings, support groups, counseling (both individual and group), anniversary remembrances, and referral to other support services. The range of services offered and the intensity of the follow-up vary widely among individual hospice programs. One-to-one contacts are frequently limited to a phone call, letter, or visit at three-month intervals for a year.

Hospice bereavement programs have much in common with mutual support groups. In fact, most hospice programs can be characterized as mutual support offered under the umbrella of a newly institutionalized health care option. As with mutual support efforts, hospice bereavement programs are targeted for the vast majority of bereaved people who can be expected to work through their grief without needing professional help. Like mutual support groups, hospices emphasize education and support. Because they are formal health care institutions, however, there is usually some involvement of health care professionals—not necessarily mental health professionals—in the bereavement programs. As described during the site visit to the Boulder County Hospice and as reflected in its written materials, grief is seen as a complex time of need rather than an illness. The goals of follow-up bereavement services are: ''to provide family members with information about the normal grief process; to provide grieving family members an opportunity to review and reflect on the experience of caring for their loved one and their loss experience; to assess and monitor individual coping ability, stress levels, and available support; to encourage family members to utilize existing support systems or to seek and create additional sources of support.''[22]

Although some hospices offer limited psychotherapeutic counseling, most do not. They typically make assessments and refer people to other community resources if they are experiencing abnormal grief reactions. The staff of the Boulder County Hospice estimates that less than 5 percent of bereaved individuals in their program have needed to be referred to mental health professionals. Perhaps because of the extensive family involvement required in hospices, those who are psychologically less healthy do not choose this mode of care.

Although until recently there has been little third-party reimbursement for hospice care, in 1982, as part of the Tax Equity and Fiscal Responsibility Act (P.L. 97-248, Section 122), the Social Security Act was amended to provide federal reimbursement for hospices under Medicare. The legislation calls for a three-year experiment, through October 1986, with requirements for quality assessment and evaluation of cost impact as the prerequisites for deciding whether to continue the hospice benefit further. Although it is too early to assess the impact of this legislation, certain provisions seem likely to alter what has been thought of as hospice care, including the bereavement services involved.[25] Hospices are required to provide bereavement services for families, yet they cannot be reimbursed for such programs. Without direct support for these services, there is growing concern that bereavement care, one of the hallmarks of hospices, may be reduced to whatever minimal level will meet formal requirements.

The Impact of Hospice Bereavement Programs

Hospices offer a rich opportunity for addressing a number of important questions on bereavement, including the effects of caring for a dying patient at home on the subsequent bereavement reactions of families, the nature of anticipatory grieving and its effect on subsequent bereavement, and the relative effectiveness of different approaches to bereavement support. Hospices that are affiliated with prepaid or other closed health plans provide a unique opportunity to study family reactions over time.

With the advent of Medicare reimbursement for hospices, a number of federal agencies and private foundations have become interested in studying the effects of this type of care. Although their principal interest seems to be on the cost of care for the terminally ill, studies of the preventive implications of bereavement interventions for survivors should not be overlooked. If effective, such interventions for the bereaved could have significant long-term implications for medical care costs and productivity in the workplace that would far outstrip the cost implications for medical care of the dying person in the last few months of life. Thus, hospices provide not only intrinsically interesting sites in which to examine various aspects of bereavement and approaches to interventions, but also an unusual opportunity to study questions of cost-effectiveness that have been virtually overlooked in bereavement research.

Perhaps because of their grass-roots beginnings and desire to be separate from the mainstream of medical care, hospices initially were unwilling to be evaluated. Much of the early literature on hospices from England and the United States simply stated that these programs were providing good and necessary services that benefited patients and families while avoiding all the perceived evils of modern medical institutions. To the extent that research was being done, it focused on symptom control, especially on analgesics for pain management.

In the last several years, the resistance to formal evaluation of hospices has lessened. This is due in large part to the need to demonstrate the cost-effectiveness of hospices in order to secure continuing funding. Before passage of the Medicare amendment, the Health Care Financing

Administration, in conjunction with the John A. Hartford and Robert Wood Johnson Foundations, sponsored a major national hospice evaluation. Twenty-six hospices were eligible to receive Medicare reimbursement for three years. These 26 waivered hospices were compared with 14 nonwaivered hospices and with conventional care. Unfortunately only a very small part of this multimillion dollar study was devoted to an examination of bereavement services and their impact on surviving families.

As part of the National Hospice Study,[6] the principal care persons (PCPs) of cancer patients who died in hospital-based hospices (N = 580), home-based hospices (N = 780), and conventional care settings (N = 270) were interviewed twice prior to bereavement (at intake and three weeks later) and at three and one-half months after bereavement. The mean age of these groups was 58, approximately half were surviving spouses, and 72 percent were women.

Although it had been hypothesized that there would be significantly better outcomes for the survivors of both hospice groups than for conventional care survivors, the data on a number of different measures generally indicate more differences between the two types of hospices than between hospices and conventional care. Before and after bereavement, PCPs from hospital-based hospices were significantly less distressed emotionally, felt less burdened by patient care, and reported greater satisfaction with patient care than survivors in home-care hospices. Following bereavement, however, home-care PCPs—although more distressed—scored significantly better on a scale of social reengagement than hospital-based PCPs. It is not known whether this reflects a response to the higher level of emotional distress, and hence a reaching out for more help, or whether it merely represents a return to normal social involvement that was cut back because of the time spent caring for the terminally ill patient in the home. There were no significant differences between the three groups in the number of doctor visits made in the first three months of bereavement. Although it is not clear what proportion of bereavement assistance and counseling was sought by the PCPs and what proportion was offered by the programs on an outreach, preventive basis, hospice survivors (especially those from home-care programs) received significantly more bereavement assistance than the PCPs from conventional care settings.[41]

Because survivors were followed for only a few months, the long-term effects of the different modalities of hospice and conventional care on bereavement outcomes are not known. However, this study is important because it begins to document the impact of hospice care on survivors and points the way to research hypotheses deserving further study.

It is unfortunate that funds have not been made available to continue this aspect of the study, so that outcome measures could be refined and the long-term effects of different contexts of dying and different interventions could be documented on an already identified, large sample of bereaved individuals.

Parkes[33] reports on the use of trained lay volunteers to provide support and practical advice to "high-risk" survivors whose relative (mostly spouses) or close friend died at St. Christopher's Hospice in London. One hundred and eighty-one recently bereaved individuals were divided into three groups: imperative need, high-risk, and low-risk; the high-risk people were then further divided into an intervention or nonintervention group by random assignment. Data on the two high-risk groups were presented. At 20 months postbereavement the groups were compared on a number of measures, including physical symptoms, depression, habit changes (smoking, alcohol, and drug use), an index of worry, and a general health index. As in Raphael's study,[35] significant differences were found between the two high-risk groups. Those in the intervention group had become like the low-risk individuals; the differences in outcomes were even more significant for men than for women.

Unlike most hospices, the Palliative Care Unit (PCU) at the Royal Victoria Hospital in Montreal has been actively engaged in research and evaluation since its inception in 1975. This ongoing interest in research may be due to the fact that the Royal Victoria is a teaching hospital. A bereavement intervention study began when the hospice first opened.[3] Twenty close adult relatives of patients who died of cancer during a six-month period in the hospice were matched with 20 relatives of patients who died in the active treatment part of the hospital. The PCU families received total hospice care including predeath support before the death and bereavement counseling. Open expression of grief and communication between family members were encouraged before the death. After the death a nurse offered reassurrance and active listening for six months (in person and by telephone). None of the hospital families received any of these services.

All subjects were contacted for a telephone evaluation interview 54 weeks after the death. The questionnaire assessed current living arrangements and changes in lifestyle following bereavement, anniversary activities, grief reactions, and adjustment as measured by physical and psychological health and social behavior. The hospice group showed significantly more signs of adjustment and reorganization and the control group showed significantly more signs of grief and counterproductive coping strategies. The authors commented that hospice subjects sounded calm while control subjects appeared agitated and upset on the telephone.

In 1978, a major study began at the Royal Victoria to assess the impact of hospice care generally and bereavement interventions specifically. The study, which is not yet completed, is being directed by Dr. Margaret Kiely, a psychologist from the University of Montreal. A site visit was made to Montreal to learn the details of this study. Subsequently, preliminary results were presented at a conference.[15] The study's objectives were to evaluate the effectiveness of bereavement support compared with no support, and the effectiveness of support by trained lay volunteers as compared with nurses. Efforts were made to standardize the content of the intervention, although the intensity and duration could vary according to need. For those who received bereavement support, usually one to five home visits were made during the first four months of bereavement. The study also compared results for bereaved subjects from three settings—the PCU, other parts of the Royal Victoria, and a hospice unit in a chronic care hospital.

A detailed evaluation instrument was designed to measure physical and emotional health, social and emotional adjustment, changes in life style and habits, and demographic data. Evaluation interviews of all subjects were conducted in person at 6, 13, and 25 months following bereavement.

Preliminary analyses show different patterns of bereavement reactions between men and women and between French- and English-speaking families. Some other impressions from the data are unexpected. Experimental subjects reported twice as many physical symptoms as controls. Subjects from the PCU did worse on several outcome measures than people from the other settings where less attention was paid to anticipatory grieving. Data from one year after bereavement suggest that interventions were helpful, but at two years after bereavement those people who had had interventions were significantly worse off.

It should be noted that it is not at all clear what has been assessed—the bereavement process, the effects of hospice care generally, the effects of a bereavement intervention, or even the evaluation process, which itself became an intervention. In this study, as in others that do multiple assessments in person, evaluation interviews themselves may facilitate grieving because they provide an opportunity to interact with a compassionate person and to review feelings about the loss. Further analyses may shed some additional light on these questions but may never be able to establish completely the impact of each of these components on the course of bereavement.

PSYCHOTHERAPEUTIC INTERVENTIONS FOR THE BEREAVED

For individuals who feel overwhelmed by the painful emotions attributable to grieving or who are experiencing pathologic or distorted grief reactions, psychotherapeutic intervention may be warranted. As used here, psychotherapy refers to verbal techniques used by mental health professionals to assist the bereaved. Psychotherapeutic methods and approaches encompass a wide range.

- The service providers most commonly are psychiatrists, psychiatric social workers, or clinical psychologists, who may practice either independently or as part of teams in medical centers, in counseling agencies, or in programs specifically aimed at helping the bereaved.
- In certain settings assistance may also be provided by psychiatric nurses and specially trained counselors, including pastoral counselors.
- Individuals may refer themselves or may be referred by friends, clergy, or medical personnel.
- Treatment may be brief and time-limited—ranging from 6 sessions (often described as "crisis intervention") to 20 or 30 sessions—or it may be long-term and open-ended.
- Therapy may be dynamic, behavioral, or systems-oriented and may be offered to individuals, families, or groups of similarly bereaved persons.

As discussed in Chapter 3, a number of theories guide psychotherapy with the bereaved. The particular training and orientation of the clinician, as well as an assessment of the individual client's or patient's needs, usually determine the type of help that is offered. Despite the individuality of methods and approaches, mental health practitioners generally share certain characteristics: nonjudgmental support and compassion and a wish to help the bereaved person or family resume adequate functioning and sense of well-being.

Psychotherapists with a psychodynamic or psychoanalytic perspective may be inclined to focus on the individual. They may help the bereaved patient to uncover, in a safe and self-accepting way, hostile feelings toward the deceased that had been kept out of awareness but that had taken a toll on the individual's psychologic well-being. They may also assist the bereaved to modify extremely negative self-perceptions that go beyond the relationship with the deceased. Typically these clinicians assume that pathologic grief reactions derive largely from preexisting factors in the bereaved person and features of the relationship with the deceased, such as inappropriate or immature defensive and coping strategies, preexisting emotional instability, a history of unresolved prior losses, and an especially ambivalent or dependent relationship. The treatment goal is to clarify any neurotic conflicts that have rendered the person vulnerable to pathologic grief, and to help the person work through troubling emotions and trains of thought.[23,59]

A behaviorist may conceptualize the problem in a similar way, but focus less attention on the internal personality characteristics of the patient and more attention on specific behaviors. The therapist may try to "desensitize" the bereaved person who seems incapable of accepting and mourning the loss. The therapist may help the person construct and gradually accomplish a scale of increasingly difficult tasks (e.g., facing photographs of the deceased or visiting the gravesite) that imply an increased ability to relinquish the deceased.

Cognitive approaches are designed to remove obstacles to normal grieving by assisting the bereaved to "re-grieve" the loss in their own imagination.[27,54] By reliving the loss and reexperiencing feelings toward the deceased, the bereaved are helped to revise their images and to restructure the meaning of the loss.

There are a number of different interpersonal approaches to psychotherapy that deal directly with a family system or that focus on the psychosocial context of the individual patient. For example, therapists with a family or systems approach are primarily concerned with the impact of the loss on the family system, that is, how the death affects roles and communication patterns among the survivors. They are likely to treat the couple (in the case of a child's death, for example) or surviving family as the "patient," helping to identify and ameliorate patterns of communication and behavior that are putting strain on individual family members.

By contrast, the newly developed Interpersonal Therapy is designed to treat individual patients who have depression associated with abnormal grief reactions. This "is a focused, short-term, time-limited therapy that emphasizes the current interpersonal relations of the depressed patient while recognizing the role of genetic, biochemical, developmental, and personality factors in causation of and vulnerability to depression."[18] Proponents of this therapy point out that it is similar to other therapies in terms of techniques but different in terms of specific strategies for accomplishing tasks. Treatment proceeds in three stages. First, the depression is explained to the patient and related to current and past interpersonal relationships, and major problem areas are identified. The goals of the second phase are to facilitate the grieving process, to assist the patient in developing relationships to substitute for what has been lost, to make the necessary role transitions, and to restore self-esteem.

Finally, the end of therapy is discussed explicitly and the patient is helped to recognize his or her independent competence.

Although the training and theories that guide the work of mental health professionals may differ from those of others (nontherapists) who work with the bereaved, there is likely to be considerable overlap in practice. In both psychotherapy and the mutual support model described earlier, there is provision of support, an attempt to facilitate and manage grief reactions, and an effort toward improving family relationships. Both approaches may work with the bereaved to develop new coping skills or to modify existing ones. Differences lie in the depth and scope of intervention. Whereas nontherapists may be proficient at helping those who are experiencing "normal" or "normative" grief, they are usually not prepared to cope with extreme distress or those highly disturbed reactions that suggest underlying mental illness.

In addition, nontherapists do not use bereavement as an opportunity to do more extensive psychotherapeutic work, whereas dynamically oriented therapists, in particular, may explore basic aspects of the personality, aiming at modification of defenses and working through of neurotic conflicts or developmental difficulties. How ambitious the goals of treatment are to be depends on the particular agreement and wishes of the therapist and patient.

Three of the site visits made by the committee and staff were to psychotherapeutic programs for the bereaved. The diversity of their approaches is illustrative of some of the professional models that have been used with the bereaved.

The St. Francis Center in Washington, D.C., includes a professional counseling service as well as a lay support component. Counseling is done by clinical psychologists or psychiatric social workers on a one-to-one basis and in groups. Clients may refer themselves to this service, be referred by the volunteer service if their problems seem too extensive to be handled by laypeople, or be referred by their physicians or clergy. Some of the clients in the counseling program are basically healthy people who are experiencing normal grief reactions but who have nonsupportive families and friends, but most have preexisting personality problems that were exacerbated by the loss or are experiencing especially acute or prolonged grief.

Individual counseling is usually held once or twice a week, for as little as two weeks or as long as two years if needed. Clients are given permission to grieve, to tell their story repeatedly if they need to, and to express their feelings. Information about the bereavement process helps the bereaved understand that often even very strong negative feelings are normal. Group therapy also is offered. Currently there are groups for young widows and widowers, each with four to five people who need help in alleviating the painful and confusing responses to the loss of a spouse.

The Center for the Study of Neuroses at the Langley-Porter Institute, University of California at San Francisco, is a major psychotherapy research center. Two studies of bereavement responses have been conducted using psychodynamically oriented brief therapy (12 sessions) for self-referred clients who are experiencing difficulty. According to staff, people who experience extreme difficulty following bereavement or other trauma are those who have a "history of maladaptive attitudes and beliefs that prior to the event had lain dormant."[20] During therapy the patient is confronted with transference interpretations about anger and other emotions, and the pending termination of treatment is explicitly raised as part of the way to work through the loss. Negative self-concepts, which may be activated by the trauma of bereavement, and the nature of the attachment to the deceased are reviewed in therapy and patients are helped to detach themselves from the deceased.

The Center for Preventive Psychiatry in White Plains, N.Y., is intended primarily for the treatment of young children. Many bereaved children are seen each year in the Situational Crisis Service. Staff workers at the Center believe that bereavement places a child at increased risk for the rest of his or her life if not properly attended to. Their approach is to treat both child and parent(s). Parents are helped to understand the nature of bereavement in children, are given guidance about how to communicate with their child and about symptoms that deserve attention, and are supported in their own grief. Children are typically in therapy twice a week for about a year following bereavement and are then seen annually thereafter for many years. This periodic mental health checkup is believed to be an important way to make certain that the child is progressing normally and to offer additional brief therapy if new problems have emerged.

The Impact of Psychotherapy with the Bereaved

Lack of comparability across the various psychotherapeutic approaches and therapists, along with a shortage of appropriate and quantifiable measures of outcome, have stymied past efforts to evaluate psychotherapy in general. In addition, for a number of practical reasons the research that has been done on the efficacy of psychotherapy has focused mainly on short-term treatment, and the patients have been highly selected. Most studies currently funded by the National Institute of Mental Health focus on behavior therapy, although most psychotherapy provided in the United States is psychodynamically oriented; most studies are of outcomes rather than the processes and mechanisms that lead to particular outcomes; most research is conducted on patients whose diagnoses are clearly agreed upon and fit neatly into a category in the American Psychiatric Association's *Diagnostic and Statistical Manual*; and relatively few studies have been conducted on children or adolescents. These limitations of psychotherapy research generally apply to bereavement intervention research as well.

In fact, most psychotherapy in general as well as for bereavement in particular is provided by individual practitioners in private offices where the content of the interactions and outcomes are kept confidential. Individual case studies and clinical reports attest to the efficacy of certain kinds of therapeutic interventions for people who are at high risk for or who have experienced pathologic reactions to bereavement; such reports usually describe a particular individual therapist's work, however, which may be largely idiosyncratic and, therefore, not readily generalizable.

Much progress has been made recently in improving the reliability of outcome measures[55] and in developing more standardized psychotherapies that will lend themselves to evaluation. Increasing attention is being paid to the development of short-term therapies and manuals to describe and instruct therapists in their conduct.[18] These training tools permit greater comparability in treatment across therapists, thereby facilitating more replicable evaluation research. This work is well developed for studies of depression,[56] but very few research studies involving quantitative methods and control groups have been conducted so far in the area of bereavement (see Table 2).

Gerber et al.[5] report on a controlled, prospective, longitudinal study that offered brief therapy to the aged bereaved. A group of nonpatient elderly individuals, members of a prepaid medical plan, who had lost a spouse either from cancer (40 percent of sample) or cardiovascular disease (60 percent of sample) were followed for a minimum of three years; 169 individuals were randomly assigned to an intervention group (containing 116 people) or to a control group (containing 53 people). Weekly meetings with a psychiatric social worker or psychiatric nurse were offered for six months to individuals or to all family members who were part of the same household. Although originally it was planned that these meetings would be in the home or office, many preferred weekly telephone contact and occasional office or home sessions. Therapy focused on moral support, grief work, and environmental manipulation.

A variety of measures were used to document the impact of intervention on the surviviors' medical, psychologic, and social adjustment ini-

TABLE 2 Summary of Intervention Research on Psychotherapy With the Bereaved

Study Author and Year of Publication	Type of Intervention	Study Population	Type of Evaluation	Measures Used	Results
Gerber et al., 1975[5]	Telephone and 1 : 1 support by psychiatric social workers and nurses during first 6 months of bereavement. Support, emotional expression, and practical assistance.	Aged bereaved spouses from a Health Maintenance Organization randomly assigned to support group (N = 116) and control group (N = 53).	Controlled prospective longitudinal study with interviews at 2, 5, 8, and 15 months following bereavement.	Variety of measures of medical, social, and psychologic adjustment, including review of medical records. Only medical data reported.	1. Most of the significant differences were at 5 and 8 months. 2. Supported people had fewer prescription drugs, fewer doctor visits, and felt ill less often than controls. 3. No significant differences in major illnesses. 4. Those who were healthy at time of bereavement benefited more from intervention.
Polak et al., 1975;[34] Williams et al., 1976;[57] and Williams and Polak, 1979[58]	Immediate crisis intervention by mental health professionals in home with additional telephone and face-to-face sessions (2–6) for 1–10 weeks. Counseling focused on family coping.	Intact families following sudden death. Thirty-two experimental vs. 54 not very well matched bereaved controls vs. 40 nonbereaved controls.	Three × two repeated measures design—3 groups examined at 6 and 18 months postbereavement.	Medical and psychiatric ratings and self-reported health status.	1. Two-stage impact of sudden death. At 6 months, bereaved subjects had more illness, coping problems, and disturbed social functioning than nonbereaved. At 18 months, more practical problems. 2. Short-term crisis intervention produced no major differences between experimental subjects and bereaved controls at 6 or 18 months. 3. Intervention may have delayed or interfered with normal bereavement process.

Study	Intervention	Design/Sample	Measures	Results
Raphael, 1977[35]	1:1 by psychiatrist. Support, emotional expression, and review of relationship. 1–9 home interviews at 6–12 weeks postbereavement.	High-risk recent widows randomly allocated to intervention (N = 31) and control (N = 33) groups and low-risk (N = 138) to another control group.	Index of health change at 13 months postbereavement.	1. Very significant differences between supported and unsupported high-risk widows at 13 months, especially for symptoms and doctor visits. 2. At 13 months, high-risk widows with support look like low-risk widows. 3. Perceived supportiveness of social network is key predictor.
Rosenheim and Ichilov, 1979[38]	Prebereavement support for children whose parent was dying. 10–12 consecutive weekly meetings with psychology graduate student. Focus on reactions to parent's illness and home life in effort to avoid adjustment problems.	24 children, ages 10–14, randomly assigned to treatment (E) or control (C) group. No history of psychiatric disturbance.	Manifest anxiety scale, teacher questionnaire, and semistructured interviews with well parent.	1. Significant decrease in anxiety in E group. 2. Insignificant decrease in psychophysiologic symptoms. 3. Significant improvement in scholastic and social functioning in E group and worsening of these functions in C group.
Mawson et al., 1981[26]	Behavioral therapy comparing maximum exposure to stimuli with avoidance and distraction from painful thoughts and getting on with life. Three 1–1½ hour sessions/week for 2 weeks with psychiatrist or nurse therapist.	12 patients with "morbid grief" (persistent distress for at least 1 year following loss) randomly allocated to exposure vs. avoidance therapy.	Self-ratings at 0, 2, 4, 8, 12, and 28 weeks.	Several measures of pathology of grief (bereavement avoidance, physical symptoms, anger, guilt, attitudes toward self and deceased), depression, anxiety, and social adjustment.	1. Exposure group showed significant improvement on some measures and an improved trend on other measures. 2. Improvement maintained at 28 weeks. 3. Avoidance group showed no significant improvement or trends in that direction.

263

TABLE 2 Summary of Intervention Research on Psychotherapy With the Bereaved (*Continued*)

Study Author and Year of Publication	Type of Intervention	Study Population	Type of Evaluation	Measures Used	Results
Forrest et al., 1982[4]	Support and up to 4 hours of counseling over 2–6 week period.	50 mothers of stillborns and babies who died within 7 days of birth randomly assigned to support and counseling vs routine hospital care immediately following the death.	Assessment interviews at 6 and 14 months postbereavement.	Goldberg General Health Questionnaire; Leeds anxiety scale; self-rating scales for social and emotional functioning for fathers and mothers.	1. At 6 months, supported group was significantly better than controls. 2. Among controls, fathers were better than mothers at 6 months. 3. At 14 months, no significant differences between groups.
Kupst et al., 1982[21]	Anticipatory grief work. Intervention by master's degree social workers and counselors to help understand illness, manage emotional distress, and facilitate family communication during each phase of illness.	64 families of leukemic children randomly allocated to intensive, moderate, or no support groups.	Family coping at time of diagnosis and 3, 6, 12, and 24 months thereafter for each of the three groups.	Ratings by medical, nursing, and psychosocial staff and self-reports.	No major differences between the intervention and nonintervention groups.
Horowitz et al., 1984[10]	Time-limited (12 hours) dynamic psychotherapy for stress response syndromes.	52 adults with postbereavement adjustment disorder following death of spouse or parent.	Independent systematic interviews before and after therapy, rating scales by evaluator and patient, and review with ratings of videotapes by additional independent clinicians.	Stress and general symptom measures; measures of personal attitude and social and work functions; ratings of therapy processes.	Significant improvement in most patients.

| Horowitz et al., 1984[11] | Time-limited (12 sessions) dynamic psychotherapy focusing on review of relationship with deceased and facilitation of grieving. | 35 adult patients who sought treatment following parental bereavement and 37 bereaved controls who had not sought treatment. | Nonequivalent contrast group design with evaluations at 2, 7, and 13 months after bereavement. | Nine different self-administered and clinical assessment instruments were used to assess stress-specific and general signs and symptoms of distress and current levels of adjustment. | 1. Patients had higher initial distress levels than nonpatients. 2. At 13 months, patients' distress was markedly reduced. No significant differences between patients and controls on self-administered measures. 3. Clinical ratings of patients showed more depression and anxiety than controls at 13 months. 4. Perceived social support and most demographic variables were not related to outcomes. 5. Loss of mother was associated with negative outcomes. |

tially and at 2, 5, 8, and 15 months following bereavement. Only the medical indicators are reported.

During and shortly after the intervention, the supported people reported less drug use, less illness, and fewer visits to their doctors than the controls. By the time of the final evaluation, 15 months after bereavement, there were few significant differences in these measures and no significant differences in major illnesses. The authors report that those who benefited most from the intervention were people who were physically healthy at the time of bereavement.

Horowitz et al.[9,11] studied the impact of brief, dynamically oriented psychotherapy on self-referred adults who had lost a parent through death. Twelve therapy sessions focused on the relationship with the deceased and facilitation of grief. Thirty-five patients were compared with 37 volunteer subjects who had also been parentally bereaved but who had not sought treatment. Assessments were done at 2, 7, and 13 months to examine changes within and between groups over time. A number of self-administered instruments and clinical rating scales were used to assess symptoms of psychologic distress, adjustment, functioning, self-concept, life events, perceived social support, and sociodemographic variables.

Not surprisingly, initial levels of distress were significantly higher for patients than for controls. At the 13-month follow-up, patients' distress was substantially reduced on most measures. The predictive value of a number of intervening variables was examined. Contrary to the findings in many other reports, perceived social support was not related to outcomes. Death of a mother, cumulative life events, social class, and development of self-concept were related to outcomes.

The outcome of brief treatment was also reported for a group of 52 bereaved patients who were treated for adjustment reactions or posttraumatic stress disorders following the death of a spouse or parent.[11] The treatment was dynamic psychotherapy, limited to a maximum of 12 weekly sessions. Patients were assessed by independent evaluators several months after the last therapy session. While the majority of patients had major reductions in stress-specific and general symptoms, as well as improvements in personal and social functioning, a range on all these outcome measures was noted. The authors found that pretreatment levels of impairment and distress were significantly related to outcome, but that demographic variables were not. Aspects of the therapists' techniques interacted with two "dispositional" variables—organizational level of the self-concept, and motivation for dynamic psychotherapy—in predicting outcome of treatment. More exploratory techniques seemed to be more suitable for highly motivated and better organized patients, while more supportive actions were more suitable for patients at lower dispositional levels.[10]

Raphael[35] tested the effectiveness of brief supportive psychiatric therapy for widows judged be at high risk for morbidity. Two hundred recently bereaved women under the age of 60 were identified when they applied for widows' pensions. "High risk" was defined as perceived lack of social support and ambivalence in their marital relationships, two previously confirmed predictors of poor bereavement outcomes. Sixty-four high-risk widows were randomly allocated to an intervention group (N = 31) or nonintervention group (N = 33). The low-risk widows formed a residual control group. Psychotherapeutic interventions designed to support and facilitate the grieving process, and review of the marital relationship was offered by Raphael, a psychiatrist, in the widows' homes during the initial three-month crisis period of bereavement.

Widows in all three groups were assessed at 13 months after bereavement by a self-administered general health questionnaire sent through the mail. The therapy resulted in a significant reduction in the level of risk. At 13 months, there were significant differences in health status between the experimental and control group on such measures as physical symptoms, physician visits, weight loss, smoking, drinking and medicine use, depression, and ability to work. By this time the high-risk experimental subjects looked like their low-risk counterparts.

Polak and his colleagues studied the effects of immediate crisis intervention beginning within hours after the sudden death of a family member and continuing for 10 weeks.[34,57,58] Counseling by mental health professionals focused on family coping. The outcome measures used were medical and psychiatric ratings of individuals and families and self-reported health status. The authors found that short-term crisis intervention produced no major differences between the experimental group and the bereaved controls at 6 or 18 months after bereavement. In fact, they suggest that such very immediate intervention may have delayed or interfered with the normal bereavement process and that the counselors felt they were intruding on these families. Although this study has been severely criticized for the lack of comparability between the groups and other methodological shortcomings,[2] it nonetheless raises important questions about the timing of interventions. As discussed earlier in this chapter, experience from the original widow-to-widow program suggested that intervention was not appropriate for at least several weeks after bereavement. That professional services provided in the first hours of bereavement had no positive effects and may have upset family functioning is, therefore, not so surprising.

Mawson et al.[26] report on the effectiveness of a "guided mourning" intervention to assist patients who were stuck in their grieving. Twelve patients who complained of persistent distress for at least a year following bereavement were randomly allocated to one of two treatment conditions. Guided mourning focused on exposure to avoided and painful memories of the deceased. The control treatment encouraged the patient to avoid thinking of the deceased and to get on with life. This treatment condition was designed to mimic what the authors perceived to be the usual experience of the bereaved in their social encounters with family and friends. Individual patients in both groups were treated by a psychiatrist or nurse therapist for three 90-minute sessions over two weeks. Self-ratings before therapy, immediately after treatment, and at 4, 8, 12, and 28 weeks after treatment measured pathology of grief (physical symptoms, avoidance, hostility-anger-guilt, attitude toward self and the deceased), depression, anxiety, and social adjustment. Immediately after the two-week treatment and at the subsequent follow-up times, guided mourning patients showed improvement on most measures (sometimes statistically significant improvement) while control patients either did worse or showed no trend toward change.

There appear to be only two controlled studies in the literature on the effects of psychotherapeutic support for parents whose child has died or is dying. In an effort to assist parents in adjusting to their child's probable death, Kupst et al.[21] randomly allocated 64 families of children with leukemia who were being treated at Children's Memorial Hospital in Chicago to one of three groups: intense, moderate, and no support (from social workers and master's level counselors). No major differences were found between the groups on self-reports or professional ratings at 3, 6, 12, or 24 months after the initial diagnosis. Forrest et al.[4] offered immediate support and counseling for up to six weeks to mothers of stillborns and of babies who died within a week of birth. The social and emotional functioning of the experimental group was significantly better than that of the controls at 6 months after bereavement; by 14 months there were no significant differences between the groups. This finding is consistent with Vachon's findings[51] from her intervention with widows, namely, that support may speed up the recovery process but that in the long run most people recover on their own.

Finally, although there are no controlled studies of therapeutic interventions for bereaved children, there is one Israeli study of an intervention designed to assist children whose parent was dying.[38] Two to three months of weekly counseling during the parent's illness resulted in a significant decrease in children's anxiety and significant improvement in scholastic performance and social functioning at school, while matched unsupported controls did worse during this time. Unfortunately the children were not followed after the parent's death, so the long-term effects of anticipatory bereavement support are not known.

THE ROLE OF MEDICATIONS

Medications (pharmacologic interventions) may be used alone or in conjunction with any of the psychosocial approaches just described. Pharmacologic interventions have potential clinical value as well as important theoretical implications regarding the nature of the bereavement process. The medications used to assist the bereaved are almost always psychopharmacologic agents from three classes of drugs: (1) anti-anxiety drugs, (2) hypnotics, and (3) antidepressants.

Anti-Anxiety Drugs

These drugs also are known as "minor tranquilizers," "anxiolytics," and "sedatives." The most commonly prescribed drugs in this class are benzodiazepines, which are most often prescribed by primary care physicians to relieve symptoms of anxiety, fear, tension, "stress," or psychic pain. Controlled studies indicate they are of value in reducing distress in acute stress and situational neurotic reactions. However, no controlled studies have yet been conducted specifically on bereaved persons. Numerous surveys (see Chapter 2) report that bereaved persons use these drugs rather frequently, particularly during the early weeks of grief when subjective distress is greatest.

Hypnotics

Since insomnia is one of the common symptoms of grief, it is not surprising that many studies report use of hypnotics (sleeping pills) by many bereaved persons. Some of these hypnotics require a prescription (especially barbiturates and hypnotic benzodiazepines) while others do not. No studies have been directed specifically at evaluating the efficacy of any of these drugs in bereaved persons.[12,49]

Antidepressants

Tricyclic antidepressants and monoamine oxidase inhibitors have been shown to be effective in relieving symptoms and other manifestations of clinical depression in a large number of controlled studies.[19,28] Because the symptoms of grief may include sadness, hopelessness, bodily complaints, insomnia, and other features similar to clinical depression, it is not surprising that these drugs are prescribed for some grieving persons. In actual clinical practice, however, they are used relatively infrequently—far less frequently than anti-anxiety drugs and hypnotics.

Theoretical Issues

As indicated above, the possible value of psychopharmacologic medication for relieving the symptoms of acute grief is not substantiated by current evidence. But even if systematic studies were to demonstrate the efficacy of any of these drugs in reducing some of the distressing symptoms of grief, controversy would continue over their appropriate use. This controversy derives from different theoretical perspectives as to the "normality" or adaptive value of grief.

Many clinicians and theorists who view grief as normal believe that the use of drugs to reduce distress will interfere with the adaptive value of "grief work," and that failing to grieve or suppressing grief predisposes the individual to later mental disorder or medical disease.[28] Little evidence has been systematically collected to support this view (see Chapter 2).

Other clinicians and theorists are concerned over the possible impact of the intense distress of grief on biologic processes and functional activity. Viewing grief itself as a stressor, they support the use of psychopharmacologic drugs to relieve discomfort and to promote coping skills. However, even these clinicians tend to recommend caution—"The final resolution of loss is better accomplished by psychological help than by the use of drugs. Although drugs may be helpful in treating the . . . bereaved, their use is adjunctive, symptomatic, and limited in time."[8]

Recommendations for Clinical Practice

In the absence of scientific evidence, the committee is not able to make firm recommendations for clinical practice. The majority of clinicians who report using psychopharmacologic drugs for bereaved persons do so in the early phases of intense distress. However, concern has been expressed over possible adverse effects of these compounds. In particular, use of benzodiazepines or barbiturate-like drugs entails some risk of developing patterns of habitual use or frank drug dependence; in suicidal overdose, especially in combination with alcohol, all of these drugs may be lethal; and certain long-acting sleeping medications (e.g., flurazepam) and most tranquilizers carry risks of impaired daytime motor coordination and mental acuity—problems that can be especially hazardous to the elderly.[12,49]

Concern about adverse effects of certain benzodiazepines on elderly patients was also embodied in the recommendations made by a recent National Institutes of Health/National Institute of Mental Health consensus panel on drugs and insomnia.[30] The panel asserted that "short-term insomnia is usually associated with a situational stress (e.g., acute personal loss). . . . If drug treatment is elected, the smallest effective dose should be used . . . for a treatment period usually of not more than 3 weeks. Intermittent use of the drug is advisable, with skipping of nightly dosage after 1 or 2 good nights' sleep. . . . Aged patients, who tend to clear drugs more slowly and who are more sensitive to a given blood level of benzodiazepines, are more likely to develop cognitive and motor impairments when given the more slowly eliminated benzodiazepines [e.g., flurazepam and diazepam]. Ataxia and problems with memory and thinking are possible complications that may not appear until several weeks after beginning treatment. . . . Dosages for these populations must be carefully adjusted, and more rapidly eliminated drugs [e.g., temazepam, triazolam, and oxazepam] are preferable."

Although the committee is aware that antidepressants are sometimes used for bereaved persons, it does not recommend their use for individuals whose grief remains within "normal" bounds of intensity and duration. It should be noted that the use of antidepressants for grief (as opposed to depression) would be novel practice and, technically speaking, a new indication not currently approved by the Food and Drug Administration. If a bereaved individual were to meet the criteria of persistent symptoms and impaired function for a diagnosis of clinical depression, this diagnosis in itself would justify consideration of prescribing antidepressants.[13] However, even then it should be noted that although antidepressant drugs are of demonstrated value for many forms of clinical depression, not all diagnosed patients should automatically be prescribed drugs.

As discussed in earlier chapters, many bereaved individuals have depression-like symptoms during the early phase of grief. After a year, 10–20 percent still have persistent symptoms of depression. Some committee members argued that because of excessive caution about the treatment of depressive symptoms early in grieving, those who are truly depressed will be treated later than desirable. However, it is usually not possible to predict in the acute phase of grief who will remain depressed, and other committee members pointed out, therefore, that early drug therapy would result in the unnecessary treatment of a very substantial portion of bereaved individuals.

Recommendations for Research

In view of the lack of systematic controlled studies and the continuing controversy, the committee recommends that the National Institute of Mental Health sponsor and support studies on the impact of medications on the grieving process, especially the efficacy and adverse effects of benzodiazepines and tricyclic antidepressants. Such studies would examine the ability of drugs to reduce distress and promote social functioning as well as their potential for negative consequences, such as masking grief reactions that may appear later in distorted form.

Studies should be conducted to evaluate the short-term efficacy of drugs on specific symptoms as well as on coping abilities and on social, occupational, familial, and psychologic functioning. Studies involving long-term follow-up are also desirable to test hypotheses about the relationship between delayed, "absent," or suppressed grief and the subsequent development of medical illness, depression, alcoholism, and other emotional problems.

The committee notes the importance and difficulty of conducting methodologically and ethically sound drug studies. Since grief is not an illness and there is no established "treatment of choice," some may feel that drug trials in this area raise special ethical considerations. As is true of all human research, subjects will need to be well informed of the study goals, methods, possible adverse consequences, and remedies should these adverse consequences occur. For example, the adverse effects of antidepressant medications when used properly for limited time periods (up to six months) are relatively minor and somewhat predictable. When used for more extended periods, their effects are less well known. Subjects involved in drug trials would need to be informed of uncertainties such as these.

SUMMARY AND CONCLUSIONS

This chapter has described four types of programs for helping the bereaved and has analyzed the scant research evidence for the efficacy of each in an effort to address several basic questions.

Should All Bereaved People Be in an Intervention Program?

The evidence suggests that everyone needs support, reassurance, and some education and information following bereavement. This may be provided by family, friends, or clergy in an informal way, by laypeople in similar circumstances, by a community support group, or by health professionals. As discussed in the preceding chapter, health professionals have a responsibility to offer support, to inform the bereaved of additional resources in the community (such as mutual support groups), and to monitor their progress and make referrals to mental health professionals as appropriate.

There is no evidence that all bereaved people need or want formal interventions, though mutual support groups may fill a gap for those who have little other social support. There is some evidence to suggest that intervention programs help people to move faster through the grieving process, but ultimately most people get through it regardless of whether they have formal support. Still, shortening a process that is painful for an individual and for those around that person may be of considerable intrinsic value and deserves further study.

Which Programs Are Appropriate for Whom? And When?

The answer to this question is not entirely clear from the existing evidence. Furthermore, because most people do not experience enduring negative consequences or suffer ill health following bereavement and because of the paucity of outcome data regarding the efficacy of interventions, it would be unwise to make recommendations about the applicability of specific interventions. Nonetheless, some guidance can be offered about the appropriateness of the general approaches under various circumstances.

Experience from the widow-to-widow programs suggests that immediately following bereavement people are not generally ready to seek help outside their immediate social network or to benefit from it; for at least several weeks they are likely to feel more or less numb and to have the support of family and friends. Experiences from mutual support groups and hospices suggest that after several weeks one-to-one support from someone who has experienced bereavement may be useful. By this time family and friends may have returned to their usual activities and some of the reality of the loss may have begun to sink in. The opportunity to talk with another person who has had the same experience, can offer practical advice, and can assure the newly bereaved person that things will seem better soon is often very reassuring. Not until several months after bereavement do most widows feel ready to join a support group of other widows.

There is some evidence suggesting that a formal program during the very early period of crisis can be helpful for widows who are at high risk[35] or for mothers who lose newborns.[4] The latter point was also discussed at the site visit to the Boulder hospice, which sponsors a support group for parents who lose newborns. The experience of staff working with this group is that these parents want and need support and guidance immediately after the death, because there typically is no one in their social network who has shared the experience of the birth or who knew the infant.

For people who experience normal reactions and who are not seen as being at particularly high risk for adverse consequences of bereavement, the support of family and friends, perhaps augmented by some type of mutual support intervention, will generally be sufficient. However, for people who define themselves or who are seen by others in the community as continuing to be overwhelmed by their grief (or unable to grieve), psychotherapeutic interventions may be warranted. In addition, certain categories of people may be at such high risk following bereavement that they should perhaps be evaluated by mental health professionals and followed for some period of time, with psychotherapeutic interventions as indicated. These groups include young children who have lost a parent or sibling, people with a history of psychiatric disorders (especially depression), and people related or close to someone who committed suicide.

How Effective Are the Various Interventions?

As indicated above, very little is known about the ability of any intervention to reduce the pain and stress of bereavement, to shorten the normal process, or to mitigate its long-term negative consequences. While the few controlled studies that have been conducted report contradictory findings, subjective reports attesting to the helpfulness of interventions abound.

All intervention strategies, from well-meaning words of comfort offered by friends to professionally rendered psychotherapy, have a potential for both positive and negative consequences. Yet the possibility of iatrogenic effects (poor outcomes due to the interventions) is rarely discussed, and their occurrence in psychosocial interventions has never, to our knowledge, been rigorously studied. For example, although numerous anecdotal reports and a few controlled studies attest to the positive features of mutual support, it is possible that peer pressure exerted on individuals who are psychologically vulnerable following bereavement could lead to some poor outcomes, such as feelings of failure for not living up to group expectations or changing in ways that, while consistent with group norms, are ultimately not helpful to the individual. Perhaps those who are vulnerable to these potential problems are the ones who choose not to participate in these programs. Little is known about the selection biases that predispose some people to seek help and others not to, on what bases people choose specific modalities of help, or about how people would have fared without interventions.

Recommendations for Future Preventive Intervention Research

Before recommendations can be made about the appropriateness of specific interventions under particular circumstances, a considerable amount of research is needed. All such studies should be conducted within a context that acknowledges the normal variability in individual responses and adaptation to bereavement, cultural diversity, respect for grief as a normative process, and awareness of the dangers of seeing variations within a normal range as health problems. As discussed in several previous chapters, there is a great need to reach consensus about what constitutes appropriate outcomes of the bereavement process and how to measure them. Broad categories of outcomes for which measures are needed include diminished distress levels such as decline in depressive symptomatology; inappropriate or excessive use of cigarettes, alcohol, sedatives, and medical care; physical health effects including exacerbation of previous illnesses; social role performance; and intrapsychic processes, such as changes in self-image and attributions. In order to be meaningful, intervention research must be specific to the age and sex of the survivor, the nature of the lost relationship, the nature of the death, and the phase of bereavement. These basic variables and other modifiers of responses, such as the actual and perceived availability and adequacy of social support, must be adequately controlled for in the research designs and analyses before conclusive statements can be made about the impact of interventions. Research on preventive interventions should be designed to test hypotheses generated from basic research on the grieving process and its multiple outcomes. With the new Medicare funding, hospices provide a natural opportunity for large-scale studies of bereavement and the impact of a variety of different interventions on outcomes.

With these general considerations in mind, several specific areas would be useful to study:

- the differential impact of interventions aimed at assisting the bereaved during various phases of the grieving process (such as before and immediately after death) and designed to assist with different aspects of bereavement (such as immediate distress or longer-term social adaption and reorganization)
- the differential impact of interventions aimed at specific elements of the stress model: the context of the event, modifiers such as personality variables, coping styles, and social support networks

• the impact of interventions on high- versus low-risk people, including identification of the level of risk, ameliorative measures, and specific outcomes

• the characteristics of different mutual support and psychotherapeutic approaches and their ability to effect recovery, diminish psychologic distress, and promote social functioning

• the relative benefits of one-to-one versus group support at various phases of the bereavement process

• the relationship between self-reported and objectively measured outcomes

• the use of medications (sedatives, hypnotics, and antidepressants) and their effects on the course of bereavement

• the effects of different types of interveners on outcomes

• the effects of psychosocial and pharmacologic interventions on basic biologic processes involved in the course and outcomes of bereavement in animals and human beings

• the impact of information about bereavement processes on the behavior of professionals and on the behavior, course of grieving, and outcomes of bereaved individuals

REFERENCES

1. Barrett, C.J. Effectiveness of widows' groups in facilitating change. *Journal of Consulting and Clinical Psychology* 46:20–31, 1978.
2. Bloom, B.L. *Community Mental Health: A General Introduction*. Belmont, Calif.: Wadsworth Publishing, 1975.
3. Cameron, J., and Brings, B. Bereavement outcome following preventive intervention: a controlled study. In: *The R.V.H. Manual on Palliative/Hospice Care* (Ajemian, I., and Mount, B.M., eds.). New York: Arno Press, 1980.
4. Forrest, G.C., Standish, E., and Baum, J.D. Support after perinatal death: a study of support and counselling after perinatal bereavement. *British Medical Journal* 285:1475–1479, 1982.
5. Gerber, I., Wiener, A., Battin, D., and Arkin, A.M. Brief therapy to the aged bereaved. In: *Bereavement: Its Psychosocial Aspects* (Schoenberg, B., and Gerber, I., eds.). New York: Columbia University Press, 1975.
6. Greer, D., Mor, V., Sherwood, S., Morris, J.N., and Birnbaum, H. (eds.) *Final Report of the National Hospice Study*. Submitted to the Health Care Financing Administration, Washington, D.C., 1984.
7. Hamburg, B.A., and Killilea, M. Relation of social support, stress, illness and use of health services. In: *Healthy People: The Surgeon General's Report on Disease Prevention and Health Promotion*, Vol. II. Washington, D.C.: U.S. Government Printing Office, 1979.
8. Hollister, L. Psychotherapeutic drugs in the dying and bereaved. *Journal of Thanatology* 2:623–629, 1972.
9. Horowitz, M.J., Krupnick, J., Kaltreider, N., Wilner, N., Leong, A., and Marmar, C.

Initial psychological response to parental death. *Archives of General Psychiatry* 38:316–323, 1981.

10. Horowitz, M.J., Marmar, C., Weiss, D., DeWitt, K., and Rosenbaum, R. Brief psychotherapy of bereavement reactions: the relationship of process to outcome. *Archives of General Psychiatry* (in press), 1984.

11. Horowitz, M.J., Weiss, D.S., Kaltreider, N., Krupnick, J., Wilner, N., Marmar, C., and Dewitt, K. Response to death of a parent: a follow up study. *Journal of Nervous and Mental Diseases* (in press), 1984.

12. Institute of Medicine, National Academy of Sciences. *Sleeping Pills, Insomnia and Medical Practice.* Washington, D.C.: National Academy of Sciences, 1979.

13. Jacobs, S. Questions and answers. *Hospital and Community Psychiatry* 33:532, 1982.

14. Katz, A.H. Self-help organizations and volunteer participation in social welfare. *Social Work* 15:51–60, 1970.

15. Kiely, M.C. Royal Victoria Hospital bereavement study evaluation report. Paper presented at Palliative Care Conference on Bereavement: New Horizons, Philadelphia, September 1983.

16. Killilea, M. Mutual help organizations: interpretations in the literature. In: *Support Systems and Mutual Help* (Caplan, G., and Killilea, M., eds.). New York: Grune and Stratton, 1976.

17. Killilea, M. Interaction of crisis theory, coping strategies and social support systems. In: *The Modern Practice of Community Mental Health* (Schulberg, H.C., and Killilea, M., eds.). San Francisco: Jossey-Bass, 1982.

18. Klerman, G., Weissman, M., Rounsaville, B., and Chevron, E. *Interpersonal Psychotherapy of Depression.* New York: Basic Books, 1984.

19. Kolb, L., and Brodie, H. *Modern Clinical Psychiatry* (10th edition). Philadelphia: W.B. Saunders, 1982.

20. Krupnick, J., and Horowitz, M. Stress response syndromes: recurrent themes. *Archives of General Psychiatry* 38:428–435, 1981.

21. Kupst, M.J., Tylk, L., Thomas, L., Mudd, M.E., Richardson, C., and Schulman, J.L. Strategies of intervention with families of pediatric leukemia patients: a longitudinal perspective. *Social Work in Health Care* 8:31–47, 1982.

22. Lattanzi, M.E. Hospice bereavement services: creating networks of support. *Family and Community Health* 5(3):54–63, 1982.

23. Lazare, A. Unresolved grief. In: *Outpatient Psychiatry: Diagnosis and Treatment* (Lazare, A., ed.). Baltimore: Williams & Wilkins, 1979.

24. Lieberman, M.A., and Borman, L.D. Researchers study THEOS: report group's effect big help to members. *THEOS* 20:3–6, 1981.

25. Lynn, J., and Osterweis, M. Ethical issues arising in hospice care. In: *Hospice Programs and Public Policy* (Torrens, P.R., ed.). Chicago: American Hospital Association (in press), 1984.

26. Mawson, D., Marks, I.M., Ramm, L., and Stern, R.S. Guided mourning for morbid grief: a controlled study. *British Journal of Psychiatry* 138:185–193, 1981.

27. Melges, F.T., and DeMaso, D.R. Grief resolution therapy: reliving, revising, and revisiting. *American Journal of Psychotherapy* 34:51–60, 1980.

28. Morgan, D. Not all sadness can be treated with antidepressants. *West Virginia Medical Journal* 76(6):136–137, 1980.

29. Munley, A. *The Hospice Alternative: A New Context for Death and Dying.* New York: Basic Books, 1983.

30. National Institutes of Health Consensus Development Conference Panel. Confer-

ence on Drugs and Insomnia November 15–17, 1983. *Conference Summary*, Vol. 4, No. 10. Bethesda, MD: NIH Office of Medical Applications Research, 1983. Also, *Journal of the American Medical Association* (in press), 1984.

31. Osterweis, M., and Champagne, D.S. The U.S. hospice movement: issues in development. *American Journal of Public Health* 69:492–496, 1979.

32. Parkes, C.M. Bereavement counselling: does it work? *British Medical Journal* 281:3–6, 1980.

33. Parkes, C.M. Evaluation of a bereavement service. *Journal of Preventive Psychiatry* 1:179–188, 1981.

34. Polak, P.R., Egan, D., Vandenbergh, R., and Williams, W.V. Prevention in mental health. *American Journal of Psychiatry* 132:146–149, 1975.

35. Raphael, B. Preventive intervention with the recently bereaved. *Archives of General Psychiatry* 34:1450–1454, 1977.

36. Riessman, F. The helper therapy principle. *Social Work* 10:27–32, 1965.

37. Rogers, J., Vachon, M.L.S., Lyall, W.A., Sheldon, A., and Freeman, S.J.J. A self-help program for widows as an independent community service. *Hospital and Community Psychiatry* 31:844–847, 1980.

38. Rosenheim, E., and Ichilov, Y. Short term preventive therapy with children of fatally ill parents. *Israeli Annals of Psychiatry and Related Disciplines* 17:67-73, 1979.

39. St. Christopher's Hospice. *St. Christopher's Hospice Annual Report, 1974-75*, London, England, 1975.

40. Saunders, C. Control of pain in terminal cancer. *Nursing Times* 72:1133–1135, 1976.

41. Sherwood, S., Morris, J.N., and Wrights, S.M. Primary care persons' bereavement outcomes. In: *Final Report of the National Hospice Study* (Greer, D., Mor, V., Sherwood, S., Morris, J.M., and Birnbaum, H., eds.). Submitted to the Health Care Financing Administration, Washington, D.C., 1984.

42. Silverman, P.R. Services to the widowed during the period of bereavement. In: *Social Work Practice: Proceedings*. New York: Columbia University Press, 1966.

43. Silverman, P.R. The widow as caregiver in a program of preventive intervention with other widows. *Mental Hygiene* 54:540–547, 1970.

44. Silverman, P.R. Widowhood and preventive intervention. *Family Coordinator* 21:95–102, 1972.

45. Silverman, P.R. *If You Will Lift the Load, I Will Lift It Too: A Guide to Developing Widow-to-Widow Programs*. New York: Jewish Funeral Directors of America, 1976.

46. Silverman, P.R. Bereavement as a normal life transition. In: *Social Work With the Dying Patient and the Family* (Prichard, E., Collard, J., Orcutt, B., Kutscher, A., Seeland, I., and Lefkowitz, N., eds.). New York: Columbia University Press, 1977.

47. Silverman, P.R., and Cooperband, A. On widowhood: mutual help and the elderly widow. *Journal of Geriatric Psychiatry* 8:9–27, 1975.

48. Silverman, P.R., MacKenzie, D., Pettipas, M., and Wilson, E.W. (eds.). *Helping Each Other in Widowhood*. New York: Health Sciences Publishing, 1974.

49. Solomon, F., White, C., Parron, D.L., and Mendelson, W. Sleeping pills, insomnia, and medical practice. *New England Journal of Medicine* 300:803–808, 1979.

50. Spiegel, D. The recent literature: self-help and mutual support groups. *Community Mental Health Review* 5:15–25, 1980.

51. Vachon, M.L.S., Sheldon, A.R., Lancee, W.J., Lyall, W.A.L., Rogers, J., and Freeman, S.J.J. A controlled study of self-help intervention for widows. *American Journal of Psychiatry* 137:1380–1384, 1980.

52. Vachon, M.L.S., Sheldon, A.R., Lancee, W.J., Lyall, W.A.L., Rogers, J., and Freeman, S.J.J. Correlates of enduring distress patterns following bereavement: social network, life situation and personality. *Psychological Medicine* 12:783–788, 1982.
53. Videka-Sherman, L. Effects of participation in a self-help group for bereaved parents: Compassionate Friends. *Prevention in Human Services* 1:69–77, 1982.
54. Volkan, V.D. ''Re-grief'' therapy. In: *Bereavement: Its Psychological Aspects* (Schoenberg, B., and Gerber, I., eds.). New York: Columbia University Press, 1975.
55. Waskow, I.E., and Parloff, M.B. (Eds.) *Psychotherapy Change Measures.* Rockville, MD: National Institute of Mental Health, DHEW Pub. No. (ADM)74–120, 1975.
56. Waskow, I.E., Parloff, M.B., Hadley, S.W., and Autry, J.H. *Treatment of Depression Collaborative Research Program: Background and Research Plan.* Rockville, MD: National Institute of Mental Health (in press), 1984.
57. Williams, W.V., Lee, J., and Polak, P.R. Crisis intervention: effects of crisis intervention on family survivors of sudden death situations. *Community Mental Health Journal* 12:128–136, 1976.
58. Williams, W.V., and Polak, P.R. Follow-up research in primary prevention: a model of adjustment in acute grief. *Journal of Clinical Psychology* 35:35–45, 1979.
59. Worden, J.W. *Grief Counseling and Grief Therapy: A Handbook for the Mental Health Practitioner.* New York: Springer, 1982.

Conclusions and Recommendations

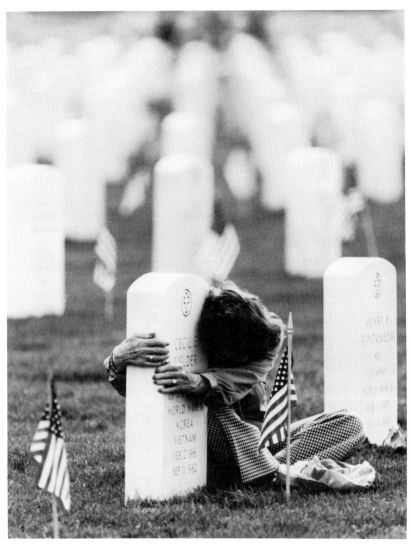

ANTHONY SUAU/THE DENVER POST

CHAPTER 11

Conclusions and Recommendations

In this chapter, the committee recapitulates its major conclusions and suggests directions for clinical practice and future research. These conclusions and recommendations are organized around the three questions mandated for study.

WHAT CAN BE CONCLUDED FROM AVAILABLE RESEARCH EVIDENCE ABOUT THE HEALTH CONSEQUENCES OF BEREAVEMENT?

The evidence from clinical experience and several kinds of research—epidemiologic, case follow-up, clinical, and social science—leads to several important conclusions. First, bereavement is associated with appreciable distress in virtually everyone. Second, the distress, which can vary greatly in intensity and in the extent of interference with function, is long lasting. A survivor's way of life can be altered for as long as three years and commonly is disturbed for at least one year. Third, there is tremendous variation in individuals' reactions to bereavement. These reactions consist of a number of intertwined processes—psychologic, social, and biologic. They cannot be neatly plotted in a series of well-defined stages, nor is movement from the impact of the death to the resolution of bereavement likely to be in a straight path. Individuals will vary in terms of speed of recovery and in the amount of back-and-forth movement between phases. Fourth, as has been recorded in myth and literature over the centuries, and as suggested by individual clinical experience, some bereaved persons are at increased risk for illness and even death.

Most bereaved individuals do not become seriously ill or die following the loss of someone close, but there is good evidence linking bereavement to a number of adverse health outcomes for some people. These health consequences include premature mortality, some medical and psychiatric morbidity, and health-damaging behaviors. Following conjugal bereavement, young and middle-aged widowers who do not remarry are at increased risk of mortality for a number of years, especially during the first year. For women, there is some evidence suggesting increased mortality in the second year (but not the first) following bereavement. Higher mortality rates in men are due to increases in the relative risk of death by suicide, accidents, cardiovascular disease, and some infectious diseases. In widows, the relative risk of death from cirrhosis and perhaps suicide increases. The bereaved's increased alcohol consumption, smoking, and use of tranquilizers and other medicines are well documented, especially among people who used these substances prior to the loss. Thus, bereavement appears to exacerbate and precipitate health-compromising behaviors.

During the early, "acute" phase of bereavement, most adults suffer a variety of symptoms, some of which also are characteristic of depression. Yet the constant, painful awareness of loss, together with the relative absence of self-blame, makes it clear that ordinary grief is distinct from depression. Grief may, however, give way to depression; approximately 10 to 20 percent of the widowed are still sufficiently symptomatic a year or more after their loss to suggest real clinical depression. Although this proportion is relatively small, out of the approximately 800,000 people who are widowed each year, this means that 80,000 to 160,000 people suffer serious depression in any given year. The number of depressed individuals following other types of bereavement—death of a child, sibling, or parent—is not known.

There are few good controlled studies linking bereavement to specific disorders. But the diagnosis-specific mortality rates, symptoms, and health behaviors just discussed suggest that bereavement may exacerbate existing illnesses, precipitate depression leading to suicide, aggravate or lead to alcohol abuse that can result in cirrhosis of the liver, and leave people vulnerable to infectious diseases.

Like adults, children exhibit a range of responses immediately following bereavement. Although some researchers have reported that children do not grieve in the same way as adults, a number of grief-like reactions have been noted, such as appetite and sleep disturbances and difficulty in concentrating. Like adults, bereaved children may complain of physical symptoms, especially abdominal pain. They may also withdraw and regress in their behavior. There is general agreement that school functioning—both academic performance and social behavior—are adversely affected by bereavement. Not surprisingly, the way children react to death depends on their age and stage of development.

Enduring psychologic symptoms of neurosis and depression have been observed in community and patient samples of children who have lost a parent or sibling. Several studies report a relationship between childhood bereavement and mental illness, especially depression, in adult life, as well as increased risk of suicide. There is evidence suggesting a link between this type of early loss and adult impairment in sexual identity, capacity for intimacy, and development of autonomy. Thus, at least some bereaved children are at increased risk for a number of adverse consequences. However, current data do not support the impression that the negative results are as widespread or as inevitable as formerly thought. Although the full impact of death on children may not be realized until many years later, many factors subsequent to the death—including the normal developmental push and the adequacy of caretakers—will have major effects on ultimate outcomes.

Almost everyone—adults and children—is distressed when someone close dies, yet the nature of the distress and its manifestations depend on a host of factors relating to characteristics of the bereaved individual and of the deceased, the nature of the death, the nature and meaning of the relationship, and perceptions about the availability and adequacy of social support before and after the death. These factors also influence the outcomes of the bereavement process, including the health outcomes just discussed. Certain biologic, psychologic, social, and situational factors that place individuals at risk or protect them from adversity are apparent prior to the loss, others are related to the death itself, and some become apparent in the early aftermath of bereavement.

Although rigorous studies of these many risk factors have not been conducted, there are several that appear to be good predictors of certain outcomes of bereavement. Poor previous physical health is associated with poor physical health following bereavement. Mental illness, especially depression, is likewise likely to be exacerbated following bereavement and to interfere with normal grieving. Perceived social support is the best replicated predictor of psychosocial adjustment. However, like marriage—which appears to be a protective factor for men against poor health following a spouse's death—it is not clear whether the mere presence of social support leads to good outcomes, or whether people who were emotionally healthy to begin with are able to elicit social support to meet their needs following bereavement.

ARE THERE PREVENTIVE INTERVENTIONS THAT SHOULD BE MORE WIDELY ADOPTED IN THE HEALTH CARE SYSTEM?

Viewed in its broadest sense, the term "preventive intervention" includes education, assessment, and primary, secondary, and tertiary prevention. From that perspective, there are a number of informal and formal activities that the committee felt should be undertaken with the bereaved in the community and as a part of humane and professionally responsible practice. As discussed in Chapter 9, the committee's views in this area are based more on its own collective judgment and upon clinical case reports than on definitive research findings.

The committee was struck by the large amount of advice in the literature directed to the public and to health professionals, and by the enormous growth of lay and professional programs to assist the bereaved. Although much of the advice and many of the programs seem to rest on solid conceptual ground, very few studies have been conducted to determine whether these concepts have been translated into appropriate intervention strategies or even to test their effects.

Because of this lack of evidence on the efficacy of the many intervention strategies, the committee cannot recommend that as a matter of public policy any particular approach be more widely adopted at this time. However, the efforts to devise conceptually sound programs to assist the bereaved are to be commended and certainly should not be discontinued. In fact, as discussed in Chapter 10 and in the final section of this chapter, the committee believes it is time to subject various intervention strategies to rigorous study so as to determine their benefit to particular groups of bereaved individuals.

Practice Recommendations

In the committee's view, the well-being of the family and others close to a dying patient is part of health professionals' responsibility in terminal illness. Furthermore, as indicated in Chapter 9, the committee believes that health care professionals and institutions have a continuing responsibility to assist the bereaved. The education of health care professionals should prepare them to provide information, offer emotional support, recognize the red flags that may signal a need for professional mental health intervention, and be knowledgeable about both lay and professional community resources to which the bereaved can be referred as appropriate and desired. Routine history taking in primary care settings should include questions about recent losses and attention to the individual's adjustment to them.

This is not to suggest that health professionals must routinely engage in long-term counseling of the bereaved. The committee does suggest, however, that within the context of ongoing medical care, professionals have some responsibility—beyond simple human compassion—to become knowledgeable about bereavement and skilled in dealing with it. Unfortunately, in most reimbursement schemes there is a strong disincentive to provide the kind of follow-up activities described in this volume as desirable. The committee hopes that, while progress is being made toward remedying this, institutions will recognize the importance of such activities and will permit health professionals to spend time with the bereaved, even in the absence of direct reimbursement.

That nursing and medical education should prepare health professionals for this role is not a new proposal. It has been a matter of public and professional concern for a number of years. The committee thus endorses efforts to devise training methods that will better equip health professionals to deal with sensitive psychosocial issues, to be aware of their own limitations, and to have the necessary knowledge and skills to make appropriate referrals.

In the committee's view, these skills must rest on the broader foundations that health and mental health education and preparation for the ministry provide in order to be effective. The committee cannot endorse the development and certification of a new profession for ''grief counseling'' that is separate from existing health and social services.

Until better data are available on variations in grief responses among the members of ethnic and minority groups, health professionals should be aware that the phases, timing, and significance of grieving by individuals of different backgrounds may vary from those reported in studies of persons in the mainstream population. In particular, as discussed in Chapter 8, the likelihood of the distress following bereavement taking the form of physical symptoms, and the particular bodily complaints, may vary substantially by cultural group and social class. If they are unaware of this possibility, health professionals might conduct needless and costly tests or prescribe unnecessary and potentially harmful treatment. Thus, the committee urges that caution be used in determining deviance from norms, almost all of which have been based on the mainstream Caucasian culture.

It is readily apparent that most bereaved individuals do not need professional mental health treatment. Yet, there are certain symptoms and circumstances of bereavement that are likely to warrant professional intervention for people in all cultural groups. For both adults and children, a prior history of mental illness, especially depression, and the suicide of someone close are likely to render them especially vulnerable and therefore candidates for close professional monitoring following bereavement. Persistent somatic complaints or depressive symptoms that do not lessen in intensity over time may also be signs of difficulty. In children, repeated aggressive or hostile behavior toward others, a prolonged drop in school performance, or regressive and insecure behaviors that persist over time are additional signs that help may be needed. For adults, drug and alcohol abuse, other health-injurious behaviors, difficulty in maintaining social relationships, and an individual's own perception that he or she is not doing well should trigger a professional referral for evaluation. Furthermore, if the occurrence of an individual's symptoms is associated with family dysfunction, it is logical to include family assessment and treatment when dealing with abnormal bereavement states.

In the case of bereaved children, it seems clear there is a potential for long-term, enduring consequences. Whether the best way to handle this vulnerability is with routine, periodic ''mental health check-ups'' is not clear. Such check-ups might lead both parents and child to believe there will be problems—potentially contributing to a self-fulfilling prophecy. Thus, in the committee's view, it would be better to educate those who interact with children (parents, teachers, pediatricians) to recognize the signs that indicate a need for professional mental health intervention than to have mental health workers routinely involved.

As discussed in Chapters 2 and 10, a number of drugs are rather commonly prescribed to help ease the pain of bereavement. Many physicians have been hesitant to prescribe medication, particularly tricyclic antidepressants, for patients experiencing grief reactions, even when these are intense, distressing, and disabling. The view is widely held that to suppress the grief experience will have later adverse consequences. Yet no controlled trials have been reported in the literature to assess the long-term or short-term, positive or negative effects of antidepressants on grief. The absence of such trials is all the more striking in view of the fact that clinical reports indicate a substantial proportion of bereaved individuals are often prescribed sedatives and minor tranquilizers, primarily for insomnia. Again, there are no controlled trials of the efficacy of such prescriptions. Quite clearly such studies are needed. In the absence of such data, the committee urges clinicians to exercise caution in prescribing medications for bereaved individuals.

The committee noted with interest the various efforts of health care institutions to assist the bereaved and to support health professionals in their activities in settings made stressful by frequent death. Examples of institutional responses to the soon-to-be bereaved and recently bereaved that appear to be conceptually sound practices include the availability of well-trained social workers and chaplains to assist dying patients and their families, hospital-based support groups for parents who lose a newborn and for relatives surviving other kinds of deaths, liberal visiting hours to allow families to spend time with dying patients, efforts to work with families and patients who prefer to be at home, and sensitivity to families' wishes regarding their presence at the time of death.

Not only must health care institutions be concerned with the well-being of patients and their families. They must also pay attention to staff needs, especially in such stressful settings as intensive care units, emergency rooms, and cancer wards, and to the impact of management and organizational practices on staff functioning in such settings. Some mechanisms for monitoring staff emotional response to their work should be formalized. Regular meetings at which staff are encouraged to air their concerns, adequate back-up support from mental health professionals, and clearly delineated roles on health care teams may help alleviate the sense of isolation and overwhelming burden of individual responsibility so commonly reported.

Public Education

Because of the fairly recent historical changes noted in this volume, including institutional care of the dying and geographic mobility of families, most people have little direct contact with death and may not be prepared for its impact on their families. That the public wants information about bereavement is evidenced by the amount of attention paid to this topic in the mass media. In recent years there have been numerous articles, television shows, and radio programs dealing with people's reactions to bereavement. Although there are no studies to document the effects of information on the bereavement process, the committee was struck by the widespread view that thorough information of several types can be beneficial and often seems to be lacking. As discussed in several chapters, people's reactions to bereavement often are so varied, intense, and unexpected that they and those around them may be caught off guard. People expect to feel sad; they do not expect to be angry at the deceased. And yet anger is common. They may be surprised at how quickly their emotions swing from one feeling to another and at their inability to control their moods. Knowing how they are feeling, they may be surprised that others in the family seem to be reacting so differently. Numerous anecdotes are reported in the literature about the inappropriateness of well-meaning comments offered by friends of the bereaved.

These examples and many others discussed in this volume suggest that people need information to prepare themselves for the death of someone close and to respond sensitively to others in similar situations. As discussed in Chapter 10, this has been a major activity of many mutual support groups. Because bereavement is and should be handled largely by families and other informal social networks, public education about reactions to bereavement and how they might differ for adults and children, and for mothers and fathers, should be encouraged so that families and friends can provide the best possible support for the bereaved.

WHAT FURTHER RESEARCH WOULD BE ESPECIALLY PROMISING TO PURSUE?

Throughout this volume, gaps in current understanding about the bereavement process, its outcomes, and the methods to assist the bereaved have been pointed out. Inadequacies in the data base, such as the narrow scope of research, lack of good multidisciplinary studies, and some pervasive methodologic problems, have hampered the development of definitive conclusions. In this section, the committee draws together its key recommendations regarding future research directions that seem especially promising.

Research on the Processes and Outcomes of Bereavement

Important health consequences of bereavement do exist, although they are not evenly distributed in the general population of bereaved people. As discussed in Chapters 2 through 5 and in Chapter 8, a large number of psychologic, social, situational, and biologic factors have been implicated as contributors to increased risk of adverse consequences. Few of these risk factors have been well studied. Their relative importance is not known, nor is much understood about which factors contribute to which outcomes. These influences are likely to interact in complex ways to place individuals at risk in some ways and protect them in others.

In the committee's view, high priority should be given to research aimed at better documentation and refinement of those factors that place particular individuals or groups at high risk following the death of someone close. Current hypotheses about subpopulations that are at risk for particular adverse consequences should be tested, and prospective studies should be designed to identify characteristics of new subgroups. More definitive knowledge about individual risk factors and their interplay holds the promise of identification of high-risk individuals and the design of interventions to prevent or mitigate specific negative outcomes.

To accomplish this goal, the scope of research must be broadened. Although there is a vast literature from many different disciplines, most of it is on conjugal bereavement in adults and parental bereavement in children. There are very few data on the nature and consequences of bereavement following the death of a sibling at any age, of a child at any age, or of parents during adult life. Research on specific losses would clarify understanding of the special problems of each. Current understanding of the relationship between bereavement and the nature of the death is also very limited.

Second, the health consequences of bereavement, especially the medical ones, are less well researched for children than for adults who have lost a spouse. Most studies of children are retrospective and have not used control groups. Most are based on responses of children receiving mental health care or, in the case of very young children, are based on observations of institutionalized children. Controlled studies of community samples of bereaved children should be conducted. Professionals' current knowledge does not clearly indicate whether it is bereavement itself or the way a child is dealt with and cared for subsequently that has the most effect on long-term outcomes. Prospective longitudinal studies that follow children for many years could shed some light on this issue.

Third, most of what is known about bereavement comes from observations made in the United States, the United Kingdom, Australia, and Israel. The American literature, but for a few descriptive accounts, is limited almost exclusively to studies of white, usually middle-class, persons. How other socioeconomic, racial, and ethnic groups react psychologically, socially, and biologically to bereavement is not known. Thus, it is unclear how generalizable the current knowledge base is; this makes it difficult to develop intervention strategies that are appropriate to the needs of minority groups. Indeed, as pointed out in Chapter 8, there is reason to suspect that impoverished ethnic minority group members, recent refugees, and migrants may be at especially high risk for negative health outcomes of bereavement. This topic should be investigated. Such research would benefit from interdisciplinary collaboration of health researchers with anthropologists and with health professionals who share a cultural identity with the groups being studied. Research on these three groups—individuals who have experienced various types of losses, children, and various sociocultural groups—would greatly expand the scope of current knowledge of the impact of bereavement upon specific subpopulations.

To refine this knowledge, research on the biology of grieving is also needed. As discussed in Chapter 6, grief produces major perturbations in the respiratory, autonomic, and endocrine systems and may substantially alter cardiovascular and immune function as well. Much of the existing biologic research has been concerned simply with documenting these changes in animals and humans. In the committee's view, it is time now to focus on clinically relevant physiologic changes in humans in order to understand better the mechanisms by which reactions to bereavement might result in actual illness.

In particular, more information is needed on the long-term effects of loss in order to understand how physiologic responses change over the course of grieving and how responses to loss compare with other responses to stress. Additional studies are needed on the basic neurophysiologic parameters of grief responses in order to understand more fully the susceptibility of bereaved subjects to disease. The relationship between the responses to loss and responses to other life stresses, and detailed comparisons of neuroendocrine and other biologic changes accompanying grief and depression are needed. Multidisciplinary studies should be conducted of the relationships between the intertwined but not fully congruent behavioral, psychosocial, and biologic processes. This expanded knowledge of physiologic processes following bereavement and their relationship to other responses will contribute to the development of appropriate preventive interventions.

Most studies, whether biologic or psychologic, focus on the first year of bereavement. But because most people now die of chronic illness with forewarning for their families, the period of anticipatory grieving before the death deserves rigorous study. Furthermore, because it seems clear that for many people the grieving process continues beyond a year, studies should track bereaved individuals for a longer period of time. Thus, more prospective longitudinal studies that begin before and run for several years after bereavement are needed.

Traditionally, health consequences have been studied in individuals, but there is a growing realization that the individual's reactions may be based partly on interactions with the individual's most intimate group, which usually is the family. The death of one member will affect each and every other member as well as the family system as a whole. Thus, following bereavement, the changes in roles, relationships, and functioning within the family could lead to symptoms or disease in one or more members. In order to fully understand this process, prospective studies of entire families are needed.

Finally, all research in this field has suffered from certain methodological shortcomings. It has been hampered by the lack of agreement concerning predictor variables and outcomes—what things are appropriate to measure, how to measure them, and what to consider as endpoints. This problem is evident in the epidemiologic, psychosocial, and intervention studies. So long as researchers make idiosyncratic decisions about these issues, comparisons across studies can be made only tentatively. The committee therefore recommends that the National Institute of Mental Health (NIMH) sponsor a conference of scientists from the many professional disciplines involved in bereavement research to develop a consensus about predictors and outcomes so that future studies will be more fully comparable.

Although a great deal is known about various aspects of bereavement and its consequences, most of it is discipline-specific. Isolated findings from psychology and psychiatry and from the biologic, medical, and social sciences each tell part of the story. But until more good multidisciplinary studies are done, the bereavement process and the mechanisms that explain it cannot be fully understood. Without such studies, the interactions between risk factors will remain unclear and it will not be possible to confidently identify groups at high risk. Good cross-disciplinary longitudinal studies also will provide the foundations for intervention strategies that are appropriate to the range of needs of bereaved individuals.

The committee recognizes the difficulties involved in long-term multidisciplinary research. It is hard to get and keep a team of researchers together, and the research is expensive. There are special problems inherent in studying people over time: the situation is not static, many intervening variables cannot be controlled, and there are practical difficulties involved in tracking people for years. Nonetheless, in the committee's view, funding agencies should give high priority to such research because it is only through well-designed, long-term, prospective, multidisciplinary studies that the impact of bereavement will really be understood.

Research on Intervention Strategies

The committee strongly urges that a broad research initiative be undertaken to study the impact of various psychosocial and pharmacologic interventions on the course and consequences of bereavement. Such research should be conducted in the awareness of cultural diversity and individual variations in reaction to bereavement. It should be specific to age, sex, social class, ethnicity, nature of the loss, and phase of bereavement. The impact of interventions on the acute distress of bereavement, on social as well as biologic functioning, and on health are some of the outcomes that deserve study.

Current knowledge about the four major types of interventions discussed in Chapter 10—mutual support, hospices, psychotherapy, and drug therapy—does not yield conclusions about the applicability and effectiveness of specific interventions. There is a paucity of good outcome data regarding their efficacy, apparently for several reasons. In the case of the psychotherapeutic approaches, confidentiality and small sample sizes have constrained research. In the case of mutual support groups and hospices, there is typically no one associated with the programs who has research skills and there has sometimes been a reluctance to expose the programs to scrutiny.

Although the committee does not wish to single out any one approach as more deserving of study than another, it notes that there is currently an opportunity to study hospice bereavement programs that should not be ignored. With the amendment of the Social Security Act in 1982, hospice patient care services will now be reimbursed by Medicare for a three-year period. Although bereavement services for families will not be directly reimbursed, hospice programs must include these services in order to qualify for Medicare. Increasingly large numbers of people are being served by hospices and standardized data collection requirements are being established. The diversity of programs should enable the study of various approaches to bereavement intervention in a naturally occurring experiment.

In the committee's view, the Health Care Financing Administration and other branches of the federal government should make bereavement studies one of the priority areas for research during this experimental period. To focus only on terminal care and its costs would be to ignore an integral part of the hospice program and to pass up a rare opportunity to conduct major studies of the preventive possibilities of bereavement support and its associated savings potential. In designing such studies, attention should be paid to possible distinguishing characteristics of families who choose the hospice option; those characteristics could have particular significance following bereavement and, if not identified and controlled for, could confound the results of the efficacy of bereavement interventions.

Although each of the major forms of intervention has certain distinctive features, there is a great variation within each type as well as some similarities among the different approaches. This makes it difficult to draw conclusions about the applicability or efficacy of mutual support groups, hospices, or psychotherapy in general. In addition, the literature often does not specify enough details about the nature of a particular intervention or enough precision about its goals to permit valid comparisons even within one of the broad approaches. Here, as elsewhere, the lack of agreement about which outcomes to measure, and when and how to measure them, has further limited the usefulness of the data that have been collected.

Research initiatives in this area should encourage cooperation between program administrators, clinicians, and researchers from several disciplines so that carefully controlled studies can be conducted. In the case of drug therapies, the lack of research is striking. There have been virtually no controlled trials on the efficacy of commonly prescribed hypnotics and minor tranquilizers or on the use of antidepressants with the bereaved. Neither the immediate nor long-term effects of using drug therapy alone or in conjunction with psychosocial intervention are known.

Finally, the committee recommends that the NIMH establish a special ad hoc research review committee to deal with bereavement studies of all kinds. A broad research initiative in this area requires a review committee that understands the nature and complexity of bereavement; the state of the art in research on the process, outcomes, and interventions; the value of different methods of studying bereavement; and the problems involved in conducting good longitudinal, multidisciplinary research in this area. Although currently many specific gaps exist in our understanding of the bereavement process, it is time to begin to put the entire puzzle together—to link research on mechanisms, processes, and outcomes to the identification of groups at high risk for adverse outcomes, and to determine the best way to help individuals who have lost someone with whom they had close emotional ties.

Subject Index

A

in death of parent, 26, 84
in death of spouse, 25–26, 39
sociocultural influences on, 209
bereavement reactions after, 24,
87–92, 125–126
guilt in, 88
psychotherapeutic interventions in, 274
in spouse, 24, 87, 88
in depression, 168
family patterns of, 89–90, 126
notes left in, blaming survivors, 89
of parent, 90
childhood bereavement reactions in, 125–126
repeated threats of, 88
research issues on, 92
social stigma of, 90–91
Support system, 5, 8, 202–204, 285
in childhood bereavement, 112,
123–124, 126
parental role in, 128–132
continuing after death of patient,
224–229
during dying period, 217–220
elements of, 203
enhancing self-esteem, 203
health professionals and institutions in, 215–236
for health professionals working
with dying patients, 229–231,
234, 289
in hospice programs, 251, 252
perceived lack of, 39, 40
personality affecting, 58–59
self-help groups in, 240–249
sociocultural variations in, 204
after suicide of relative, 90, 91
around time of death, 220–224
of widows and widowers, 74
Surrogate mothers, artificial,
emotional attachment to, in
monkeys, 189–190

Symptomatology of bereavement,
151–152, 169

T
Terminal illness. *See also* Cancer
anticipatory grief in. *See* Anticipatory grief
hospice services in, 249–257
mutual support groups related to,
241
of parent, childhood bereavement
in, 125, 127
roles of health professionals during
dying period in, 217–220
suicide in, 88–89, 92
transfer to regional facility in, 227
Thyroid gland, in bereavement, 31,
151
Tranquilizer use, associated with
bereavement, 29, 35, 40, 269,
270, 288
Twins, death of one of, 78

V
Visiting policies in health institutions, 219, 220, 234, 289

W
War casualities, 222–223
Widow-to-Widow Program, 242–245
Widows and widowers, bereavement
reactions of, 71–75. *See also*
Conjugal bereavement
Work
maternal, animal models of infant response to, 188
return to, after bereavement, 18,
202
shift change in, 166, 167